Teen Health Series

Allergies
SOURCEBOOK
Third Edition

Health Reference Series

Third Edition

Allergies
SOCCEBOOK

*Basic Consumer Health Information about
Allergic Disorders, Such as Anaphylaxis, Hives,
Eczema, Rhinitis, Sinusitis, and Conjunctivitis, and
Their Triggers, Including Pollen, Mold, Dust Mites,
Animal Dander, Insects, Chemicals, Food, Food
Additives, and Medications*

*Along with Advice about the Diagnosis and
Treatment of Allergy Symptoms, a Glossary
of Related Terms, a Directory of Resources
for Help and Information, and Suggestions
for Additional Reading*

Edited by
Amy L. Sutton

Omnigraphics

615 Griswold Street • Detroit, MI 48226

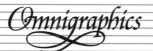

Bibliographic Note

Because this page cannot legibly accommodate all the copyright notices, the Bibliographic Note portion of the Preface constitutes an extension of the copyright notice.

Edited by Amy L. Sutton

Health Reference Series

Karen Bellenir, *Managing Editor*
David A. Cooke, M.D., *Medical Consultant*
Elizabeth Collins, *Permissions and Research Coordinator*
Cherry Stockdale, *Permissions Assistant*
EdIndex, Services for Publishers, *Indexers*

* * *

Omnigraphics, Inc.

Matthew P. Barbour, *Senior Vice President*
Kay Gill, *Vice President—Directories*
Kevin Hayes, *Operations Manager*
David P. Bianco, *Marketing Director*

* * *

Peter E. Ruffner, *Publisher*

Frederick G. Ruffner, Jr., *Chairman*

Copyright © 2007 Omnigraphics, Inc.

ISBN 978-0-7808-0950-5

Library of Congress Cataloging-in-Publication Data

Allergies sourcebook : basic consumer health information about allergic disorders, such as anaphylaxis, hives, eczema, rhinitis, sinusitis, and conjunctivitis, and their triggers, including pollen, mold, dust mites, animal dander, insects, chemicals, food, food additives, and medications; along with advice about the diagnosis and treatment of allergy symptoms, a glossary of related terms, a directory of resources for help and information, and suggestions for additional reading / edited by Amy L. Sutton. -- 3rd ed.
   p. cm. -- (Health reference series)
  Summary: "Provides basic consumer health information about allergy triggers and allergic reactions, prevention, and treatment. Includes index, glossary of related terms, and other resources"--Provided by publisher.
  Includes bibliographical references and index.
  ISBN 978-0-7808-0950-5 (hardcover : alk. paper) 1. Allergy--Popular works. I. Sutton, Amy L.
  RC584.A3443 2007
  616.97--dc22

            2007011738

Table of Contents

Visit www.healthreferenceseries.com to view *A Contents Guide to the Health Reference Series*, a listing of more than 13,000 topics and the volumes in which they are covered.

Part V: Diagnosing and Treating Allergies

Part VII: Additional Help and Information

Preface

About This Book

Allergic disorders affect more than 50 million Americans, causing symptoms that range from annoying to deadly. Their treatments and diagnoses cost the U.S. health care system $18 billion dollars annually, and the prevalence of some types of allergic disorders—such as eczema and rhinitis—appears to be increasing. There is good news, however. In many cases, allergy sufferers can obtain significant relief by learning about allergy triggers and how to avoid them, using medications, and taking advantage of new allergy therapies.

Allergies Sourcebook, Third Edition provides updated information about the causes, triggers, treatments, and prevalence of common allergic disorders, including rhinitis, sinusitis, conjunctivitis, hives, dermatitis, eczema, and anaphylaxis. It discusses the immune system and its role in the development of allergic disorders and describes such commonly encountered allergens as pollen, mold, dust mites, and animal dander. Facts about allergies to foods and food additives, insect stings, medications, and chemicals are also included, along with information about allergy testing, treatments, coping strategies, and prevention efforts. The book concludes with a glossary of related terms, a directory of resources, and suggestions for additional reading.

How to Use This Book

This book is divided into parts and chapters. Parts focus on broad areas of interest. Chapters are devoted to single topics within a part.

Part I: Facts about Allergies and the Immune System identifies the immune system's role in the allergic response and details the physical and economic burden that allergic diseases place on U.S. children, adolescents, and adults. It also discusses the link between allergies and other concerns, including asthma, vaccines, and cognitive impairment.

Part II: What You Should Know about Allergic Reactions provides detailed information about a variety of allergic reactions and conditions, including allergic rhinitis (hay fever), sinusitis, allergic conjunctivitis, urticaria (hives), contact dermatitis, and eczema. This part also describes anaphylaxis, a severe, potentially life-threatening allergic reaction.

Part III: Foods and Food Additives That Trigger Allergic Reactions discusses the most common food allergies, including eggs, milk, tree nut and peanut, seafood, wheat, and soy. Information about food additives that may trigger reactions is also provided along with tips about avoiding food allergy triggers and caring for a food-allergic child.

Part IV: Airborne, Chemical, and Other Environmental Allergy Triggers offers information about indoor and outdoor airborne allergens, including pollen, ragweed, mold, dust mites, cockroach antigen, and animal dander. This part also describes allergic symptoms triggered by sensitivity to chemicals and pollutants as well as allergies to insect venom, medicines, and latex.

Part V: Diagnosing and Treating Allergies identifies skin and blood tests that aid in the diagnosis of allergies. Information about over-the-counter and prescription medications, the usefulness of allergy shots (immunotherapy), and the advisability of alternative medicine treatments for allergic symptoms is also provided.

Part VI: Avoiding Triggers and Preventing Allergy Symptoms includes tips on managing the home environment with allergen avoidance strategies, cleaning techniques, and air filtration. This part also offers tips on controlling outdoor triggers while exercising and gardening and preventing allergic reactions in child care situations or during travel.

Part VII: Additional Help and Information includes a glossary of important terms, a directory of organizations that provide allergy information, and suggestions for additional reading.

Bibliographic Note

This volume contains documents and excerpts from publications issued by the following U.S. government agencies: National Institute of Allergy and Infectious Diseases (NIAID); National Institute of Arthritis and Musculoskeletal and Skin Diseases (NIAMS); National Institute of Environmental Health Sciences (NIEHS); National Institute for Occupational Safety and Health (NIOSH); National Institutes of Health (NIH); National Women's Health Information Center (NWHIC); and the U.S. Food and Drug Administration (FDA).

In addition, this volume contains copyrighted documents from the following organizations: About, Inc.; A.D.A.M., Inc.; Alabama Cooperative Extension System/Alabama A&M and Auburn Universities; AllergicChild.com; Allergy/Asthma Information Association; Allergy and Asthma Network Mothers of Asthmatics; American Academy of Dermatology; American Academy of Otolaryngic Allergy; American Academy of Otolaryngology—Head and Neck Surgery; American Association for Clinical Chemistry; American College of Allergy, Asthma and Immunology; American Lung Association; American Partnership for Eosinophilic Disorders; American Rhinologic Society; American Society of Health-System Pharmacists; The Anaphylaxis Campaign; Asthma and Allergy Foundation of America; Better Health Channel; Canadian Food Inspection Agency; Children's Hospital of Philadelphia; The Food Allergy & Anaphylaxis Network; Food Allergy Initiative; International Food Information Council; Medical College of Wisconsin; National Jewish Medical and Research Center; National Pharmaceutical Council; Nemours Center for Children's Health Media/TeensHealth .org; Schering Corporation; University of Florida Cooperative Extension—Institute of Food and Agriculture Sciences; University of Maine Cooperative Extension; University of Pittsburgh Medical Center; University of Texas Southwestern Medical Center at Dallas; University of Vermont Extension; and the World Allergy Organization.

Full citation information is provided on the first page of each chapter or section. Every effort has been made to secure all necessary rights to reprint the copyrighted material. If any omissions have been made, please contact Omnigraphics to make corrections for future editions.

Acknowledgements

Thanks go to the many organizations, agencies, and individuals who have contributed materials for this *Sourcebook* and to medical consultant Dr. David Cooke and document engineer Bruce Bellenir.

xv

Special thanks go to managing editor Karen Bellenir and permissions and research coordinator Liz Collins for their help and support.

About the Health Reference Series

The *Health Reference Series* is designed to provide basic medical information for patients, families, caregivers, and the general public. Each volume takes a particular topic and provides comprehensive coverage. This is especially important for people who may be dealing with a newly diagnosed disease or a chronic disorder in themselves or in a family member. People looking for preventive guidance, information about disease warning signs, medical statistics, and risk factors for health problems will also find answers to their questions in the *Health Reference Series*. The *Series*, however, is not intended to serve as a tool for diagnosing illness, in prescribing treatments, or as a substitute for the physician/patient relationship. All people concerned about medical symptoms or the possibility of disease are encouraged to seek professional care from an appropriate health care provider.

A Note about Spelling and Style

Health Reference Series editors use *Stedman's Medical Dictionary* as an authority for questions related to the spelling of medical terms and the *Chicago Manual of Style* for questions related to grammatical structures, punctuation, and other editorial concerns. Consistent adherence is not always possible, however, because the individual volumes within the *Series* include many documents from a wide variety of different producers and copyright holders, and the editor's primary goal is to present material from each source as accurately as is possible following the terms specified by each document's producer. This sometimes means that information in different chapters or sections may follow other guidelines and alternate spelling authorities. For example, occasionally a copyright holder may require that eponymous terms be shown in possessive forms (Crohn's disease *vs.* Crohn disease) or that British spelling norms be retained (leukaemia *vs.* leukemia).

Locating Information within the Health Reference Series

The *Health Reference Series* contains a wealth of information about a wide variety of medical topics. Ensuring easy access to all the fact sheets, research reports, in-depth discussions, and other material contained within the individual books of the *Series* remains one of our highest priorities. As the *Series* continues to grow in size and scope, however, locating the precise information needed by a reader may become more challenging.

A *Contents Guide to the Health Reference Series* was developed to direct readers to the specific volumes that address their concerns. It presents an extensive list of diseases, treatments, and other topics of general interest compiled from the Tables of Contents and major index headings. To access *A Contents Guide to the Health Reference Series*, visit www.healthreferenceseries.com.

Medical Consultant

Medical consultation services are provided to the *Health Reference Series* editors by David A. Cooke, M.D. Dr. Cooke is a graduate of Brandeis University, and he received his M.D. degree from the University of Michigan. He completed residency training at the University of Wisconsin Hospital and Clinics. He is board-certified in Internal Medicine. Dr. Cooke currently works as part of the University of Michigan Health System and practices in Ann Arbor, MI. In his free time, he enjoys writing, science fiction, and spending time with his family.

Our Advisory Board

We would like to thank the following board members for providing guidance to the development of this *Series*:

- Dr. Lynda Baker, Associate Professor of Library and Information Science, Wayne State University, Detroit, MI

- Nancy Bulgarelli, William Beaumont Hospital Library, Royal Oak, MI

- Karen Imarisio, Bloomfield Township Public Library, Bloomfield Township, MI

- Karen Morgan, Mardigian Library, University of Michigan-Dearborn, Dearborn, MI

- Rosemary Orlando, St. Clair Shores Public Library, St. Clair Shores, MI

Health Reference Series *Update Policy*

The inaugural book in the *Health Reference Series* was the first edition of *Cancer Sourcebook* published in 1989. Since then, the *Series* has been enthusiastically received by librarians and in the medical community. In order to maintain the standard of providing high-quality health information for the layperson the editorial staff at Omnigraphics felt it was necessary to implement a policy of updating volumes when warranted.

Medical researchers have been making tremendous strides, and it is the purpose of the *Health Reference Series* to stay current with the most recent advances. Each decision to update a volume is made on an individual basis. Some of the considerations include how much new information is available and the feedback we receive from people who use the books. If there is a topic you would like to see added to the update list, or an area of medical concern you feel has not been adequately addressed, please write to:

Editor
Health Reference Series
Omnigraphics, Inc.
615 Griswold Street
Detroit, MI 48226
E-mail: editorial@omnigraphics.com

Part One

Facts about Allergies and the Immune System

Chapter 1

Understanding the Immune System and Its Role in Allergic Disease

The immune system is a network of cells, tissues, and organs that work together to defend the body against attacks by "foreign" invaders. These are primarily microbes (germs)—tiny, infection-causing organisms such as bacteria, viruses, parasites, and fungi. Because the human body provides an ideal environment for many microbes, they try to break in. It is the immune system's job to keep them out or, failing that, to seek out and destroy them.

When the immune system hits the wrong target or is crippled, however, it can unleash a torrent of diseases, including allergy, arthritis, or AIDS. The immune system is amazingly complex. It can recognize and remember millions of different enemies, and it can produce secretions and cells to match up with and wipe out each one of them.

The secret to its success is an elaborate and dynamic communications network. Millions and millions of cells, organized into sets and subsets, gather like clouds of bees swarming around a hive and pass information back and forth. Once immune cells receive the alarm, they undergo tactical changes and begin to produce powerful chemicals. These substances allow the cells to regulate their own growth and behavior, enlist their fellows, and direct new recruits to trouble spots.

"Understanding the Immune System: How It Works" is excerpted from the booklet published by the National Institute of Allergy and Infectious Diseases (NIAID, www.niaid.nih.gov), part of the National Institutes of Health, NIH Publication No. 03-5423, September 2003.

Self and Nonself

The key to a healthy immune system is its remarkable ability to distinguish between the body's own cells—self—and foreign cells—nonself. The body's immune defenses normally coexist peacefully with cells that carry distinctive "self" marker molecules. But when immune defenders encounter cells or organisms carrying markers that say "foreign," they quickly launch an attack.

Anything that can trigger this immune response is called an antigen. An antigen can be a microbe such as a virus, or even a part of a microbe. Tissues or cells from another person (except an identical twin) also carry nonself markers and act as antigens. This explains why tissue transplants may be rejected.

In abnormal situations, the immune system can mistake self for nonself and launch an attack against the body's own cells or tissues. The result is called an autoimmune disease. Some forms of arthritis and diabetes are autoimmune diseases. In other cases, the immune system responds to a seemingly harmless foreign substance such as ragweed pollen. The result is allergy, and this kind of antigen is called an allergen.

The Structure of the Immune System

The organs of the immune system are positioned throughout the body. They are called lymphoid organs because they are home to lymphocytes, small white blood cells that are the key players in the immune system.

Bone marrow, the soft tissue in the hollow center of bones, is the ultimate source of all blood cells, including white blood cells destined to become immune cells. The thymus is an organ that lies behind the breastbone; lymphocytes known as T lymphocytes, or just "T cells," mature in the thymus.

Lymphocytes can travel throughout the body using the blood vessels. The cells can also travel through a system of lymphatic vessels that closely parallels the body's veins and arteries. Cells and fluids are exchanged between blood and lymphatic vessels, enabling the lymphatic system to monitor the body for invading microbes. The lymphatic vessels carry lymph, a clear fluid that bathes the body's tissues.

Small, bean-shaped lymph nodes are laced along the lymphatic vessels, with clusters in the neck, armpits, abdomen, and groin. Each lymph node contains specialized compartments where immune cells congregate, and where they can encounter antigens.

Immune cells and foreign particles enter the lymph nodes via incoming lymphatic vessels or the lymph nodes' tiny blood vessels. All lymphocytes exit lymph nodes through outgoing lymphatic vessels. Once in the bloodstream, they are transported to tissues throughout

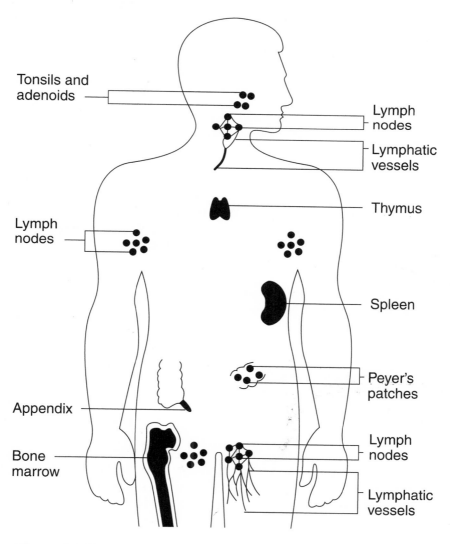

Figure 1.1. The organs of the immune system are positioned throughout the body.

the body. They patrol everywhere for foreign antigens, then gradually drift back into the lymphatic system, to begin the cycle all over again.

The spleen is a flattened organ at the upper left of the abdomen. Like the lymph nodes, the spleen contains specialized compartments where immune cells gather and work, and serves as a meeting ground where immune defenses confront antigens.

Clumps of lymphoid tissue are found in many parts of the body, especially in the linings of the digestive tract and the airways and lungs—territories that serve as gateways to the body. These tissues include the tonsils, adenoids, and appendix.

Immune Cells and Their Products

The immune system stockpiles a huge arsenal of cells, not only lymphocytes but also cell-devouring phagocytes and their relatives. Some immune cells take on all comers, while others are trained on highly specific targets. To work effectively, most immune cells need the cooperation of their comrades. Sometimes immune cells communicate by direct physical contact, sometimes by releasing chemical messengers.

The immune system stores just a few of each kind of the different cells needed to recognize millions of possible enemies. When an antigen appears, those few matching cells multiply into a full-scale army. After their job is done, they fade away, leaving sentries behind to watch for future attacks.

All immune cells begin as immature stem cells in the bone marrow. They respond to different cytokines and other signals to grow into specific immune cell types, such as T cells, B cells, or phagocytes. Because stem cells have not yet committed to a particular future, they are an interesting possibility for treating some immune system disorders. Researchers currently are investigating if a person's own stem cells can be used to regenerate damaged immune responses in autoimmune diseases and immune deficiency diseases.

B Lymphocytes

B cells and T cells are the main types of lymphocytes.

B cells work chiefly by secreting substances called antibodies into the body's fluids. Antibodies ambush antigens circulating the bloodstream. They are powerless, however, to penetrate cells. The job of attacking target cells—either cells that have been infected by viruses or cells that have been distorted by cancer—is left to T cells or other immune cells.

Each B cell is programmed to make one specific antibody. For example, one B cell will make an antibody that blocks a virus that causes the common cold, while another produces an antibody that attacks a bacterium that causes pneumonia.

When a B cell encounters its triggering antigen, it gives rise to many large cells known as plasma cells. Every plasma cell is essentially a factory for producing an antibody. Each of the plasma cells descended from a given B cell manufactures millions of identical antibody molecules and pours them into the bloodstream.

An antigen matches an antibody much as a key matches a lock. Some match exactly; others fit more like a skeleton key. But whenever antigen and antibody interlock, the antibody marks the antigen for destruction.

Antibodies belong to a family of large molecules known as immunoglobulins. Different types play different roles in the immune defense strategy.

- Immunoglobulin G, or IgG, works efficiently to coat microbes, speeding their uptake by other cells in the immune system.

- IgM is very effective at killing bacteria.

- IgA concentrates in body fluids—tears, saliva, the secretions of the respiratory tract and the digestive tract—guarding the entrances to the body.

- IgE, whose natural job probably is to protect against parasitic infections, is the villain responsible for the symptoms of allergy.

- IgD remains attached to B cells and plays a key role in initiating early B-cell response.

T Cells

Unlike B cells, T cells do not recognize free-floating antigens. Rather, their surfaces contain specialized antibody-like receptors that see fragments of antigens on the surfaces of infected or cancerous cells. T cells contribute to immune defenses in two major ways: some direct and regulate immune responses; others directly attack infected or cancerous cells.

Helper T cells, or Th cells, coordinate immune responses by communicating with other cells. Some stimulate nearby B cells to produce antibody, others call in microbe-gobbling cells called phagocytes, still others activate other T cells.

Killer T cells—also called cytotoxic T lymphocytes or CTLs—perform a different function. These cells directly attack other cells carrying certain foreign or abnormal molecules on their surfaces. CTLs are especially useful for attacking viruses because viruses often hide from other parts of the immune system while they grow inside infected cells. CTLs recognize small fragments of these viruses peeking out from the cell membrane and launch an attack to kill the cell.

In most cases, T cells only recognize an antigen if it is carried on the surface of a cell by one of the body's own MHC, or major histocompatibility complex, molecules. MHC molecules are proteins recognized by T cells when distinguishing between self and nonself. A self MHC molecule provides a recognizable scaffolding to present a foreign antigen to the T cell.

Although MHC molecules are required for T-cell responses against foreign invaders, they also pose a difficulty during organ transplantations. Virtually every cell in the body is covered with MHC proteins, but each person has a different set of these proteins on his or her cells. If a T cell recognizes a nonself MHC molecule on another cell, it will destroy the cell. Therefore, doctors must match organ recipients with donors who have the closest MHC makeup. Otherwise the recipient's T cells will likely attack the transplanted organ, leading to graft rejection.

Natural killer (NK) cells are another kind of lethal white cell, or lymphocyte. Like killer T cells, NK cells are armed with granules filled with potent chemicals. But while killer T cells look for antigen fragments bound to self-MHC molecules, NK cells recognize cells lacking self-MHC molecules. Thus NK cells have the potential to attack many types of foreign cells.

Both kinds of killer cells slay on contact. The deadly assassins bind to their targets, aim their weapons, and then deliver a lethal burst of chemicals.

Phagocytes and Their Relatives

Phagocytes are large white cells that can swallow and digest microbes and other foreign particles. Monocytes are phagocytes that circulate in the blood. When monocytes migrate into tissues, they develop into macrophages. Specialized types of macrophages can be found in many organs, including lungs, kidneys, brain, and liver.

Macrophages play many roles. As scavengers, they rid the body of worn-out cells and other debris. They display bits of foreign antigen in a way that draws the attention of matching lymphocytes. And they churn out an amazing variety of powerful chemical signals, known as monokines, which are vital to the immune responses.

Granulocytes are another kind of immune cell. They contain granules filled with potent chemicals, which allow the granulocytes to destroy microorganisms. Some of these chemicals, such as histamine, also contribute to inflammation and allergy.

One type of granulocyte, the neutrophil, is also a phagocyte; it uses its prepackaged chemicals to break down the microbes it ingests. Eosinophils and basophils are granulocytes that "degranulate," spraying their chemicals onto harmful cells or microbes nearby.

The mast cell is a twin of the basophil, except that it is not a blood cell. Rather, it is found in the lungs, skin, tongue, and linings of the nose and intestinal tract, where it is responsible for the symptoms of allergy.

A related structure, the blood platelet, is a cell fragment. Platelets, too, contain granules. In addition to promoting blood clotting and wound repair, platelets activate some of the immune defenses.

Cytokines

Components of the immune system communicate with one another by exchanging chemical messengers called cytokines. These proteins are secreted by cells and act on other cells to coordinate an appropriate immune response. Cytokines include a diverse assortment of interleukins, interferons, and growth factors.

Some cytokines are chemical switches that turn certain immune cell types on and off.

One cytokine, interleukin 2 (IL-2), triggers the immune system to produce T cells. IL-2's immunity-boosting properties have traditionally made it a promising treatment for several illnesses. Clinical studies are ongoing to test its benefits in other diseases such as cancer, hepatitis C, and HIV infection and AIDS. Other cytokines also are being studied for their potential clinical benefit.

Other cytokines chemically attract specific cell types. These so-called chemokines are released by cells at a site of injury or infection and call other immune cells to the region to help repair the damage or fight off the invader. Chemokines often play a key role in inflammation and are a promising target for new drugs to help regulate immune responses.

Complement

The complement system is made up of about 25 proteins that work together to "complement" the action of antibodies in destroying bacteria.

Complement also helps to rid the body of antibody-coated antigens (antigen-antibody complexes). Complement proteins, which cause blood vessels to become dilated and then leaky, contribute to the redness, warmth, swelling, pain, and loss of function that characterize an inflammatory response.

Complement proteins circulate in the blood in an inactive form. When the first protein in the complement series is activated—typically by antibody that has locked onto an antigen—it sets in motion a domino effect. Each component takes its turn in a precise chain of steps known as the complement cascade. The end product is a cylinder inserted into—and puncturing a hole in—the cell's wall. With fluids and molecules flowing in and out, the cell swells and bursts. Other components of the complement system make bacteria more susceptible to phagocytosis or beckon other cells to the area.

Mounting an Immune Response

Infections are the most common cause of human disease. They range from the common cold to debilitating conditions like chronic hepatitis to life-threatening diseases such as AIDS [acquired immunodeficiency syndrome]. Disease-causing microbes (pathogens) attempting to get into the body must first move past the body's external armor, usually the skin or cells lining the body's internal passageways.

The skin provides an imposing barrier to invading microbes. It is generally penetrable only through cuts or tiny abrasions. The digestive and respiratory tracts—both portals of entry for a number of microbes—also have their own levels of protection. Microbes entering the nose often cause the nasal surfaces to secrete more protective mucus, and attempts to enter the nose or lungs can trigger a sneeze or cough reflex to force microbial invaders out of the respiratory passageways. The stomach contains a strong acid that destroys many pathogens that are swallowed with food.

If microbes survive the body's front-line defenses, they still have to find a way through the walls of the digestive, respiratory, or urogenital passageways to the underlying cells. These passageways are lined with tightly packed epithelial cells covered in a layer of mucus, effectively blocking the transport of many organisms. Mucosal surfaces also secrete a special class of antibody called IgA, which in many cases is the first type of antibody to encounter an invading microbe. Underneath the epithelial layer a number of cells, including macrophages, B cells, and T cells, lie in wait for any germ that might bypass the barriers at the surface.

10

Next, invaders must escape a series of general defenses, which are ready to attack, without regard for specific antigen markers. These include patrolling phagocytes, NK cells, and complement.

Microbes that cross the general barriers then confront specific weapons tailored just for them. Specific weapons, which include both antibodies and T cells, are equipped with singular receptor structures that allow them to recognize and interact with their designated targets.

Bacteria, Viruses, and Parasites

The most common disease-causing microbes are bacteria, viruses, and parasites. Each uses a different tactic to infect a person, and, therefore, each is thwarted by a different part of the immune system.

Most bacteria live in the spaces between cells and are readily attacked by antibodies. When antibodies attach to a bacterium, they send signals to complement proteins and phagocytic cells to destroy the bound microbes. Some bacteria are eaten directly by phagocytes, which signal to certain T cells to join the attack.

All viruses, plus a few types of bacteria and parasites, must enter cells to survive, requiring a different approach. Infected cells use their MHC molecules to put pieces of the invading microbes on the cell's surface, flagging down cytotoxic T lymphocytes to destroy the infected cell. Antibodies also can assist in the immune response, attaching to and clearing viruses before they have a chance to enter the cell.

Parasites live either inside or outside cells. Intracellular parasites such as the organism that causes malaria can trigger T-cell responses. Extracellular parasites are often much larger than bacteria or viruses and require a much broader immune attack. Parasitic infections often trigger an inflammatory response when eosinophils, basophils, and other specialized granular cells rush to the scene and release their stores of toxic chemicals in an attempt to destroy the invader. Antibodies also play a role in this attack, attracting the granular cells to the site of infection.

Immunity: Natural and Acquired

Long ago, physicians realized that people who had recovered from the plague would never get it again—they had acquired immunity. This is because some of the activated T and B cells become memory cells. The next time an individual meets up with the same antigen, the immune system is set to demolish it.

11

Immunity can be strong or weak, short-lived or long-lasting, depending on the type of antigen, the amount of antigen, and the route by which it enters the body.

Immunity can also be influenced by inherited genes. When faced with the same antigen, some individuals will respond forcefully, others feebly, and some not at all.

An immune response can be sparked not only by infection but also by immunization with vaccines. Vaccines contain microorganisms—or parts of microorganisms—that have been treated so they can provoke an immune response but not full-blown disease.

Immunity can also be transferred from one individual to another by injections of serum rich in antibodies against a particular microbe (antiserum).

For example, immune serum is sometimes given to protect travelers to countries where hepatitis A is widespread. Such passive immunity typically lasts only a few weeks or months.

Infants are born with weak immune responses but are protected for the first few months of life by antibodies received from their mothers before birth. Babies who are nursed can also receive some antibodies from breast milk that help to protect their digestive tracts.

Immune Tolerance

Immune tolerance is the tendency of T or B lymphocytes to ignore the body's own tissues. Maintaining tolerance is important because it prevents the immune system from attacking its fellow cells. Scientists are hard at work trying to understand how the immune system knows when to respond and when to ignore.

Tolerance occurs in at least two ways. Central tolerance occurs during lymphocyte development. Very early in each immune cell's life, it is exposed to many of the self molecules in the body. If it encounters these molecules before it has fully matured, the encounter activates an internal self-destruct pathway and the immune cell dies. This process, called clonal deletion, helps ensure that self-reactive T cells and B cells do not mature and attack healthy tissues.

Because maturing lymphocytes do not encounter every molecule in the body, they must also learn to ignore mature cells and tissues. In peripheral tolerance, circulating lymphocytes might recognize a self molecule but cannot respond because some of the chemical signals required to activate the T or B cell are absent. So-called clonal anergy, therefore, keeps potentially harmful lymphocytes switched off. Peripheral tolerance may also be imposed by a special class of regulatory T cells that inhibits helper or cytotoxic T-cell activation by self antigens.

Vaccines

Medical workers have long helped the body's immune system prepare for future attacks through vaccination. Vaccines consist of killed or modified microbes, components of microbes, or microbial DNA [deoxyribonucleic acid] that trick the body into thinking an infection has occurred. An immunized person's immune system attacks the harmless vaccine and prepares for subsequent invasions. Vaccines remain one of the best ways to prevent infectious diseases and have an excellent safety record. Previously devastating diseases such as smallpox, polio, and whooping cough have been greatly controlled or eliminated through worldwide vaccination programs.

Allergic Diseases Are Disorders of the Immune System

The most common types of allergic diseases occur when the immune system responds to a false alarm. In an allergic person, a normally harmless material such as grass pollen or house dust is mistaken for a threat and attacked. Allergies such as pollen allergy are related to the antibody known as IgE. Like other antibodies, each IgE antibody is specific; one acts against oak pollen, another against ragweed.

Chapter 2

Allergies in the United States

Chapter Contents

Section 2.1

Allergies:
A Leading Cause of Chronic Disease

"Allergy Statistics" is a publication of the National Institute of
Allergy and Infectious Diseases (NIAID, www.niaid.nih.gov), part
of the National Institutes of Health, August 2005.

- More than 50 million Americans suffer from allergic diseases.[1]
  A recent nationwide survey found that more than half (54.6 percent) of all U.S. citizens test positive to one or more allergens;
  among specific allergens, dust mite, rye, ragweed, or cockroach
  caused sensitization in approximately 25 percent of the population.[2]

- Allergies are the 6th leading cause of chronic disease in the
  United States, costing the health care system $18 billion annu-
  ally.[1]

- Two estimates of prevalence of allergic rhinoconjunctivitis (hay
  fever) in the United States are 9 percent[3] and 16 percent.[4] The
  prevalence of allergic rhinitis has increased substantially over
  the past 15 years.[5]

- In 2002, approximately 14 million office visits to health care
  providers were attributed to allergic rhinitis.[6]

- Estimates of the prevalence of allergy to latex allergens in the
  general population vary widely, from less than 1 percent to 6 percent.[7,8]

- Certain individuals, including health care workers who wear latex gloves and children with spina bifida who have had multiple
  surgical procedures, are at particularly high risk for allergic reactions to latex. Atopic individuals (those with allergies) are at
  an increased risk of developing latex allergy.[7]

- Atopic dermatitis is one of the most common skin diseases, particularly in infants and children. The estimated prevalence in

the United States varies from 9 to 30 percent.[10,11] The prevalence of atopic dermatitis appears to be increasing.[12,13]

- Health care provider visits for contact dermatitis and other eczemas, which include atopic dermatitis, are 7 million per year.[14]

- Chronic sinusitis is the most commonly reported chronic disease, affecting 16.3 percent of people (nearly 32 million) in the United States in 1997.[3]

- In 1996, estimated U.S. health care expenditures attributable to sinusitis were approximately $5.8 billion.[15]

- Experts estimate food allergy occurs in 6 to 8 percent of children 4 years of age or under, and in 4 percent of adults.[16,21] Approximately 150 Americans, usually adolescents and young adults, die annually from food-induced anaphylaxis.[16]

- Peanut or tree nut allergies affect approximately 0.6 percent and 0.4 percent of Americans, respectively, and cause the most severe food-induced allergic reactions.[18]

- Allergic drug reactions account for 5 to 10 percent of all adverse drug reactions, with skin reaction being the most common form.[1]

- Penicillin is a common cause of drug allergy. Approximately 7 percent of normal volunteers react to penicillin allergy skin tests (IgE antibodies).[19] While the true number of deaths from drug reactions is unknown, anaphylactic reactions to penicillin occur in 32 of every 100,000 exposed patients.[9]

- Acute urticaria (hives) is common, affecting 10 to 20 percent of the population at some time in their lives. Half of those affected continue to have symptoms for more than 6 months.[1] Allergy to venom of stinging insects (honeybees, wasps, hornets, yellow jackets, and fire ants) is relatively common, with prevalence of systemic reactions in 3 percent of American and 1 percent of children.[20] Between 40 and 100 Americans have been reported to die annually from anaphylaxis to insects, although this number may be markedly under estimated.[8]

References

1. American Academy of Allergy, Asthma and Immunology (AAAAI). *The Allergy Report: Science Based Findings on the Diagnosis & Treatment of Allergic Disorders,* 1996–2001.

2. Arbes SJ et al. Prevalences of positive skin test responses to 10 common allergens in the US population: Results from the Third National Health and Nutrition Examination Survey. *Journal of Allergy and Clinical Immunology* 116:377–383. 2005.

3. CDC. Fast Stats A-Z, *Vital and Health Statistics, Series 10, no. 205*, May 2002. http://www.cdc.gov/nchs/data/series/sr_10/ sr10_205 .pdf

4. The International Study of Asthma and Allergies in Childhood (ISAAC) Steering Committee. Worldwide variation in prevalence of symptoms of asthma, allergic rhinoconjunctivitis, and atopic eczema: ISAAC. *Lancet* 351:1225–32. 1998.

5. Linneberg A et al . The prevalence of skin-test-positive allergic rhinitis in Danish adults: two cross sectional surveys 8 years apart. The Copenhagen Allergy Study. *Allergy* 55:767–772. 2000.

6. CDC. Fast Stats A-Z, *Advanced Data from Vital and Health Statistics, no. 346, Table 13*. August 26, 2004. http://www.cdc.gov/ nchs/fastats/allergies.htm

7. Poley GE and Slater JE. Latex allergy. *Journal of Allergy and Clinical Immunology* 105 (6):1054–62. 2000.

8. Neugut AL, Ghatak AT and Miller RL. Anaphylaxis in the United States: An investigation into its epidemiology. *Archives of Internal Medicine* 161 (1):15–21. 2001.

9. The International Collaborative Study of Severe Anaphylaxis. Risk of anaphylaxis in a hospital population in relation to the use of various drugs: an international study. *Pharmacoepidemiol Drug Safety* 12(3):195–202. 2003.

10. Rudikoff D and Lebwohl M. Atopic dermatitis. *Lancet* 351(9117): 1715–21. 1998.

11. Larsen F and Hanikin J. Epidemiology of Atopic Dermatitis. *Immunology and Allergy Clinics of North America.* 22:1–25. 2002.

12. Matsumoto I et al. Change in prevalence of allergic diseases in primary school children in Fukuoka City for the last fifteen years. *Arerugi* Apr 48(4):435–42.

13. Schafer T. et al. The excess of atopic eczema in East Germany is related to the intrinsic type. *British Journal of Dermatology* 143:992–998. 2000.

14. CDC. National Center for Health Statistics. *Vital and Health Statistics Series,* 1996: vol. 13, no. 134.

15. Ray NF et al. Healthcare expenditures for sinusitis in 1996: Contributions of asthma, rhinitis, and other airway disorders. *Journal of Allergy and Clinical Immunology* 103 (3 pt. 1):408–414. 1999.

16. Sampson HA. Peanut Allergy. *New England Journal of Medicine* 346:1294–1299. 2002.

17. Bock SA, Munoz-Furlong A, and Sampson, HA. Fatalities Due to Anaphylactic Reaction to Foods. *Journal of Allergy and Clinical Immunology* 107: 191–193. 2001.

18. Sicherer SH, Munoz-Furlong A, and Sampson HA. Prevalence of peanut and tree nut allergy in the United States determined by means of a random digit dial telephone survey: A 5-year follow-up study. *Journal of Allergy and Clinical Immunology* 112(6):1203–1207. 2003.

19. Nugent JS et al. Determination of the incidence of sensitization after penicillin skin testing. *Annals of Allergy, Asthma, and Immunology* 90 (4):398–403. 2003.

20. David BK and Golden MD. Stinging Insect Allergy. *American Family Physician* 67:2541–2546. 2003.

21. Sicherer SH, Munoz-Furlong A, and Sampson HA. Prevalence of seafood allergy in the United States determined by a random telephone survey. *Journal of Allergy and Clinical Immunology* 114:159–165. 2004.

Section 2.2

More Than Half the U.S. Population Is Sensitive to One or More Allergens

Excerpted from "More Than Half the U.S. Population Is Sensitive to One or More Allergens," a press release by the National Institutes of Health (www.nih.gov), August 4, 2005.

More than 50% of the U.S. population tested positive to one or more allergens, according to a large national study. The new findings, based on data from the third National Health and Nutrition Examination Survey (NHANES III), shows that 54.3% of individuals aged 6 to 59 years old had a positive skin test response to at least one of the 10 allergens tested. The highest prevalence rates were for dust mite, rye, ragweed, and cockroach, with about 25% of the population testing positive to each allergen. Peanut allergy was the least common, with 9% of the population reacting positively to that food allergen.

The findings, published in the August [2005] issue of the *Journal of Allergy and Clinical Immunology,* were conducted by researchers at the National Institute of Environmental Health Sciences (NIEHS) and the National Institute of Allergy and Infectious Diseases, both components of the National Institutes of Health.

A positive skin test result may mean the individual is more vulnerable to asthma, hay fever, and eczema. "Asthma is one of the world's most significant chronic health conditions," said David A. Schwartz, M.D., the NIEHS Director. "Understanding what may account for the rising worldwide asthma rates will allow us to develop more effective prevention and treatment approaches."

NHANES III is a nationally representative survey conducted by the Centers for Disease Control and Prevention between 1988 to 1994 to determine the health and nutritional status of the U.S. population. Approximately 10,500 individuals participated in the skin testing. During these tests, skin was exposed to allergy-causing substances (allergens) and a positive test was determined by the size of the reaction on the skin. The 10 allergens tested include: Dust mite, German cockroach, cat, perennial rye, short ragweed, Bermuda grass, Russian thistle, white oak, *Alternaria alternata,* and peanuts.

Researchers also compared skin test responses between NHANES III and the previous survey, NHANES II, conducted from 1976 to 1980. The prevalence of a positive skin test response was much higher in NHANES III than in NHANES II.

According to the lead author, Samuel J. Arbes, Ph.D. of NIEHS, "An increase in prevalence is consistent with reports from other countries and coincides with an increase in asthma cases during that time." In the United States, the prevalence of asthma increased 73.9% from 1980 to 1996. However, Dr. Arbes was quick to point out that differences in skin test procedures between the two surveys prevent the authors from definitively concluding that the prevalence of skin test positivity has increased in the U.S. population.

"There is still much we don't understand about why some people become sensitized to allergens and others do not," said Darryl C. Zeldin, M.D., senior author on the paper. "Much more research is needed in order for us to understand the complex relationships between exposures to allergens, the development of allergic sensitization, and the onset and exacerbation of allergic diseases such as asthma."

The researchers recently added an allergy component to NHANES 2005 to 2006. In addition to the other NHANES data collection components, dust samples from the homes of 10,000 individuals are being analyzed for allergens, and blood samples taken from these individuals are being examined for antibodies to those allergens.

For more information about allergens and other environmental health topics, please visit the http://www.niehs.nih.gov or http://www.niaid.nih.gov.

Section 2.3

Americans Underestimate the Consequences of Allergies

Ninety-four percent of allergy sufferers report in a recent survey that their quality of life, often including their work productivity, sleep, concentration, and even their sex lives, is affected by their allergies. However, despite this, only 50 percent of allergy sufferers consider the disease to be a serious medical condition and nearly two thirds (64 percent) did not see an allergist or other doctor the last time their symptoms acted up.

In response, the American College of Allergy, Asthma and Immunology (ACAAI), sponsor of a 2002 survey, issued a call to action for allergy sufferers to take their condition seriously and seek the advice of an allergist or personal physician to mitigate symptoms and feel good again. "Allergies and their symptoms not only cause quality of life consequences such as fatigue, impaired work performance and general malaise, but also, insufficiently treated allergies often lead to serious conditions such as sinus or ear infections, asthma and sleep problems," said Dr. Bobby Lanier, president of ACAAI. "What people need to know is that there is no need to suffer the health and quality of life consequences of allergies, and they should seek the help of a medical expert."

Each autumn, about 50 million Americans will suffer from allergic symptoms. Seasonal allergies are caused by pollens or mold spores, and year-round allergies are caused by indoor allergens. According to the ACAAI, sufferers often confuse allergy symptoms with the common cold because the conditions may mimic each other. In fact, of those sufferers surveyed, 41 percent thought they had a cold or virus when they first began suffering with allergies. Indicators of a cold include a stuffy nose, sneezing, sore scratchy throat, fatigue, and sometimes a fever.

Some of the signs of seasonal allergies can include watery eyes, runny nose, sneezing, congestion or itchy throat. Because these symptoms are easy to confuse, the ACAAI notes that it is imperative to involve an allergist or personal physician when any of these symptoms linger. This nationwide telephone survey was conducted by RoperASW from August 5 to August 14, 2002, among 300 adults, aged 18-64, who suffer from allergies.

Seeking Relief

There are a variety of allergy medications on the market, and often sufferers seek symptom relief with over-the-counter (OTC) allergy medications. The survey revealed that the most common reason to take an OTC medication was because of convenience (49 percent of those who take such medications). Yet allergy sufferers try an average of five OTC products in an effort to find one that works to satisfaction, and almost all users experience side effects from them.

"With many different allergy medications available today, people mistakenly believe this disease can be diagnosed and treated without the involvement of a medical expert," continued Dr. Lanier. "Some medications may not completely control allergy symptoms and others may have undesirable side effects. I've seen patients who have experienced years of unneeded suffering due to self-medication on a trial-and-error basis. The best way to manage allergies and lead a life that is as normal and symptom-free as possible is to see an allergist or personal physician at the onset of symptoms," concluded Dr. Lanier.

Additional Findings

Additional survey outcomes include:

- On average, allergies interfere with many aspects of quality of life, including getting a good night's sleep (68 percent), doing outdoor activities (53 percent), being able to concentrate (50 percent), being productive at work (43 percent), and sex life (13 percent).

- The majority of allergy sufferers (72 percent) agree that their allergies are annoying to them. Moreover, about one in three (35 percent) say they feel they are "always battling allergies."

- Among all allergy sufferers, it most often takes very bad symptoms (11 percent) or having symptoms progress to sinus or respiratory infection (9 percent) for them to go to a doctor.

- Drowsiness is the most common side effect (67 percent) from taking an OTC and two thirds of those experiencing drowsiness drove a car shortly after taking an OTC.

Source: The American College of Allergy, Asthma & Immunology (ACAAI).

Section 2.4

The Economic Cost of Allergies: A Closer Look at Spending for Allergy Medications

"A Closer Look at Allergies," is reprinted by permission of the National Pharmaceutical Council, © 2001. All rights reserved. Reviewed by David A. Cooke, M.D., January 5, 2007.

An allergy is an inappropriate reaction by your immune system to harmless substances.[1] These substances can trigger sneezing, wheezing, coughing, itching, and severe, potentially fatal reactions.[2] Allergens enter the body in several ways. Airborne particles such as pollen, dust, and mold spores are breathed in through the nose and mouth; insect venom is injected through stingers; foods are ingested or swallowed. Medicines that can cause allergic reactions are injected or ingested. Many people suffer needlessly from allergies because they have never sought medical diagnosis or cannot identify the specific allergen.[1] However, with proper management and patient education, allergies can be controlled and people with allergies can lead normal and productive lives.[2]

Allergies and related conditions, such as asthma, are becoming more common and can be seasonal or year-long. The American Academy of Allergy, Asthma, and Immunology (AAAAI) estimates that allergies are the sixth leading cause of chronic disease in the United States, and cost the health care system over $18 billion annually.[3] More than 50 million Americans—about one of every five adults and children—suffer from allergies, including allergic asthma.[3] Patients and physicians are now beginning to realize that allergies are serious disorders that may demand advice from a physician. Furthermore,

24

over-the-counter treatments may prove less effective and have more side effects when addressing allergic disorders.[1]

A number of diseases can appear to be allergies, but upon professional examination prove to have other causes. For example, a runny nose and nasal congestion can be a result of chronic and repeated infections, but can appear similar to allergies. However, it is important to show proof of allergy whenever it is suspected because the treatments for allergic and non-allergic disease can be quite different.[2] Treating allergies requires avoiding allergic triggers, drug therapy to relieve and prevent chronic symptoms, and in severe cases, allergy shots to desensitize the patient to specific allergic triggers. Oral antihistamines and nasal sprays are the primary forms of drug therapy. Although nasal sprays have been shown to be effective, antihistamines remain the main drug treatment for allergies.[3,4] Newer, second-generation antihistamines (currently only available by prescription) provide relief with fewer side effects than first-generation sedating antihistamines (widely available over the counter), which have been shown to cause irritability, insomnia, anxiety, depression, dry mouth, and drowsiness.

The growing prevalence of allergies highlights the importance of practice guidelines for their diagnosis and treatment.[5] AAAAI, the National Institute of Allergy and Infectious Diseases (NIAID), and 20 other medical associations, advocacy groups, and government agencies recently published a report illustrating the best practices in the treatment of allergic disorders. Treatment recommendations include avoiding allergic triggers and using less-sedating or non-sedating antihistamines, or nasal sprays.[3] Non-sedating antihistamine-decongestant combinations are recommended by the AAAAI for patients with heavy congestion, and have been shown to reduce asthma symptoms among people diagnosed with both allergies and asthma.[6] The Joint Task Force on Practice Parameters in Allergy, Asthma and Immunology also states in its guidelines that non-sedating antihistamines should be considered before sedating antihistamines because they cause fewer side effects.[7]

From an employer's perspective, these therapies appear to be cost saving. The relatively high numbers of people who suffer from allergies and the lost productivity associated with them make allergies one of the most expensive diseases for employers. However, estimates suggest that employers can save $2 to $4 for each $1 spent to increase the use of non-sedating rather than sedating antihistamines.[8] The risk of workplace injury, for example, is significantly higher among workers taking sedating antihistamines. Productivity is also reduced when workers use sedating antihistamines. According to one study, if 50 percent of workers treated for allergies use sedating antihistamines and therefore functioned at 75 percent efficiency, the estimated lost productivity cost would be $2.4 billion for men and $1.4 billion for women. The estimated cost of lost workdays would be an additional $108 million.[9]

In addition to direct medical costs of $4.5 billion per year for the treatment of allergies, there are also indirect costs associated with allergies due to absenteeism and reduced productivity from the sedating effects of older drugs used in treatment.[3,10]

Data from the 1987 National Medical Expenditure Survey suggests that:[11]

* Americans miss 811,000 days of work due to allergies;
* Americans miss 824,000 days of school due to allergies; and,
* Americans have 4.2 million days of reduced activity per year due to allergies.

More recently, a 1999 report from the American Academy of Allergy, Asthma, and Immunology (AAAAI) estimates 3.8 million lost work and school days due to allergies.[3]

Like baldness, height and eye color, the capacity to become allergic can be an inherited characteristic.[2] If one parent has allergies, there is a 50 percent chance their children will have an allergy. If both parents have allergies, it is much more likely (66 percent) that their children will have allergies.[3] Yet a genetic predisposition to allergies does not necessarily mean allergic sensitivity. Developing allergic sensitivity is dependent on genetics, exposure to one or more allergens to which there is a genetically programmed response, and the degree and length of exposure. Other allergic reactions, such as those

Table 2.1. Some Examples of Allergens by Route of Exposure[3]

Inhaled Allergens	Contact Allergens	Ingested Allergens
Pollens	Plants	Foods
Molds/fungi	Drugs	Drugs
House dust mites	Cosmetics	
Animal danders	Jewelry (e.g., nickel)	
Cockroaches	Latex products	
Latex particles	Occupational chemicals/dyes	

produced by many plants, dyes, metals, and chemicals in deodorants and cosmetics, have no genetic basis.[2]

A Closer Look at Spending for Allergy Medications

Spending on pharmaceuticals was analyzed for individuals who received health benefit coverage from large employers in 1994 and 1997. The sample included individuals who were diagnosed with allergies or conditions for which allergy medicines are often prescribed. A similar analysis was conducted for individuals enrolled in private managed care plans from 1997 to 1999.

Spending for allergy medications rose 67 percent from 1994 to 1997. Volume factors (increased numbers of people with allergies receiving antihistamines and allergy-related prescriptions, and increased intensity and duration of drug therapy) accounted for roughly four-fifths of the total increase. Price factors had a relatively modest impact on spending growth.

Table 2.2. Factors Influencing Drug Spending for Allergies 1994–1997

Factors Influencing Growth in Rx Expenditures:	% Positive Impact	% Negative Impact
Total Growth in Expenditures	+67	
Growth Due to Volume Factors	+53	
Changes in the Number of Prescriptions per Person for Established Drugs		-38
Changes in the Number of Prescriptions per Person for New Entrants	+48	
Changes in Days of Therapy for Established Drugs	+13	
Changes in Days of Therapy for New Entrants	+1	
Patients per 1000 Health Care Enrollees	+28	
Growth Due to Price Factors	+14	
Inflation	+6	
Changes in Mix of Established Drugs	+8	
Price of New Entrants	+0.1	

Source: MEDSTAT's Marketscan database.

Factors Influencing Drug Spending for Allergies 1997–1999

Spending for allergy medications rose 89 percent between 1997 and 1999. Again, volume factors (increased numbers of people with allergies receiving antihistamines and allergy-related prescriptions, and increased intensity and duration of drug therapy) accounted for the majority of the increase. Increased numbers of patients being treated alone accounted for nearly half of the overall increase in spending.

Table 2.3. Factors Influencing Drug Spending for Allergies 1997–1999

Factors Influencing Growth in Rx Expenditures:	% Positive Impact	% Negative Impact
Total Growth in Expenditures	+89	
Growth Due to Volume Factors	+77	
Changes in the Number of Prescriptions per Person for Established Drugs	+0.1	
Changes in the Number of Prescriptions per Person for New Entrants	+21	
Changes in Days of Therapy for Established Drugs	+15	
Changes in Days of Therapy for New Entrants	+0.6	
Patients per 1000 Health Care Enrollees	+40	
Growth Due to Price Factors	+11	
Inflation	+8	
Changes in Mix of Established Drugs		-0.4
Price of New Entrants	+4	

Source: Protocare Sciences managed care database.

Methodology

This study separately analyzed prescription drug spending growth for two large national claims databases, one representing managed care plan enrollees and the other representing those covered by large employer-provided health benefit plans. The study defined and assessed several factors affecting the price per day of therapy and the volume of therapy—the number of days of therapy received and the number of patients receiving drug therapy. The analysis also examined the effects of price and volume changes for established drugs on the market during the entire period of analysis and for new drugs that were first marketed during this period.

References

1. Ulene, Art and the Asthma and Allergy Foundation of America. *How to Outsmart Your Allergies*. New York: HealthPOINTS, 1998.

2. The Asthma and Allergy Foundation of America. What are Allergies? Asthma and Allergy Answers. 1999.

3. American Academy of Allergy Asthma and Immunology (AAAAI). *The Allergy Report*. Milwaukee, WI: AAAAI, 2000.

4. Weiner JM, Abramson MJ, Puy RM. Intranasal corticosteroids versus oral H1 receptor antagonists in allergic rhinitis: systematic review of randomized controlled trials. *BMJ* 1998;317(7173): 1624–1629.

5. Rachelefsky GS. National guidelines needed to manage rhinitis and prevent complications. *Annals of Allergy, Asthma, & Immunology* 1999;82:296–305.

6. Corren J, Harris A, Aaronson D, et al. Efficacy and safety of loratadine plus pseudoephedrine in patients with seasonal allergic rhinitis and mild asthma. *J Allergy Clin Immunol* 1997; 100:781–788.

7. Dykewicz MS, Fineman S, Skoner DP, Nicklas R, Lee R, Blessing-Morre J, Li JT, Bernstein IL, Berger W, Spector S, Schuller D. Diagnosis and management of rhinitis: Complete guidelines of the Joint Task Force on practice parameters in allergy, asthma, and immunology. *Ann Allergy Asthma Immunol* 1998:478–518.

8. Measuring the value of the pharmacy benefit: Allergy as a case example. William M. Mercer, Inc. 2000.

9. Fireman P. Treatment of allergic rhinitis: Effect on occupation productivity and work force costs. *Allergy and Asthma Proc* 1997, 18(2):63–67.

10. Meltzer EO, Grant JA. Impact of cetirizine on the burden of allergic rhinitis. *Ann Allergy Asthma Immunol* 1999;83(5): 455–463.

11. Malone DC, Lawson KA, Smith DH, Arrighi HM, Battista C. A cost of illness study of allergic rhinitis in the United States. *J Allergy Clin Immunol* 1997:22–27.

Chapter 3

Questions and Answers about Allergies and Allergens

What is an allergy?

Allergy is a genetic condition causing the body to respond to harmless substances in the environment as though they were dangerous invaders. This response produces symptoms that may be mild to life threatening in susceptible people.

When does an allergy begin?

It occurs after a person with allergic tendencies is repeatedly exposed to the substance in his or her environment or his or her diet.

What causes an abnormal response?

When the allergic person comes into contact with the offending substance, the body's immune system rushes to the rescue and begins to produce antibodies to fight off the invader. These antibodies alter the way in which the body reacts and may produce allergic symptoms.

Is there a name for these offending substances?

They are called allergens.

"Allergy Q&A" © American Academy of Otolaryngic Allergy. All rights reserved. Reprinted with permission. Reviewed by David A. Cooke, M.D., January 5, 2007.

What kind of things are allergens?

Anything to which a person becomes allergic is an allergen. Certain substances, because of their physical and chemical structure, are more likely to become allergens than others. Prime examples are ragweed and other pollens and penicillin. Others are dust, mold, spores, animal dander, feathers, cereal grains, some airborne chemical pollutants, drugs, and insect venom.

What are the most common allergic symptoms?

The most common allergic symptoms are hay fever, asthma, and eczema.

What is hay fever?

"Hay fever" was named because of nasal symptoms developing during hay season, but most nasal allergies are called hay fever. In hay fever, the lining of the nose becomes irritated, causing the sufferer to sneeze and the nose to become stuffed up or to run. Eyes may itch or turn watery. Sometimes the ears feel blocked up. Hay fever occurs most frequently during the spring, summer, or fall when trees, grasses, and weeds produce pollen. One of the principal offenders is the ragweed plant, which produces the pollen from late summer until frost.

What is asthma?

Asthma is a condition that affects breathing and the lungs. The patient wheezes, coughs, and is short of breath.

What is eczema?

Eczema is an inflammation of the skin. It can take the form of red patches, crusts, and scales. The affected area generally itches. The condition generally occurs from eating certain foods.

Do all allergic responses fall into one of these categories?

No. In addition to hay fever, asthma, and eczema, there can be a wide range of allergic reactions suffered in all parts of the body. For example, headaches, hives, diarrhea, and stomach distress can be the result of allergy.

Is an allergy really a serious illness?

An allergic reaction can be slight and annoying or very serious. The inflamed lining of the nose of someone who suffers from hay fever can become infected, making the symptoms worse. Most dangerous of all is a sudden, heavy dose of an allergen, especially one like a bee sting or drug injection. This can trigger a generalized allergic reaction bringing on collapse, shock, or even death.

Are allergies inherited?

Although specific allergies themselves are not inherited, the tendency toward allergies is. The more allergic one's family is, the more likely one is to develop allergies. Though the trend to develop allergies may not appear in all members of a family or even in every generation of a family, the tendency is still there.

Are allergies common?

It is estimated that at least 20% of the population is likely to develop some kind of allergy.

At what age is a person most likely to develop an allergy?

It is most common for allergies to begin in childhood, but it is quite possible for allergic symptoms to make their first appearance at any age. You're never too old to develop an allergy.

Can an allergy be outgrown?

No. It is common for people to change the way their other allergic symptoms affect them, especially in childhood. For example, a baby may develop colic or eczema or have recurrent ear infection, but as it grows older, it may develop other allergic symptoms such as hay fever, ear fluid, or asthma. Adults have many varied symptoms such as chronic postnasal drainage, rashes, and stomach and intestinal problems. Older patients still have a tendency to have allergic symptoms, although they may become less noticeable with maturity.

What causes a person to develop an allergy?

There is no standard way for an allergy to begin, and the onset may be sudden or gradual. For a person to become allergic to a substance, he or she must be exposed to it more than once, and generally that exposure is quite frequent. Often, symptoms develop after an unusual stress to the immune system, such as that following a severe viral infection.

If I have an allergy, should I be treated by an allergist?

Because allergies can produce such a wide range of symptoms, there are a number of doctors, both specialists and general practitioners, in addition to allergists, who may be qualified to treat the allergic patient. For example, a skin allergy can be effectively treated by a dermatologist (a doctor who specializes in treating skin diseases) and an infantile cow's milk allergy may be treated by the child's own pediatrician. An internist who is concerned with lung disease may also be involved with allergies that affect the lungs. An allergist may be any physician trained in the diagnosis and treatment of allergies. There are general allergists who treat allergies throughout the body and specialty allergists, such as otolaryngologists (ear, nose, and throat specialists), who specialize in a specific part of the body.

Should an otolaryngologist treat my allergies?

An otolaryngologist is a doctor specializing in the treatment of ear, nose, and throat diseases. Half of the problems he or she encounters are probably due, either directly or indirectly, to allergy. Chronic nasal congestion and postnasal drip, seasonal or constant, is often allergic and may be complicated by chronic sinus and middle ear disease. Hearing loss, dizziness, headaches, weeping ear canals, and chronic sore throats may be due to allergy. The otolaryngologist who does his or her own allergy treatment is able to follow the patient's progress with specialized examinations and nose and throat medical and surgical treatment, such as polyp removal, placement of middle ear ventilating tubes, straightening of the nasal septum, and treatment of sinus infections. An otolaryngologist not providing allergy care may refer you to a colleague for such care.

What is the first treatment for allergies?

First of all, a careful history of the allergic person is taken. The most basic treatment, once an allergen has been identified, is to eliminate it. This may mean giving away a pet, avoiding certain jewelry and cosmetics, deleting specific foods from the diet, and alerting physicians about drug allergies.

What if the allergen can't be eliminated?

In the case of an allergen in the environment, such as dust, pollen, and mold, a thorough house cleaning, along with other careful preventive measures, will cut down on the exposure. However, if the allergen is seasonal pollen, moving may not be the solution because there might be tree or weed pollens in the new location that could bring about the development of another, equally distressful allergic reaction.

Then are drugs the answer?

Drug treatment has long been a cornerstone of allergy treatment. Antihistamines and/or decongestants (for the nose) and bronchodilators (for asthma) counteract the symptoms caused by the main chemical released by the body's immune system in an allergy attack. There are other drugs, both pills and nasal sprays, which can prevent the release of these inflammatory chemicals or suppress the immune reactions themselves.

What about cortisone?

Steroids of the cortisone family can suppress allergic reactions, but often there is the risk that the patient may develop significant side effects. Newer steroid nose sprays will often relieve allergies and not cause the side effects.

What about allergy shots?

Injections (immunotherapy) have been a satisfactory treatment for many inhaled allergens (that is, pollens, dust, molds and animal dander) and for bee stings. Before immunotherapy is begun, allergy tests are done in order to determine the offending allergens.

What do allergy shots involve?

The patient is given small doses of allergens by injection on a regular basis, usually weekly.

Is there a standard dosage for everyone?

No. The appropriate allergens and their doses must be determined individually for each patient. Skin testing (placing a minute amount of the allergen under the skin) and the radioallergosorbent test (RAST, a blood test for specific allergies) are both widely used for this purpose. Both detect the substances to which a person is allergic, as well as the degree of sensitivity, which helps determine the initial treatment dose.

How long will I have to take shots?

The injections can bring significant relief within a few months, but may require longer. They are usually continued for 2 to 3 years. In some cases, unfortunately, it may be necessary to continue the treatment indefinitely.

How successful is the treatment?

Over 80% of the patients who receive regular shots experience significant improvement or complete relief of their symptoms.

Chapter 4

The Impact of Allergies on Children and Adolescents

Chapter Contents

Section 4.1

Allergies in Children

"All About Allergies" was provided by KidsHealth, one of the largest resources online for medically reviewed health information written for parents, kids, and teens. For more articles like this one, visit www.KidsHealth .org, or www.TeensHealth.org. © 2005 The Nemours Foundation. This information was reviewed by Barbara P. Homeier, M.D., June 2005.

Dust, cats, peanuts, cockroaches. An odd grouping, but one with a common thread: allergies—a major cause of illness in the United States. Up to 50 million Americans, including millions of children, have some type of allergy. In fact, allergies account for the loss of an estimated 2 million school days per year.

What are allergies?

An allergy is an overreaction of the immune system to a substance that's harmless to most people. But in someone with an allergy, the body's immune system treats the substance (called an allergen) as an invader and reacts inappropriately, resulting in symptoms that can be anywhere from annoying to possibly harmful to the person.

In an attempt to protect the body, the immune system of the allergic person produces antibodies called immunoglobulin E (IgE). Those antibodies then cause mast cells (which are allergy cells in the body) to release chemicals, including histamine, into the bloodstream to defend against the allergen "invader."

It's the release of these chemicals that causes allergic reactions, affecting a person's eyes, nose, throat, lungs, skin, or gastrointestinal tract as the body attempts to rid itself of the invading allergen. Future exposure to that same allergen (things like nuts or pollen that you can be allergic to) will trigger this allergic response again. This means every time that person eats that particular food or is exposed to that particular allergen, he or she will have an allergic reaction.

Who gets allergies?

The tendency to develop allergies is often hereditary, which means it can be passed down through your genes. However, just because you, your

38

partner, or one of your children might have allergies doesn't mean that all of your children will definitely get them, too. And a person usually doesn't inherit a particular allergy, just the likelihood of having allergies.

But a few children have allergies even if no family member is allergic. And if a child is allergic to one substance, it's likely that he or she will be allergic to others as well.

What are the most common airborne allergens?

Some of the most common things people are allergic to are airborne (carried through the air).

Dust mites are one of the most common causes of allergies. These microscopic insects live all around us and feed on the millions of dead skin cells that fall off our bodies every day. Dust mites are the main allergic component of house dust, which is made up of many particles and can contain things such as fabric fibers and bacteria, as well as microscopic animal allergens. Present year-round in most parts of the United States (although they don't live at high altitudes), dust mites live in bedding, upholstery, and carpets.

Pollen is another major cause of allergies (most people know pollen allergy as hay fever or rose fever). Trees, weeds, and grasses release these tiny particles into the air to fertilize other plants. Pollen allergies are seasonal, and the type of pollen a child is allergic to determines when he or she will have symptoms. For example, in the mid-Atlantic states, tree pollination begins in February and March, grass from May through June, and ragweed from August through October; so people with these allergies are likely to experience increased symptoms during those times. Pollen counts measure how much pollen is in the air and can help people with allergies determine how bad their symptoms might be on any given day. Pollen counts are usually higher in the morning and on warm, dry, breezy days, whereas they're lowest when it's chilly and wet. Although they're not exact, the local weather report's pollen count can be helpful when planning outside activities.

Molds, another common allergen, are fungi that thrive both indoors and out in warm, moist environments. Outdoors, molds may be found in poor drainage areas, such as in piles of rotting leaves or compost piles. Indoors, molds thrive in dark, poorly ventilated places such as bathrooms and damp basements with water leaks or floods. A musty odor suggests mold growth. Although molds tend to be seasonal, many can grow year-round, especially those indoors.

Pet allergens from warm-blooded animals can cause problems for kids and parents alike. When the animal—often a household pet—

licks itself, the saliva gets on its fur or feathers. As the saliva dries, protein particles become airborne and work their way into fabrics in the home. Cats are the worst offenders because the protein from their saliva is extremely tiny and they tend to lick themselves more than other animals as part of grooming.

Cockroaches are also a major household allergen, especially in inner cities. Exposure to cockroach-infested buildings may be a major cause of the high rates of asthma in inner-city children.

What are the most common food allergens?

The American Academy of Allergy, Asthma, and Immunology estimates that up to 2 million, or 8%, of children in the United States are affected by food allergies, and that eight foods account for most of those food allergy reactions in kids: eggs, fish, milk, peanuts, shellfish, soy, tree nuts, and wheat.

Cow's milk (or cow's milk protein): Between 1% and 7.5% of infants are allergic to the proteins found in cow's milk and cow's milk-based formulas. About 80% of formulas on the market are cow's milk-based. Cow's milk protein allergy (also called formula protein allergy) means that the infant (or child or adult) has an abnormal immune system reaction to proteins found in the cow's milk used to make standard baby formulas.

Eggs: One of the most common food allergies in infants and young children, egg allergy can pose many challenges for parents. Because eggs are used in many of the foods kids eat—and in many cases they're "hidden" ingredients—an egg allergy is hard to diagnose. An egg allergy usually begins when children are very young, but most outgrow the allergy by age 5. Most kids with an egg allergy are allergic to the proteins in egg whites, but some can't tolerate proteins in the yolk.

Fish and shellfish: The proteins in fish can cause a number of different types of allergic reactions, including a gastrointestinal reaction that leads to diarrhea and vomiting. Children can also have skin reactions to fish causing itching and dryness. Fish allergy is also one of the more common adult food allergies and one that children don't always grow out of.

Peanuts and tree nuts: Peanuts are one of the most severe food allergens, often causing life-threatening reactions. About 1.5 million people in the United States are allergic to peanuts (which are not a true nut, but a legume—in the same family as peas and lentils). Half of those allergic to peanuts are also allergic to tree nuts, such as almonds, walnuts, pecans, cashews, and often sunflower and sesame seeds.

Soy: Like peanuts, soybeans are legumes. Soy allergy is more prevalent among babies than older children; about 30% to 40% of infants who are allergic to cow's milk are also allergic to the protein in soy formulas.

Wheat: Wheat proteins are found in many of the foods we eat—some are more obvious than others. As with any allergy, an allergy to wheat can happen in different ways and to different degrees. Although wheat allergy is often confused with celiac disease, there is a difference. Celiac disease is caused by a permanent sensitivity to gluten, which is found in wheat, oat, rye, and barley. It typically develops between 6 months and 2 years of age and the sensitivity causes damage to the small intestine.

What are some other common allergens?

Insect stings: For most children, being stung by an insect means swelling, redness, and itching at the site of the bite, in addition to a few tears. But for children with insect venom allergy, an insect bite can cause more severe symptoms. Although some doctors and parents have believed that most children eventually outgrow insect venom allergy, a recent study found that insect venom allergies often persist into adulthood.

Medicines: Antibiotics—medications used to treat infections—are the most common types of medicines that cause allergic reactions. Many other medicines, including over-the-counter medications, can also cause allergic reactions.

Chemicals: Some cosmetics or laundry detergents can cause people to break out in an itchy rash. Usually, this is because the person has a reaction to the chemicals in these products. Dyes, household cleaners, and pesticides used on lawns or plants can also cause allergic reactions in some people.

Some children also have what are called cross-reactions. For example, kids who are allergic to birch pollen might have reactions when they eat an apple because that apple is made up of a protein similar to one in the pollen. Another example is that children who are allergic to latex (as in gloves or certain types of hospital equipment) are more likely to be allergic to kiwifruit or bananas.

What are the signs and symptoms of allergies?

The type and severity of allergy symptoms vary from allergy to allergy and child to child. Symptoms can range from minor or major seasonal annoyances (for example, from pollen or certain molds) to year-round problems (from allergens like dust mites or food).

Because different allergens are more prevalent in different parts of the country and the world, allergy symptoms can also vary, depending on where you live. For example, peanut allergy is unknown in Scandinavia, where they don't eat peanuts, but is common in the United States, where peanuts are not only a popular food, but are also found in many of the things we eat.

Airborne allergy symptoms: Airborne allergens can cause something known allergic rhinitis, which occurs in about 15% to 20% of Americans. It typically develops by 10 years of age and reaches its peak in the early 20s, with symptoms often disappearing between the ages of 40 and 60. Symptoms can include:

- sneezing;
- itchy nose and/or throat;
- nasal congestion; and
- coughing.

These symptoms are often accompanied by itchy, watery, and/or red eyes, which is called allergic conjunctivitis. (When dark circles are present around the eyes, they are called allergic "shiners"). Those who react to airborne allergens usually have allergic rhinitis and/or allergic conjunctivitis. If a person has these symptoms, as well as wheezing and shortness of breath, the allergy may have progressed to become asthma.

Food allergy symptoms: The severity of food allergy symptoms and when they develop depends on:

- how much of the food is eaten;
- the amount of exposure the child has had to the food; and
- the child's sensitivity to the food.

Symptoms of food allergies can include:

- itchy mouth and throat when food is swallowed (some children have only this symptom—called "oral allergy syndrome");
- hives (raised, red, itchy bumps);
- rash;
- runny, itchy nose; and
- abdominal cramps accompanied by nausea and vomiting or diarrhea (as the body attempts to flush out the food allergen).

Insect venom allergy symptoms: Being stung by an insect that a child is allergic to may cause some of the following symptoms:

- throat swelling;
- hives over the entire body;
- difficulty breathing;
- nausea; and
- diarrhea.

What's anaphylaxis?

In rare instances, if the sensitivity to an allergen is extreme, a child may experience anaphylaxis (or anaphylactic shock)—a sudden, severe allergic reaction involving various systems in the body (such as the skin, respiratory tract, gastrointestinal tract, and cardiovascular system).

Severe symptoms or reactions to any allergen, from certain foods to insect bites, require immediate medical attention and can include:

- difficulty breathing;
- swelling (particularly of the face, throat, lips, and tongue in cases of food allergies);
- rapid drop in blood pressure;
- dizziness;
- unconsciousness;
- hives;
- tightness of the throat;
- hoarse voice;

- nausea;
- vomiting;
- abdominal pain;
- diarrhea; and
- lightheadedness.

Anaphylaxis can happen just seconds after being exposed to a triggering substance or can be delayed for up to 2 hours if the reaction is from a food. It can involve various areas of the body.

Fortunately, though, severe or life-threatening allergies occur in only a small group of children. In fact, the annual incidence of anaphylactic reactions is small—about 30 per 100,000 people—although those with asthma, eczema, or hay fever are at greater risk of experiencing them. Most—up to 80%—of the anaphylactic reactions are caused by peanuts or tree nuts.

How are allergies diagnosed?

Some allergies are fairly easy to identify because the pattern of symptoms following exposure to certain allergens can be hard to miss. But other allergies are less obvious because they can masquerade as other conditions.

If your child has cold-like symptoms lasting longer than a week or 2 or develops a "cold" at the same time every year, consult your child's doctor, who will likely ask questions about your child's symptoms and when they appear. Based on the answers to these questions and a physical exam, your child's doctor may be able to make a diagnosis and prescribe medications or may refer you to an allergist for allergy skin tests and more extensive therapy.

To determine the cause of an allergy, an allergist will likely perform skin tests for the most common environmental and food allergens. Skin tests can be done in young infants, but they're more reliable in children over the age of 2 years.

A skin test can work in one of two ways:

- A drop of a purified liquid form of the allergen is dropped onto the skin and the area is pinched with a small pricking device.

- A small amount of allergen is injected just under the skin. This test stings a little but isn't extremely painful. After about 15 minutes, if a lump surrounded by a reddish area appears (like a mosquito bite) at the injection site, the test is positive.

If reactions to a food or other allergen are severe, a blood test may be used to diagnose the allergy so as to avoid exposure to the offending allergen. Skin tests are less expensive and more sensitive than blood tests for allergies. But blood tests may be required in children with skin conditions or those who are extremely sensitive to a particular allergen. Blood tests are also helpful in deciding whether a child has outgrown a food allergy, because the skin tests tend to remain positive even after the food allergy has disappeared.

Even if a skin test and/or a blood test shows an allergy, a child must also have symptoms to be definitively diagnosed with an allergy. For example, a toddler who has a positive test for dust mites and sneezes frequently while playing on the floor would be considered allergic to dust mites.

How are allergies treated?

There is no real cure for allergies, but it is possible to relieve a child's symptoms. The only real way to cope with them on a daily basis is to reduce or eliminate exposure to allergens. That means that parents must educate their children early and often, not only about the allergy itself but also about what reaction they will have if they consume or come into contact with the offending allergen.

Informing any and all caregivers (from child-care personnel to teachers, from extended family members to parents of your child's friends) about your child's allergy is equally important to help keep your child's allergy symptoms to a minimum.

If reducing exposure isn't possible or is ineffective, medications may be prescribed including antihistamines (which you can also buy over the counter) and inhaled or nasal spray steroids. In some cases, an allergist may recommend immunotherapy (allergy shots) to help desensitize your child.

And here are some things that can help your child avoid airborne allergens:

- Keep family pets out of certain rooms, like your child's bedroom, and bathe them if necessary.

- Remove carpets or rugs from your child's room (hard floor surfaces don't collect dust as much as carpets do).

- Don't hang heavy drapes and get rid of other items that allow dust to accumulate.

- Clean frequently.

- Use special covers to seal pillows and mattresses if your child is allergic to dust mites.

- If your child is allergic to pollen, keep your windows closed when the pollen season is at its peak, change your child's clothing after being outdoors, and don't let your child mow the lawn.

- Have your child avoid damp areas, such as basements, if he or she is allergic to mold, and keep bathrooms and other mold-prone areas clean and dry.

What does injectable epinephrine do?

Food allergies usually aren't lifelong (although those to peanut, tree nut, and seafood can be). Avoiding the food is the only way to avoid symptoms while the sensitivity persists. If your child is extremely sensitive to a particular food, or if he or she has asthma in addition to the food allergy, your child's doctor will probably recommend that you carry injectable epinephrine (adrenaline) to counteract any allergic reactions. He or she may also recommend carrying injectable epinephrine if your child is allergic to insect venom.

Available in an easy-to-carry container that looks like a pen, injectable epinephrine is carried by millions of parents across the country everywhere they go. With one injection into the thigh, the device administers epinephrine to ease the allergic reaction.

An injectable epinephrine prescription usually includes two auto-injections and a "trainer" that contains no needle or epinephrine, but allows you and your child (if he or she is old enough) to practice using the device. It's essential that you familiarize yourself with the procedure by practicing with the trainer. Your child's doctor can also give you instructions on how to use and store injectable epinephrine.

If your child is 12 years or older, make sure he or she keeps injectable epinephrine readily available at all times. If your child is younger than 12, talk to the school nurse, your child's teacher, and your childcare provider about keeping injectable epinephrine on hand in case of an emergency.

It's also important to make sure that injectable epinephrine devices are available at your home, as well as at the homes of friends and family members if your child spends time there. Your child's doctor may also encourage your child to wear a medical alert bracelet. It's also a good idea to carry an over-the-counter antihistamine, which can help alleviate allergy symptoms in some people. But antihistamines should not be used as a replacement for the epinephrine pen.

Kids who have had to take injectable epinephrine should go immediately to a medical facility or hospital emergency department, where additional treatment can be given if needed. Up to one third of anaphylactic reactions can have a second wave of symptoms several hours following the initial attack, so these kids might need to be observed in a clinic or hospital for 4 to 8 hours following the reaction even though they seem well.

The good news is that only a very small group of kids will experience severe or life-threatening allergies. With proper diagnosis, preventive measures, and treatment, most children will be able to keep their allergies in check and live, happy, healthy lives.

Section 4.2

Early Fevers May Affect Allergy Risk Later in Childhood

From "Early Fevers Associated with Lower Allergy Risk Later in Childhood," by the National Institute of Allergy and Infectious Diseases (NIAID), February 9, 2004.

Infants who experience fevers before their first birthday are less likely to develop allergies by ages six or seven, according to a 2004 study funded by the National Institute of Allergy and Infectious Diseases (NIAID), part of the National Institutes of Health (NIH). The study, published in the February 2004 issue of the *Journal of Allergy and Clinical Immunology*, lends support to the well-known "hygiene hypothesis," which contends that early exposure to infections might protect children against allergic diseases in later years.

"The prevalence of asthma and allergies has increased dramatically worldwide in recent years," says Anthony S. Fauci, M.D., director of NIAID. "This study provides evidence that diminished exposure to early immunological challenges could be one of the reasons for this trend."

"The hygiene hypothesis is widely recognized but largely unproven," says Kenneth Adams, Ph.D., who oversees asthma research funded

47

by NIAID. "The findings of this study strengthen the hypothesis and, after more research, could lead to preventative therapies for asthma and allergies."

The authors of the study followed the medical records of 835 children from birth to age 1, documenting any fever-related episodes. Fever was defined as a rectal temperature of 101 degrees Fahrenheit or above. At age 6 to 7 years, more than half of the children were evaluated for their sensitivity to common allergens, such as dust mites, ragweed and cats.

Researchers found that, of the children who did not experience a fever during their first year, 50 percent showed allergic sensitivity. Of those who had one fever, 46.7 percent became allergy-prone. The children who suffered two or more fevers in their infancy had greater protection, with only 31.3 percent showing allergic sensitivity by ages 6 to 7.

In particular, fever-inducing infections involving the eyes, ears, nose or throat appeared to be associated with a lower risk of developing allergies, compared with similar infections that did not result in fevers.

"We didn't expect fever to relate with such a consistent effect," says Christine C. Johnson, Ph.D., M.P.H., senior research epidemiologist of the Henry Ford Health System in Detroit, Michigan, and one of the co-authors of the study. "It also was interesting that the more fevers an infant had, the less likely it was that he or she would be sensitive to allergies."

Dr. Johnson says that more research is needed to establish if early fevers have a direct effect on allergic development in children. Additionally, she and the other authors are working to determine if early exposure to pets as well as high levels of bacteria could also lower allergy risk. "If we can uncover which environmental factors affect allergic development and why, it may be possible to immunize children against these conditions," she says.

Reference: L Keoki Williams et al. The relationship between early fever and allergic sensitization at age 6 to 7 years. *Journal of Allergy and Clinical Immunology* 113(2): 291–296 (2004).

Section 4.3

Do Childhood Vaccines Cause Allergies?

"Do Vaccines Cause Asthma, Allergies or Other Chronic Diseases?
Reviews of Scientific Data Offer Reassurances on Vaccine Safety"
© The Children's Hospital of Philadelphia 2003.

Large scientific studies do not support claims that vaccines may cause chronic diseases such as asthma, multiple sclerosis, chronic arthritis and diabetes, according to a report in the March 2003 issue of *Pediatrics*. The report's lead author, Paul A. Offit, M.D., chief of Infectious Diseases and director of the Vaccine Education Center at The Children's Hospital of Philadelphia, identifies flaws in proposed biological explanations for how vaccines cause chronic diseases and reviews current research on associations between vaccines and those diseases.

"Anecdotal reports and uncontrolled studies have proposed that vaccines may cause particular allergic or autoimmune diseases," says Dr. Offit. "Such reports have led some parents to delay or withhold vaccinations for their children. This is very unfortunate, because the best available scientific evidence does not support the idea that vaccines cause chronic diseases. Scientific studies have shown, however, that reducing vaccination rates lead to increases in preventable infectious diseases."

In the article, co-authored by Charles J. Hackett, Ph.D., of the National Institutes of Allergy and Infectious Diseases, Dr. Offit critically analyzes proposed explanations for a link between vaccines and chronic diseases, such as the "hygiene hypothesis." The hygiene hypothesis states that improved hygiene and decreased early exposure to common childhood infections may actually raise a child's risk of developing allergies. Several studies support this hypothesis, says Dr. Offit, such as findings that children who attend child care or live in large families are less likely to have allergies.

However, adds Dr. Offit, the hygiene hypothesis does not fit vaccine-related diseases. Vaccines do not prevent most common childhood infections, such as upper and lower respiratory tract infections, which form the basis of the hygiene hypothesis. On the other hand, vaccine-preventable infectious diseases such as measles, mumps, and whooping cough are easily transmitted regardless of home hygiene. "The flaws in using this biological mechanism to explain a link between vaccines and allergies are consistent with large-scale epidemiological studies," said Dr. Offit. "Those studies found no evidence that vaccines increase the risk of asthma, food allergies, or other allergic disorders."

Another set of hypotheses proposes that vaccines cause autoimmune diseases such as multiple sclerosis or type 1 diabetes by inadvertently stimulating the immune system to attack itself. The mechanism of "molecular mimicry" is based on the fact that some proteins on invading microbes are similar to human proteins. In responding to proteins from the infectious agent, the immune system may mistakenly attack similar proteins in the patient's body, and set off a disease.

Molecular mimicry may indeed allow a natural infection to trigger an autoimmune disease, as when Lyme disease leads to chronic arthritis. However, says Dr. Offit, this process cannot be extended to what happens with vaccines. Naturally occurring viruses and bacteria are much better adapted to growing in humans than vaccines, and are much more likely to stimulate potentially damaging autoimmune reactions.

"Vaccines are engineered to carry weakened or deactivated pathogens, and consequently there are critical differences between natural infection and immunization," said Dr. Offit. "These differences are reflected in the many well-controlled epidemiological studies that do not show a causal relationship between vaccines and autoimmune diseases, including multiple sclerosis, type 1 diabetes and chronic arthritis."

About the Expert

Paul A. Offit, M.D., is the director of the Vaccine Education Center and chief of Infectious Diseases at The Children's Hospital of Philadelphia. An internationally recognized expert in virology, immunology and vaccine safety, he is a member of the Advisory Committee on Immunization Practices to the Centers for Disease Control and Prevention. In addition to publishing more than 90 peer-reviewed scientific papers, Dr. Offit is co-author of the book *Vaccines: What Every Parent Should Know*. He frequently lectures to national and international health care organizations about vaccine safety and efficacy.

Under the direction of Dr. Offit, The Children's Hospital of Philadelphia established The Vaccine Education Center in October 2000 to respond to the rapidly growing need for accurate, up-to-date, science-based information about vaccines and the diseases they prevent. The Center is a nationally recognized educational resource for health care professionals and parents, providing information on the full spectrum of vaccine-related topics. Approximately 400 people per day visit the Center's comprehensive website (vaccine.chop.edu).

Section 4.4

Allergies Linked to Poor Grades, Missed School, and Less Sleep

Allergic rhinitis can impede a child's learning, mental function, and classroom performance if not properly managed, according to data presented at the annual meeting of the American College of Allergy, Asthma and Immunology (ACAAI) in Boston.

A multidisciplinary panel report on the impact of allergic rhinitis in school children presented at the ACAAI meeting indicated 40 percent of the pediatric population suffers from allergic rhinitis. Allergies also result in absenteeism with more than two million missed school days a year. If left untreated, allergies can lead to more serious conditions such as asthma, chronic sinusitis, and other respiratory conditions.

"Children with allergic rhinitis can be more irritable and tired, which can lead to inattentiveness and difficulty concentrating in class," said Michael Blaiss, M.D., Memphis, ACAAI president 2003 to 2004, and lead author on the paper. "They may be distracted by their symptoms and become unresponsive and disinterested in activities."

Unfortunately, many children still remain undiagnosed and untreated, which is why it is important for school nurses, teachers, and parents to work together to identify children with allergic rhinitis so they can receive proper diagnosis and treatment.

The report also noted that most over-the-counter (OTC) and some prescription antihistamines can negatively impact cognitive function and learning, due to their sedating properties. Since children may be

51

more prone to sedation than adults, it is important to consider the potential impairing effects of medications when choosing appropriate treatment.

"It's clear from available research that allergic rhinitis can negatively impact school performance and learning for school-aged children, which is why accurate diagnosis and treatment of the condition is critical," Dr. Blaiss said. "One of the primary goals in treating allergic rhinitis in children is to manage the symptoms without altering their ability to function. If symptoms can be controlled with nonsedating medications, medications with the potential to cause sedation should be avoided."

According to Henry Milgrom, M.D., of the National Jewish Medical and Research Center in Denver, allergies are the most prevalent chronic condition in patients under 18 years of age. More often than not, an allergy diagnosis is clouded by a second health issue such as eczema, asthma, eustachian tube dysfunction, or sleep apnea. Sleep disorders are far more prevalent in children with seasonal allergies than children without allergies. Poor control of night-time symptoms often results in daytime fatigue, increasing learning impairment.

Allergic rhinitis also impairs cognitive function. "Both the acquisition and application of knowledge are slowed in allergic children compared with healthy children," said Dr. Milgrom. "Fatigue, irritability, intermittent hearing loss, and frequent nose wiping are all factors in contributing to a child's inattentiveness and inability to concentrate," said Dr. Milgrom.

Most of the available information focuses on antihistamines even though there are other treatment options, according to Diane E. Schuller, M.D., Penn State University, Milton S. Hershey Medical College in Hershey, Pennsylvania. "Antihistamines are just the first line of defense against allergic symptoms in children," Dr. Schuller said. "Many questions remain regarding decongestants, intranasal corticosteroids, and newer approaches including leukotriene receptors, anticholinergics, and mast cell stabilizers."

Dr. Schuller dispelled some myths about antihistamines, such as they do not lose their effectiveness over time and people do not become accustomed to their sedative or impairing effects. Second and first generation histamines are distinctly different. For example, first generation antihistamines cross the blood-brain barrier. In other words, the blood circulation to the brain is, in a sense, filtered and some chemicals float through and some do not. First generation antihistamines impair learning and cognitive processing. Second generation antihistamines do not cross the blood brain barrier.

"Differences also exist between the five second-generation-histamines approved by the FDA [U.S. Food and Drug Administration] relative to efficacy and safety. Sedation, though to a lesser extent with second generation agents, is still a concern. It's important that each patient have an individualized approach to treatment, because reactions to medication may vary," Dr. Schuller said.

Social adjustment can also be an issue in children with allergic rhinitis. In a study of almost 2,000 patients ages 12 to 65, with mild to moderate allergic rhinitis, nearly three quarters of the patients reported feeling embarrassed and troubled by their symptoms some or all of the time. Almost all of the patients reported that they were troubled by a practical problem related to dealing with allergies, such as itchiness or the inconvenience of carrying tissues.

Section 4.5

Over-the-Counter Allergy Treatments Can Hinder Learning

The number of allergic children is on the rise. And it's not just homework they're allergic to. In a recent study, more than 20 percent of the population of school children were found to be suffering from allergies. Allergies cause students in the United States to miss 2 million school days a year and to suffer a significantly reduced ability to learn, researchers have found.

There are many consequences of allergy conditions in children. Functional impairment is one of the most debilitating. These functions include hearing and speech problems, as related to otitis media with effusion, and attention and alertness problems, which can be caused by allergies as well as by some sedating medications used to treat allergic symptomatology. Inability to concentrate may affect learning, behavior, and overall school performance.

Many parents treat a child's allergies with over-the-counter anti-histamines, but they can produce significant drowsiness. The sedation caused by over-the-counter (OTC) products can reduce a child's ability to remember facts and analyze concepts. The United States is the only industrialized nation that still uses sedating antihistamines as the primary treatment for allergies in children.

The sedation associated with first-generation OTC antihistamines can also significantly hinder a child's ability to learn. Because one of the most important aspects of learning is attentiveness, the chronic use of sedating antihistamines for allergic rhinitis can also alter a child's learning potential over time. Furthermore, children may also suffer from stimulatory effects such as excitation, hyperactivity, irritability, or insomnia.

Before treating a child for allergies and asthma, a physician should be consulted. A child's condition should be discussed with the school nurse, teachers, coaches, and any other people with whom the child has regular contact. These people should be informed of the triggers that can impact the child's condition, such as animals, dust, pollen, and freshly cut grass.

A treatment plan developed by a health care provider with the input of parents, caregivers, and educators can ensure that children with allergies enjoy a full, productive school day, and take an active part in after school activities on par with their non-allergic peers.

The Allergy Report, the first multi-disciplinary consensus document on the diagnosis and treatment of allergies, was developed by 21 major health care organizations to provide health care professionals, including the school nurse, with an accessible patient management reference tool to help understand, diagnose, and manage allergic disorders.

Chapter 5

The Relationship between Allergies and Asthma

Chapter Contents

Section 5.1

Asthma and the Allergic Response

Immunoglobulin E (IgE) is a type of antibody that is present in minute amounts in the body but plays a major role in allergic diseases. IgE binds to allergens and triggers the release of substances from mast cells that can cause inflammation. When IgE binds to mast cells, a cascade of allergic reaction can begin.

- **Allergen exposure:** Repeated exposure to a particular allergen can be the first step in developing a reaction to it. Some allergens trigger strong allergic reactions, while others trigger milder reactions.

- **T cell action:** Allergens induce T cells to activate B cells, which develop into plasma cells that produce and release more antibodies.

Binding of IgE to Mast Cells

The surfaces of mast cells contain special receptors for binding IgE. The IgE antibody fits to this receptor like a module docking with the mother ship. This arrangement is such that when two adjacent mast-cell-linked IgE antibodies are in place, the allergen is drawn to both and attaches itself to both, cross-linking the two IgEs. When a critical mass of IgEs become cross-linked, the mast cell releases histamine and other inflammatory substances, and the allergic cascade begins.

The Allergic Cascade

Following exposure to an allergen, a series of initial reactions in the immune system occurs. This early-phase response is followed by a second, more severe reaction known as a late-phase response.

Typically, the allergic cascade follows this pattern:

1. Sensitization to an allergen

2. Early-phase response upon re-exposure to an allergen

3. Late-phase response to an allergen

1. Sensitization to an allergen: Being exposed for the first time.

You might be initially exposed to an allergen by:

- Inhalation (of pollen, mold, dust mites, etc.);

- Ingestion (swallowing a type of food or medication);

- Touch (coming into contact with poison ivy, latex, or certain metals, such as nickel);

- Injection (receiving a medication or being stung by an insect).

Your body produces IgE designed specifically for that particular allergen, but you won't experience a reaction yet.

- If you are atopic (meaning, you've inherited a predisposition toward allergic disease), your T cells are quick to stimulate B cells.

- When stimulated, B cells develop into plasma cells.

- Plasma cells produce IgE antibodies, which are targeted to that specific allergen.

- The IgE binds to special receptors on mast cells.

- Your system is now sensitized. Your mast cells are like little bombs that are armed and ready for detonation.

2. Early-phase response upon re-exposure to an allergen.

When you are re-exposed to an allergen:

- The IgE of mast cells binds to the allergen, cross-linking the IgE.

- When enough cross-linking occurs, the mast cells explode with histamine and other inflammatory substances, called mediators. The mediators speed through your system.

- It happens. You wheeze, sneeze, cough, get itchy eyes, have a runny nose, become short of breath—in other words, you experience the whole unpleasant range of symptoms known as the allergic response.

And all of this occurs within an hour after initial exposure.

3. Late-phase response to an allergen.

The late-phase response actually begins at the same time as the early-phase response, but it takes longer to see. In some individuals, the body rallies its immune system for this second phase, which can happen relatively soon after the initial reaction—anywhere from about three to 10 hours later). Often, this late-phase response involves immune cells known as eosinophils and it can last for 24 hours or so before subsiding. During the late-phase response, congestion and certain other symptoms can be more severe than those seen during the initial response.

Consequences of Chronic Allergic Reaction in Asthma

With repeated allergen exposure and allergic response, some damage can be done to the tissues involved. To remedy this damage, researchers are exploring the issue of airway remodeling, or scarring of the airways in the lungs of asthma patients. Long-term controller medications that aggressively attack inflammation and maintain maximum lung function are also believed to reduce the risk of permanent damage.

Although allergic disease is not curable, it is treatable enough to live with. Health care providers can be significant allies in this effort—particularly allergists, pulmonologists, and certain other specialists. In addition, many research organizations make studying allergic disease their top priority, and can be excellent sources of information on the immune system. The more you know about how an allergic response occurs, the better armed you'll be to meet its challenges.

Section 5.2

Do Allergies Cause Asthma?

This information was provided by KidsHealth, one of the largest resources online for medically reviewed health information written for parents, kids, and teens. For more articles like this one, visit www.KidsHealth.org, or www.TeensHealth.org. © 2004 The Nemours Foundation. This information was reviewed by Elana Pearl Ben-Joseph, M.D., October 2004.

Although allergies and asthma are separate conditions, they are related. People who have allergies—particularly those that affect the nose and eyes—are more likely to have asthma. If you have allergies or asthma, your child is more likely to have it, too, because the tendency to develop these conditions is often inherited.

But not everyone who has allergies has asthma, and not all cases of asthma are related to allergies. About 75% of kids who have asthma also have upper respiratory allergies. And most people who have asthma find their symptoms get worse when they're exposed to specific allergens (anything that causes an allergic reaction).

With any kind of allergy, the immune system overreacts to normally harmless allergens. Those substances, such as pollen, can cause allergic reactions in some people. As part of this overreaction, the body produces an antibody of the immunoglobulin E (IgE) type, which specifically recognizes and attaches to the allergen when the body is exposed to it.

If that happens, it sets a process in motion that results in the release of certain substances in the body. One of them is histamine, which causes allergic symptoms that can affect the eyes, nose, throat, skin, gastrointestinal tract, or lungs. When the airways in the lungs are affected, symptoms of asthma can occur.

Future exposure to the same allergens will cause the reaction to happen again. So if your child has asthma, it's a good idea to explore whether allergies may be triggering some of the symptoms. Talk with your child's doctor about how to identify possible triggers, which can be things other than allergens, such as cold air or tobacco smoke. Your doctor might also recommend visiting an allergist for allergy tests. If you find out your child is allergic to something, that substance may be causing or contributing to asthma symptoms (coughing, wheezing, and trouble breathing).

If it does look like allergens are an important trigger for your child's asthma symptoms, do what you can to help your child avoid exposure to the allergens involved. If this doesn't control your child's asthma symptoms adequately, the doctor may also prescribe medications or allergy shots.

Chapter 6

The Hygiene Hypothesis: Exposure to Diseases May Prevent Allergy Development

Increased hygiene and a lack of exposure to various microorganisms may be affecting the immune systems of many populations—particularly in highly developed countries like the United States—to the degree that individuals are losing their bodily ability to fight off certain diseases.

That's the essence of the "hygiene hypothesis," a fairly new school of thought that argues that rising incidence of asthma, inflammatory bowel disease, multiple sclerosis and perhaps several other diseases may be, at least in part, the result of lifestyle and environmental changes that have made us too "clean" for our own good.

"Medicine has a lot of history behind it related to why certain diseases are so widespread and certain diseases are not widespread," said Subra Kugathasan, M.D., Medical College of Wisconsin Associate Professor of Pediatrics (Gastroenterology), who has made a study of developments in hygiene hypothesis research.

"The immune system is there for a reason," said Dr. Kugathasan. "It's there to recognize 'the bad guys.' The immune system allows your body to kill those bad guys and allows you to survive. In order to harden the immune system, the immune system requests some kind of stimuli all the time."

"The hygiene hypothesis suggests that the more hygienic one becomes, the more susceptible one is to various autoimmune diseases.

"Hygiene Hypothesis: Are We Too 'Clean' for Our Own Good?" September 2004. © 2004 Medical College of Wisconsin. Reprinted with permission of Medical College of Wisconsin HealthLink, www.healthlink.mcw.edu.

The autoimmune diseases, the diseases that result from all the activation of your immune system, are increasing. The hygiene hypothesis—and we don't yet have a proof of it—acknowledges that the maturation of the immune system needs some kind of hardening, some kind of resistance. Put another way, you cannot really build up good muscles without doing exercise."

From Pet Dander to Pig Worms

The common belief that has driven medicine, as well as public perception and hygiene practices, is that when we get sick it is because of something we ate, or inhaled, or were exposed to in other ways. The hygiene hypothesis points in a different direction, proposing that in many diseases it is a lack of exposure to the "bad guys" that causes harm.

While the evidence was by no means clear-cut, one study indicated that in some cases contact with certain pet dander in the home actually decreases a child's risk of wheezing from asthma later in life. Other studies show that children who lived on farms when they were very young have reduced incidence of asthma, which has led several researchers to conclude that organisms in cattle dust and manure may be the stimuli that their immune systems needed to fight off asthma.

In another study, conducted by University of Iowa Division of Gastroenterology director Dr. Joel Weinstock, intestinal worms were shown to have a very dramatic effect on mice in offering protection from inflammatory bowel disease. This was followed up using whipworms from pigs, *Trichuris suis*, in a small number of humans. The worms were selected because they are "safe," as many pig farmers come in contact with them every day, they do not enter the human bloodstream, and they cannot live in the human intestine for more than a week.

All of the six patients who were given the worm treatment for their bowel disease eventually went from chronic illness to complete remission with no diarrhea, no abdominal pain and no joint problems. In very general terms, this small-scale test of the hygiene hypothesis worked because microorganisms from the worms positively affect the body's immune response to bacteria and viruses.

"Think about countries in Africa like Gambia, a country that has been studied very well," said Dr. Kugathasan. "Ninety to ninety-nine percent of people in Gambia have intestinal worms at some point in their lives. But the chronic immune diseases like asthma, Crohn disease, or multiple sclerosis are not heard of, never even mentioned in their life. They don't know anything about such diseases in those countries. While one may argue that maybe their population is genetically not predisposed to these diseases, other factors appear to be in play."

"What has happened now, with globalization and human migration, people move to areas that are very, very clean. Within one generation we have moved into a different environment. What we have been finding out is that in the second generation of Asian, Latin American and African children, where the first generation had been exposed to those kinds of parasites and early childhood infections, the second generation that has moved to 'cleaner' countries has not been exposed. The incidence of Crohn disease, multiple sclerosis, and chronic asthma is as common in the second generation from the third world as in those with European or North American backgrounds, and in some cases even higher."

Playing in the Dirt

Dr. Kugathasan and others interested in hygiene hypothesis have not proposed that "playing in the dirt," or making society less hygienic in general, are useful goals in medicine. But they do propose that taking the impact of reduced immunological strength into account for certain diseases could be beneficial.

For example, researchers who are looking into the impact of microorganisms produced by cattle on asthma in children maintain that the more they learn about how cattle exposure relates to asthma, the closer they will come to developing an effective preventive treatment.

"Over the years, what's happened with modern medicine is that we have become more aware of the disease process, so we are avoiding diseases by learning more about how they spread," said Dr. Kugathasan. "We are becoming much cleaner and learning how to prevent many diseases by immunization. And we are isolating ourselves by not going into epidemic areas. Now we don't even allow kids to play in the yard barefoot. Children playing in the dirt barefoot are exposed to a lot of microorganisms and worms and everything else, and that's not happening the way it used to."

"So the hygiene hypothesis doesn't only apply to Crohn disease and inflammatory bowel disease," Dr. Kugathasan says. "It applies to many other conditions. This doesn't mean children should roll around in the dirt or necessarily change medical practice in the United States. But to keep the immune system working properly, you need controlled stimulus or else it doesn't know how to recognize the bad guys. Treatment is meant to suppress the system, while the hygiene hypothesis suggests that it doesn't always hurt in the long run to give stimulus the other way around."

It's important that a child go through normal childhood illness, for example, notes Dr. Kugathasan. "When we visit the doctor to suppress a lot of things like colds, rather than, in effect, letting nature run its course, we're making immediate treatment the priority rather than long-term prevention, using the analogy of immunological 'muscle-building.' We know that antibiotics wipe out normal cells, too, but you don't want to destroy what medical science has accomplished. Maybe there's no going back, but it's important that we take what the hygiene hypothesis is telling us into account when treating our children."

Chapter 7

The Link between Allergic Diseases and Cognitive Impairment

Sneezing, wheezing, watery eyes, and runny nose aren't the only symptoms of allergic diseases. Many people with allergic rhinitis also report feeling "slower" and drowsy. When their allergies are acting up, they have trouble concentrating and remembering.

For instance, allergic rhinitis can be associated with:

- decreased ability to concentrate and function;
- activity limitation;
- decreased decision-making capacity;
- impaired hand-eye coordination;
- problems remembering things;
- irritability;
- sleep disorders;
- fatigue;
- missed days at work or school;
- more motor vehicle accidents; and
- more school or work injuries.

Many parents of children with allergic rhinitis observe increased bad moods and irritability in their child's behavior during the allergy season. Since children cannot always express their uncomfortable or painful symptoms verbally, they may express their discomfort by acting up at school and at home. In addition, some kids feel that having an allergic disease is a stigma that separates them from other kids.

It is important that the irritability or other symptoms caused by ear, nose, or throat trouble are not mistaken for attention deficit disorder. With proper treatment, symptoms can be kept under control and disruptions in learning and behavior can be avoided.

Causes

Experts believe the top two culprits contributing to cognitive impairment of people with allergic rhinitis are sleep interruptions and over-the-counter (OTC) medications.

Secondary factors, such as blockage of the eustachian tube (ear canal), also can cause hearing problems that have a negative impact on learning and comprehension. Constant nose blowing and coughing can interrupt concentration and the learning process, and allergy-related absences can cause people to miss school or work and subsequently fall behind.

Sleep Disruption

Chronic nasal congestion can cause difficulty in breathing, especially at night. Waking is a hard-wired reflex to make you start breathing again. If you have bad allergic rhinitis, you may wake a dozen times a night. Falling back asleep can be difficult, cutting your total number of sleep hours short.

The average person needs about eight hours of sleep per night to function normally the next day. Losing just a few hours of sleep can lead to a significant decrease in your ability to function. Prolonged loss of sleep can cause difficulty in concentration, inability to remember things, and can contribute to automotive accidents. Night after night of interrupted sleep can cause serious decreases in learning ability and performance in school or on the job.

Over-the-Counter Medications

Most allergy therapies don't take into account the effects of allergic rhinitis on mental functioning—they treat the more obvious physical symptoms. Some allergy therapies may even cause some cognitive or mental impairment.

In a recent poll in which allergy sufferers were asked how they treat their symptoms, about 50 percent responded that they use over-the-counter (OTC) medications. The most commonly used OTC medications for allergy symptoms are decongestants and antihistamines—both of which can cause sleep disturbances.

Decongestants

Decongestants constrict small blood vessels in the nose. This opens the nasal passageways and lets you breathe easier. Some decongestants are available over the counter, while higher-strength formulas are available with a prescription. In some people, oral decongestants can cause problems with getting to sleep, appetite loss, and irritability, which can contribute to allergy problems. If you have any of these symptoms, discuss them with your doctor.

Antihistamines

Antihistamines block the effects of histamine, a chemical produced by the body in response to allergens. Histamine is responsible for the symptoms of allergic rhinitis, including an itchy runny nose, sneezing, and itchy eyes. OTC antihistamines are an inexpensive choice when it comes to treating the symptoms of an allergy—but all OTC antihistamines available in the United States also can cause drowsiness. Regularly taking OTC antihistamines can lead to a feeling of constant sluggishness, affecting learning, memory, and performance.

Non-sedating antihistamines, such as Allegra® (fexofenadine) and Claritin® (loratadine), are available with a prescription. [*Note:* Claritin® is now available as an over-the-counter medication.] These antihistamines are designed to minimize drowsiness while still blocking the effects of histamine.

Solutions

With all the allergic diseases, the best way to control your symptoms is to avoid coming into contact with your triggers—the substances that cause you to have an allergic reaction. This is often easier said than done. Sometimes it is impossible to avoid the substances that cause symptoms, especially when you are not in control of your environment.

If your allergens can't be avoided, your doctor can help you to create an allergy treatment plan. People who are allergic to indoor things like dust mites or animal dander may need medication on a daily basis, while people who have seasonal symptoms may only need treatment at certain times during the year. An allergist/immunologist can help you determine to which substances you are allergic.

Several types of non-sedating medications are available to help control allergies. One nonsedating nasal spray, NasalCrom® (cromolyn), is available without a prescription. In addition to the newer antihistamines discussed above, your doctor may also prescribe nasal steroid sprays to treat nasal inflammation. Nasal steroid sprays are highly effective in treating allergy symptoms. The most common side effect associated with nasal sprays is headache.

If medications are not effective or cause unwanted side effects, your doctor may suggest immunotherapy, or allergy shots. Immunotherapy is used to treat allergy to pollen, ragweed, dust mites, animal dander, and other allergens. This process gradually desensitizes you to these substances by changing the way that your body's immune system responds to them. For example, if you are allergic to ragweed, immunotherapy treatments would involve injecting a tiny amount of ragweed pollen extract under your skin every week. Immunotherapy treatments usually last three to five years or longer. Once your body is able to tolerate the substance without producing the symptoms of an allergy, immunotherapy can be stopped, and the need for oral medications should be gone or greatly reduced.

Remember

If allergies are affecting your ability to concentrate or function, several treatment options may be beneficial. Getting allergy symptoms under control can help you sleep at night and function during the day.

If you suspect that you or a family member may have an allergic disorder, make an appointment with your doctor for proper diagnosis. Treating allergies sooner rather than later can help prevent disruptions in learning and behavior.

For more medical information, please contact an allergist in your area.

Part Two

What You Should Know about Allergic Reactions

Chapter 8

Allergic Rhinitis (Hay Fever)

Chapter Contents

Section 8.1

Facts about Allergic Rhinitis

"Runny Nose, Sneezing, Itchy Eyes . . . I gotta get some relief!"
© 2006 Alabama Cooperative Extension System—Alabama A&M and
Auburn Universities. Reprinted with permission.

Allergic rhinitis, sometimes referred to as allergies or hay fever, is a common airway disorder that affects 20 to 40 million people in the United States annually, including 10 to 30 percent of adults and 40 percent of children. It is estimated that 3.5 million workdays and 2 million school days are missed each year due to allergic rhinitis, with an estimated annual prescription cost of $6 billion. Although much discomfort and expense are associated with this disorder, nonprescription and prescription medications are effective in relieving symptoms and in lessening the disorder's impact. However, before medication is used, an understanding of types of allergies, causes, risk factors, and signs and symptoms is needed.

Two types of allergic rhinitis exist: season and perennial. Seasonal allergies are generally more common and cause problems only at certain times of the year. Usually, seasonal allergies are caused by airborne plant pollens. Since pollinating seasons vary geographically, the occurrence of seasonal allergies largely depends on location of residence. In Alabama, tree pollen is generally at its peak March through May whereas grass pollen peaks April through November. Weeds, such as ragweed, pollinate in Alabama during the months of April through October. Therefore, the most common times of seasonal allergy flares occur during early spring to late fall. In contrast to seasonal allergies, perennial allergies cause symptoms continuously throughout the year due to constant allergen exposure. Household allergens are typically the causative agents of perennial allergies and include such things as house dust mites, cockroaches, mold spores, cigarette smoke, and pet danders. Occupational aeroallergens, such as wool dust, latex, resins, biological enzymes, organic dusts such as flour, and various chemicals, can also cause symptoms associated with allergic rhinitis. Avoidance of the causative allergen is essential to reduce symptoms. Techniques to avoid triggers include keeping doors and windows closed to keep out outdoor allergens, reducing first- or secondhand exposure to cigarette smoke, eliminating common sources of dust (rugs, stuffed animals, carpet, etc.), and venting moisture generating areas to reduce mold. While two types of allergic rhinitis exist, it is important to note that the types may overlap causing an individual to have continuous symptoms but experience flares or an increase in symptoms during certain times of the year.

In both seasonal and perennial allergies, an exposure to an allergen causes an inflammatory response in the mucous membranes that line the nose and sinuses. The inflammatory response is complex and involves many cells and mediators. The most important mediator is histamine, which causes vascular enlargement resulting in nasal congestion and increased mucus secretion. Other mediators that cause the inflammatory response include kinins, prostaglandins, and leukotrienes. After exposure to an allergen, symptoms often present in two distinct phases: an early and a late phase. Early phase symptoms occur within minutes of the exposure and include itching of the eyes, nose or mouth, sneezing, and rhinorrhea (runny nose). A late phase response may occur hours later, with the main symptoms of congestion and nasal obstruction. Other symptoms that may occur include an impaired sense of smell, postnasal drip, sore throat, hoarseness, and watery eyes. Some individuals also experience fatigue or tiredness, irritability, loss of appetite, and difficulty sleeping. Although these symptoms are certainly bothersome, effective nonprescription and prescription medications are available to lessen the severity of these reactions.

Oral antihistamines and intranasal corticosteroids are the two predominant classes of medications used to combat allergic rhinitis. Severity and duration of a patient's symptoms may determine if one or more medications should be used. Alternative agents, such as mast cell stabilizers, decongestants, and antileukotrienes, can also be considered. Since allergic rhinitis cannot be "cured," treatment goals are to lessen the symptoms to improve the patient's quality of life.

Oral antihistamines are generally considered first-line therapy for allergic rhinitis due to their effectiveness in reducing sneezing, itching, and watery nose and eyes. Antihistamines are separated into two classes: first generation and second generation. First generation products include chlorpheniramine (Chlor-Trimeton), diphenhydramine (Benadryl), clemastine (Tavist), phenindamine (Nolahist) as well as numerous others. First generation antihistamines are generally available without a prescription and are relatively inexpensive. Although first generation antihistamines are effective, the main disadvantage to their use is the drowsiness and sedation that they cause. The second generation antihistamines are newer medications that cause little to no sedation and still maintain efficacy. Second generation antihistamines include fexofenadine (Allegra), loratadine (Claritin), and desloratadine (Clarinex). The recent nonprescription availability of loratadine gives patients the opportunity to practice self-care with a nonsedating second generation antihistamine. Adverse reactions that may be associated with all antihistamines include drowsiness, dizziness, fatigue, headache, and dry mouth. Second generation antihistamines have a lower incidence of these side effects compared to the side effects of first generation products. These are susceptible to individual variation and may still cause side effects. Antihistamines should not be used by individuals who are hypersensitive to the drug, by nursing mothers, or by patients with narrow-angle glaucoma, stenosing peptic ulcers, symptomatic prostatic hypertrophy, asthma attacks, bladder neck obstruction, or pyloroduodenal obstruction. Antihistamines should not be used concurrently with monoamine oxidase inhibitors (MOAI) or administered to newborn or premature infants.

For more severe symptoms of seasonal allergies or treatment of perennial allergic rhinitis, intranasal corticosteroids are the primary drugs of choice. Corticosteroids are beneficial in allergic rhinitis due to their ability to decrease inflammation caused by exposure to an allergen. Common nasal corticosteroids include beclomethasone (Beconase AQ), budesonide (Rhinocort), fluticasone (Flonase), and flunisolide (Nasarel), all of which are available by prescription only. Topical corticosteroids are generally associated with only minor side effects, such as sneezing, stinging, headache, and nosebleeds. Patients should know that peak effects will not be seen until after 2 to 3 weeks of continuous use. Patients should also be warned that proper administration techniques must be used for the medication to be effective. Therefore, all patients should be shown the appropriate administration techniques for nasal steroids.

Alternative agents for allergic rhinitis include mast cell stabilizers, decongestants, and antileukotrienes. Cromolyn is a mast cell stabilizer, which is sold over-the-counter as NasalCrom. By stabilizing the mast cell, this drug prevents the release of mediators, particularly histamine, that cause the symptoms of allergic rhinitis. Because of this unique mechanism, it must be initiated before the onset of symptoms; once symptoms appear, this drug is no longer beneficial. One disadvantage to this drug is that it requires dosing 4 times daily. Although the dosing schedule is tedious, it is one of the first-line therapies for

Table 8.1. Selected Medications Dosing and Adverse Effects

Medication Name	Usual Adult Dosing	Adverse Effects	Legend Status
First Generation Antihistamines			
chlorpheniramine (Chlor-Trimeton)	4 mg every 4 to 6 hours	Drowsiness, headache, tiredness	OTC
diphenhydramine (Benadryl)	25 to 50 mg every 6 to 8 hours	Decreased blood pressure, increased heart rate, severe drowsiness	OTC
clemastine (Tavist)	1.34 mg twice daily to 2.68 mg 3 times daily	Incoordination, sedation	OTC
phenindamine (Nolahist)	25 mg every 4 to 6 hours	Drowsiness, dizziness	OTC
Second Generation Antihistamines			
fexofenadine (Allegra)	60 mg twice daily or 180 mg once daily	Headache, dizziness	RX Only
loratadine (Claritin)	10 mg once daily	Headache, tiredness	OTC
desloratadine (Clarinex)	5 mg once daily	Headache, tiredness	RX Only
Nasal Corticosteroids			
beclomethasone (Beconase AQ)	1 to 2 inhalations in each nostril once daily	Nasal burning or stinging, nosebleeds	RX Only
budesonide (Rhinocort)	2 sprays in each nostril in the morning and evening	Nosebleeds, nasal stinging	RX Only
fluticasone (Flonase)	2 sprays per nostril twice daily	Headache, fever	RX Only
flunisolide (Nasarel)	2 sprays in each nostril twice daily	Nosebleeds, nasal stinging	RX Only
Mast Cell Stabilizers			
cromolyn (NasalCrom)	1 spray in each nostril 3 to 4 times daily	Increase in sneezing, nasal burning, or stinging	OTC
Decongestants			
pseudoephedrine (Sudafed)	30 to 60 mg every 4 to 6 hours	Increased blood pressure, increased heart rate, excitability, headache	OTC
Antileukotrienes			
montelukast (Singulair)	10 mg daily in the evening	Headache, dizziness, tiredness	RX Only

children due to its safety profile. Decongestants, such as pseudoephedrine (Sudafed), are occasionally beneficial for nasal congestion associated with allergic rhinitis, but do not improve other symptoms such as sneezing, itchy or watery eyes, or runny nose. Decongestants are available without a prescription in intranasal or oral dosage forms. Although decongestants are effective, they are often inadvisable and have warnings that limit their use in certain populations. Always consult a pharmacist before initiating therapy with any decongestant.

Montelukast (Singulair) is another treatment option for allergic rhinitis and is currently available by prescription only. Montelukast works by blocking the leukotriene receptor, which ultimately results in decreased allergic symptoms. Efficacy of montelukast as single drug therapy is still being investigated.

In summary, allergic rhinitis is an inflammatory disorder that affects millions in the United States and results in numerous missed work and school days. The usual symptoms of allergic rhinitis include runny nose; sneezing; itchy, watery eyes; and nasal congestion. These symptoms can be alleviated using effective medication, including antihistamines and nasal corticosteroids. The length and severity of symptoms will dictate what product should be used. Generally, for mild to moderate seasonal allergies, a first or second generation antihistamine, such as chlorpheniramine or loratadine, should be effective. If symptoms are severe or last year-round, see your pharmacist or physician to determine what treatment option is most appropriate. Alternative agents may be considered as necessary. Table 8.1 provides an overview of types of medications as well as usual adult dosages and side effects. Always feel free to discuss your condition with your local pharmacist. He or she will be able to help you choose a medication tailored to treat your specific symptoms.

References

1. Rosenwasser LJ. Treatment of Allergic Rhinitis. *Am J Med.* 2002 Dec 16;113(9A): 17S–24S.

2. Covington TR, editors. *Nonprescription Drug Therapy: Guiding Patient Self-Care.* 2nd ed. St. Louis: Wolters Kluwer Health; 2003.

3. Fioravante RJ. Pollen Allergy. Available at : http://www.allergyescape.com/Pollen-Allergy.html. 2003. Date Accessed: March 14, 2005.

4. Tietze KJ. Disorders Related to Cold and Allergy. In: Berardi RR, editor. *Handbook of Nonprescription Drugs.* 14th ed. Washington D.C.: American Pharmacist Association; 2004. p. 239–69.

5. Pray WS. *Nonprescription Product Therapeutics.* Baltimore: Lippincott Williams & Wilkins; 1999.

6. Dipiro JT, Talbert RL, Yee GC, Matzke GR, Wells BG, Posey LM, editors. *Pharmacotherapy: A Pathophysiologic Approach.* New York: McGraw-Hill; 2002.

7. Salib RJ, Drake-Lee A, Howarth PH. Allergic rhinitis: past, present and the future. *Clin Otolaryngol* 2003; 28: 291–303.

8. Wang D. Treatment of Allergic Rhinitis: H1-Antihistamines and Intranasal Steroids. *Curr Drug Targets Inflamm Allergy* 2002; 1(3): 215–220.

9. Simons FER. Advances in H1-Antihistamines. *N Engl J Med.* 2004 Nov 18; 351(21): 2203–17.

10. CRL Online. Lexi-Comp, Inc. Hudson City, Ohio. URL: http://crlonline.com/crlsql/servelet/crlonline. 2005. Date Accessed: March 15, 2005.

Note: Trade and brand names used in the Alabama Cooperative Extension System and the Auburn University Harrison School of Pharmacy publications are given for information purposes only. No guarantee, endorsement, or discrimination among comparable products is intended or implied by Extension or the Harrison School of Pharmacy.

Section 8.2

Nasal Wash Treatment for
People with Allergic Rhinitis

Many people with allergic rhinitis, allergic asthma, or other lung problems also have nasal and sinus symptoms. Drainage from your nose and sinuses can make rhinitis and asthma worse, especially at night. A saltwater nasal wash, or nasal irrigation, can help reduce this. A nasal wash:

- cleans mucus from the nose so medication is more effective;
- cleans allergens and irritants from the nose, reducing their impact;
- removes bacteria and viruses from the nose, reducing the frequency of infection; and
- decreases swelling in the nose and increases air flow.

What is the correct nasal wash technique?

- Wash your hands.
- Make the nasal wash solution.
  - Make the saltwater, or saline, solution fresh for every nasal wash, using a clean glass.
  - To make the saltwater solution, mix one-half teaspoon un-iodized salt in an 8-ounce glass of warm water. Un-iodized salt is used because iodized salt may be irritating when used over a long period of time.
  - Add a pinch of baking soda. A pinch is a small amount you can pick up between two fingers.
  - If you are congested, use the entire 8 ounces of saltwater during the nasal wash; otherwise, 4 ounces should be enough.

- Discard any unused saltwater and prepare a new saltwater solution before the next nasal wash.

What is the correct position for the nasal wash?

- Adults and older children—Lean far over the sink with your head down.

- Younger children—If possible, have your child lean as far over the sink as possible. A small child may have trouble cooperating with a nasal wash and may need to be held and assisted. Ask your health care provider about ways to hold a small child when doing a nasal wash. One technique is to wrap your small child in a blanket or towel with arms down while holding him or her on your lap.

Ask your health care provider to discuss which of these techniques may be best for you.

Which technique is best for me?

Ask your clinician.

Techniques for adults and older children.

- *Sinus Rinse Kit Technique:* The Sinus Rinse Kit comes with a Sinus Rinse bottle and mixture packets. When using the Sinus Rinse Kit you can use the prepared mixture packets that come with the kit or you can make your own nasal wash solution described above. The Sinus Rinse bottle is filled with salt water. The bottle is placed against the nostril. After the bottle is squeezed, salt water comes out the opposite nostril and may come out the mouth. The nose is then blown lightly. The procedure is then repeated with the other nostril.

- *Bulb Syringe Technique:* Use a large all-rubber ear syringe. An ear bulb syringe can be purchased at most pharmacies. Fill the syringe completely with the saltwater. Insert the syringe tip just inside your nostril and pinch your nostril around the tip of the bulb syringe to keep the solution from running out your nose. Gently squeeze the bulb to swish the solution around in your nose; then blow your nose lightly. Repeat the procedure with the other nostril.

- *Waterpik® Technique:* Use a Waterpik® with a Sinus or Grossan Original Sinus Irrigator Tip®. Pour the salt water into the water reservoir and set the Waterpik® at the lowest possible pressure. Insert the tip just inside your nostril and allow the fluid to run out of your mouth or other nostril. Blow your nose lightly. Repeat the procedure with the other nostril.

- *Hand Technique:* Use your hands for this technique. Pour some salt water into your palm. Sniff the liquid up your nose, one nostril at a time. Blow your nose lightly. This technique may not be as effective but may be used in some situations.

Techniques for babies.

- *Babies:* We recommend using an eyedropper or syringe (without the needle) for doing a nasal wash with a baby. Place 10 to 20 drops of the salt water in your baby's nostril. Use a bulb syringe to suction the mucus from your baby's nose. Repeat the procedure with the other nostril.

With any technique, the saltwater solution may get into the mouth during the nasal wash and leave a salty taste. You may want to rinse the mouth with water after the nasal wash.

How do you clean the equipment?

You must thoroughly clean the equipment used for a nasal wash to prevent the growth of bacteria. It is important for each family member to have his or her own bulb syringe or nasal adaptor.

Cleaning the Sinus Rinse bottle.

- After each use, rinse the bottle, cap, and tubing. Shake off any excess water and allow the pieces to dry on a clean towel. If you feel the system is contaminated, clean the bottle, cap, and tubing with rubbing (70 percent isopropyl) alcohol or white, distilled vinegar (1 part vinegar to 3 parts water). After the use of either solution, rinse the pieces well with water and shake off the excess water. Again, allow the pieces to dry on a clean towel.

- The Sinus Rinse bottle is not dishwasher safe.

Cleaning the bulb syringe (dropper, syringe, or nasal spray bottle).

- After each use (which may be several times a day), fill the bulb syringe with hot water, swish the hot water around, and empty the bulb syringe completely. Always suspend the bulb syringe tip down in a clean glass to allow the bulb syringe to drain completely. Do not allow the bulb tip to sit in a puddle of water.

• In addition to rinsing the bulb after each use, clean the bulb daily with rubbing (70 percent isopropyl) alcohol. Draw the rubbing alcohol into the bulb syringe. Swish the liquid around, and empty the bulb syringe. Again, suspend the bulb syringe tip down in a clean glass to allow it to drain completely.

Cleaning the Grossan® Nasal Adapter.

• Refer to the package insert for cleaning directions.

If you have any questions about these nasal wash techniques please ask your health care provider. Your health care provider can discuss which technique is best for you.

Section 8.3

Nasal Sprays: How to Use Them Correctly

"Nasal Steroid Sprays," © University of Pittsburgh Medical Center. Reprinted with permission. This document was published in 2000; reviewed by David A. Cooke, M.D., January 5, 2007.

Nasal steroid sprays such as Beconase, Beconase AQ, Vancenase, Vancenase AQ, Flonase, Nasalide, Nasarel, Nasacort, Nasacort AQ, Nasonex, Rhinocort, Rhinocort Aqua, and Tri-Nasal are helpful in the management of allergic rhinitis, and in some cases, of vasomotor rhinitis (this is essentially a nose that reacts by swelling more than most people's noses). Nasal steroid sprays may require a week's use as directed before they become maximally effective. Nasal steroid sprays work best if use is begun before exposure to allergens. If you are allergic to trees and your symptoms seem to start in early April, then you would be well advised to begin your nasal steroid spray the end of March.

You will not become addicted (suffer rebound swelling) from nasal steroid sprays. Addiction or rebound does occur with the over-the-counter nasal decongestant sprays such as Afrin, Duration, or Neo-Synephrine if used for more than three or four days. Once you are using the nasal steroid sprays on a regular basis, you are often able to cut down to once a day. When your allergy season is over, then you may stop the nasal steroid spray. Patients who have nasal polyps or perennial (year-round) allergic rhinitis may require the use of nasal steroid sprays for years.

How to apply your nasal steroid spray: If the spray is aerosolized, you may need to prime the bottle first. Aim the nozzle toward the side of your nose and up (not toward the middle of the septum). Some people get better delivery of the steroid spray, particularly the aqueous sprays, if they use them with the head down technique and hold that position for half a minute.

Side Effects

Side effects of nasal steroid sprays include sneezing with administration, burning, rarely septal perforation, and nosebleeds. Exacerbation of chickenpox and reversible glaucoma are very rare side effects. If you are over 60, you should have an eye exam after being on the nasal steroid spray for a month or so. If you are exposed and susceptible to chickenpox, stop your nasal steroid spray. Children should not use the beclomethasone nasal spray products because these can cause a very small amount of growth suppression, whereas the newer less systemically bioavailable nasal sprays such as Flonase and Nasonex do not cause this.

Nasalide often causes intense burning for 15 or 30 seconds after its use. Pinching the nose for 15 seconds after spraying Nasalide may control this. If irritation persists after using the nasal spray, then stop using the nasal steroid spray. Nasal steroids are quite safe to use and at the recommended doses are not absorbed systemically.

To be effective, all nasal steroid sprays require regular use; however, you may be able to maintain symptomatic control with lower doses than initially recommended. Decrease the dose to one spray once symptoms are controlled. If symptoms return at the lower dose, increase the dose to the point that symptoms are again controlled. If your symptoms are completely controlled, then you may come off the nasal steroid spray until symptoms return, then restart. If you have nasal polyps, do not come off the nasal steroid spray, even if you feel fairly normal, unless your doctor directs you to. Polyps can start to

Table 8.2. Types of Nasal Steroid Sprays

Trade (Brand) Name	Number of Puffs Per Nostril	Frequency of Dose	Fragrance	Maximum Puffs Per Nostril Per Day
Beclomethasone (Vancenase Pockethaler)	1–2 puffs each nostril	2–4 times per day	Yes	8
Beclomethasone AQ (Beconase AQ) (Vancenase DS)	1–2 puffs each nostril	2 times per day	Yes	8
	1 time per day	1 time per day	Yes	4
Budesonide (Rhinocort Aqua)	1 spray per nostril once a day	1–2 times per day	No	4
Fluticasone (Flonase)	2 puffs each nostril for one week, then 1 puff each nostril	1 time per day	Yes	4
Flunisolide (Nasalide)	1–2 puffs each nostril	2–3 times per day	No	8
Flunisolide (Nasarel) Only 5% propylene glycol	1–2 puffs each nostril	2–3 times per day	No	8
Triamcinolone Acetonide (Nasacort, *Nasacort AQ, Tri-Nasal)	2 puffs each nostril for one week, then 1 puff each nostril	1 time per day	No	4
Mometasone furoate (Nasonex)	2 puffs each nostril	1 time per day	Yes	4

*Note: Nasacort: After 100 doses, the amount of steroid delivered diminishes and the canister should be discarded even though it may appear to deliver the spray.

grow with very few symptoms and may get too big to be likely to get smaller with the reinstitution of the nasal steroid spray.

Chapter 9

Sinusitis and Related Conditions

Chapter Contents

Section 9.1

What Is Sinusitis?

From "Sinusitis," a fact sheet published by the National Institute
of Allergy and Infectious Diseases (NIAID, www.niaid.nih.gov), part
of the National Institutes of Health, January 2006.

Overview

You're coughing and sneezing and tired and achy. You think that
you might be getting a cold. Later, when the medicines you've been
taking to relieve the symptoms of the common cold are not working
and you've now got a terrible headache, you finally drag yourself to
the doctor. After listening to your history of symptoms, examining your
face and forehead, and perhaps doing a sinus x-ray, the doctor says
you have sinusitis.

Sinusitis simply means your sinuses are infected or inflamed, but
this gives little indication of the misery and pain this condition can
cause. Health experts usually divide sinusitis cases into:

- acute, which last for 4 weeks or less;

- subacute, which lasts 4 to 8 weeks;

- chronic, which usually last up to 8 weeks but can continue for
  months or even years; and

- recurrent, which are several acute attacks within a year, and
  may be caused by different organisms.

Health experts estimate that 37 million Americans are affected by
sinusitis every year. Health care providers report nearly 32 million
cases of chronic sinusitis to the Centers for Disease Control and Prevention annually. Americans spend $5.8 billion each year on health
care costs related to sinusitis.

What Are Sinuses?

Sinuses are hollow air spaces in the human body. When people say,
"I'm having a sinus attack," they usually are referring to symptoms

in one or more of four pairs of cavities, or sinuses, known as paranasal sinuses. These cavities, located within the skull or bones of the head surrounding the nose, include:

- frontal sinuses over the eyes in the brow area;
- maxillary sinuses inside each cheekbone;
- ethmoid sinuses just behind the bridge of the nose and between the eyes; and
- sphenoid sinuses behind the ethmoids in the upper region of the nose and behind the eyes.

Each sinus has an opening into the nose for the free exchange of air and mucus, and each is joined with the nasal passages by a continuous mucous membrane lining. Therefore, anything that causes a swelling in the nose—an infection, an allergic reaction, or another type of immune reaction—also can affect the sinuses. Air trapped within a blocked sinus, along with pus or other secretions, may cause pressure on the sinus wall. The result is the sometimes intense pain of a sinus attack. Similarly, when air is prevented from entering a paranasal sinus by a swollen membrane at the opening, a vacuum can be created that also causes pain.

Some Causes of Acute Sinusitis

Most cases of acute sinusitis start with a common cold, which is caused by a virus. These viral colds do not cause symptoms of sinusitis, but they do inflame the sinuses. Both the cold and the sinus inflammation usually go away without treatment in 2 weeks. The inflammation, however, might explain why having a cold increases your likelihood of developing acute sinusitis. For example, your nose reacts to an invasion by viruses that cause infections such as the common cold or flu by producing mucus and sending white blood cells to the lining of the nose, which congest and swell the nasal passages.

When this swelling involves the adjacent mucous membranes of your sinuses, air and mucus are trapped behind the narrowed openings of the sinuses. When your sinus openings become too narrow, mucus cannot drain properly. This increase in mucus sets up prime conditions for bacteria to multiply.

Most healthy people harbor bacteria, such as *Streptococcus pneumoniae* and *Haemophilus influenzae,* in their upper respiratory tracts with no problems until the body's defenses are weakened or drainage from the sinuses is blocked by a cold or other viral infection. Thus, bacteria that may have been living harmlessly in your nose or throat can multiply and invade your sinuses, causing an acute sinus infection.

Sometimes, fungal infections can cause acute sinusitis. Although fungi are abundant in the environment, they usually are harmless to healthy people because the human body has a natural resistance to fungi. Fungi, such as *Aspergillus*, can cause serious illness in people whose immune systems are not functioning properly. Some people with fungal sinusitis have an allergic-type reaction to the fungi.

Chronic inflammation of the nasal passages also can lead to sinusitis. If you have allergic rhinitis, also called hay fever, you can develop episodes of acute sinusitis. Vasomotor rhinitis, caused by humidity, cold air, alcohol, perfumes, and other environmental conditions, also may be complicated by sinus infections. (Rhinitis simply means runny nose.)

Acute sinusitis is much more common in some people than in the general population. For example, sinusitis occurs more often in people who have reduced immune function (such as those with primary immune deficiency diseases or HIV infection) and with abnormality of mucus secretion or mucus movement (such as those with cystic fibrosis).

Causes of Chronic Sinusitis

It can be difficult to determine the cause of chronic sinusitis. Some health experts think it is an infectious disease, but others are not certain. It is an inflammatory disease that often occurs in people with asthma. If you have asthma, which is an allergic disease, you may have chronic sinusitis, which may make it worse. If you are allergic to airborne allergens, such as house dust mites, mold, and pollen, which trigger allergic rhinitis, you may develop chronic sinusitis. An allergic reaction to certain fungi may be responsible for at least some cases of chronic sinusitis. In addition, people who are allergic to fungi can develop a condition called allergic fungal sinusitis.

If you are prone to getting chronic sinusitis, damp weather, especially in northern temperate climates, or pollutants in the air and in buildings also can affect you.

If you have an immune deficiency disorder or an abnormality in the way mucus moves through and from your respiratory system (for example, primary immune deficiency, HIV infection, or cystic fibrosis), you might develop chronic sinusitis with frequent bouts of acute sinusitis due to infections. In addition, if you have severe asthma, nasal polyps (small growths in the nose), or a severe asthma attack caused by aspirin and aspirin-like medicines such as ibuprofen, you might have chronic sinusitis.

Symptoms

The location of your sinus pain depends on which sinus is affected.

- Headache when you wake up in the morning is typical of a sinus problem.

- Pain when your forehead over the frontal sinuses is touched may mean that your frontal sinuses are inflamed.

- Infection in the maxillary sinuses can cause your upper jaw and teeth to ache, and your cheeks to become tender to the touch.

- The ethmoid sinuses are near the tear ducts in the corner of your eyes. Therefore, inflammation of these cavities often causes swelling of the eyelids and tissues around your eyes, and pain between your eyes. Ethmoid inflammation also can cause tenderness when you touch the sides of your nose, a loss of smell, and a stuffy nose.

- Infection in the sphenoid sinuses can cause earaches, neck pain, and deep aching at the top of your head, although these sinuses are less frequently affected.

Most people with sinusitis, however, have pain or tenderness in several locations, and their symptoms usually do not clearly show which sinuses are inflamed.

Other symptoms of sinusitis can include:

- fever;
- weakness;
- tiredness;
- a cough that may be more severe at night; and
- rhinitis or nasal congestion.

In addition, the drainage of mucus from the sphenoid or other sinuses down the back of your throat (postnasal drip) can cause you to have a sore throat. Mucus drainage also can irritate the membranes lining your larynx (upper windpipe). Not everyone with these symptoms, however, has sinusitis.

On rare occasions, acute sinusitis can result in brain infection and other serious complications.

Diagnosis

Because your nose can get stuffy when you have a condition like the common cold, you may confuse simple nasal congestion with sinusitis. A cold, however, usually lasts about 7 to 14 days and disappears without treatment. Acute sinusitis often lasts longer and typically causes more symptoms than just a cold.

Your health care provider can usually diagnose acute sinusitis by listening to your symptoms and doing a physical examination, which includes examining your nasal tissues. If your symptoms are vague or persist, your health care provider may order a CT (computed tomography) scan to confirm that you have sinusitis.

Laboratory tests to diagnose chronic sinusitis may include:

* blood tests to rule out other conditions associated with sinusitis like an immune deficiency disorder or cystic fibrosis;
* cultures (special blood tests) to detect bacterial or fungal infection; or
* biopsy to determine the health of the cells lining the nasal cavity.

Treatment

After diagnosing sinusitis and identifying a possible cause, your health care provider can suggest treatments that will reduce your inflammation and relieve your symptoms.

Acute Sinusitis

If you have acute sinusitis, your health care provider may recommend:

* decongestants to reduce congestion;
* antibiotics to control a bacterial infection, if present; and
* pain relievers to reduce any pain.

You should, however, use over-the-counter or prescription decongestant nose drops and sprays for only few days. If you use these medicines for longer periods, they can lead to even more congestion and swelling of your nasal passages.

If bacteria cause your sinusitis, antibiotics used along with a nasal or oral decongestant will usually help. Your health care provider can prescribe an antibiotic that fights the type of bacteria most commonly associated with sinusitis.

Many cases of acute sinusitis will end without antibiotics. If you have allergic disease along with sinusitis, however, you may need medicine to relieve your allergy symptoms. If you already have asthma and then get sinusitis, you may experience worsening of your asthma and should be in close touch with your health care provider.

In addition, your health care provider may prescribe a steroid nasal spray, along with other treatments, to reduce your sinus congestion, swelling, and inflammation.

Chronic Sinusitis

Health care providers often find it difficult to treat chronic sinusitis successfully, realizing that symptoms persist even after taking antibiotics for a long period. Many health care providers treat sinusitis with steroids such as steroid nasal sprays. Many health care providers treat chronic sinusitis as though it is an infection, by using antibiotics and decongestants. Others use both antibiotics along with steroid nasal sprays. Further research is needed to determine what the best treatment is.

Some people with severe asthma are said to have dramatic improvement of their symptoms when their chronic sinusitis is treated with antibiotics.

Health care providers commonly prescribe steroid nasal sprays to reduce inflammation in chronic sinusitis. Although they occasionally prescribe these sprays to treat people with chronic sinusitis over a long period, health experts don't fully understand the long-term safety of these medicines, especially in children. Therefore, health care providers will consider whether the benefits outweigh any risks of using steroid nasal sprays.

If you have severe chronic sinusitis, your health care provider may prescribe oral steroids, such as prednisone. Because oral steroids are powerful medicines and can have significant side effects, you should take them only when other medicines have not worked.

Although home remedies cannot cure sinus infection, they might give you some comfort.

- Inhaling steam from a vaporizer or a hot cup of water can soothe inflamed sinus cavities.

91

- Saline nasal spray, which you can buy in a drugstore, can give relief.

- Gentle heat applied over the inflamed area is comforting.

When medical treatment fails, surgery may be the only alternative for treating chronic sinusitis. Research studies suggest that most people who undergo surgery have fewer symptoms and better quality of life.

In children, problems often are eliminated by removing adenoids obstructing their nasal-sinus passages.

Adults who have had allergies and infections over the years sometimes develop nasal polyps that interfere with proper nasal drainage. Removal of these polyps and/or repair of a deviated septum to ensure an open airway often gives them considerable relief from sinus symptoms.

The most common surgery done today is functional endoscopic sinus surgery, in which the natural openings from the sinuses are enlarged to allow drainage. This type of surgery is less invasive than conventional sinus surgery, and serious complications are rare. Surgery should be considered only after failure of medical treatment.

Prevention

Although you cannot prevent all sinus disorders—any more than you can avoid all colds or bacterial infections—you can do certain things to reduce the number and severity of the attacks and possibly prevent acute sinusitis from becoming chronic.

- You may get some relief from your symptoms with a humidifier, particularly if room air in your home is heated by a dry forced-air system.

- Air conditioners help to provide an even temperature.

- Electrostatic filters attached to heating and air conditioning equipment are helpful in removing allergens from the air.

If you are prone to getting sinus disorders, especially if you have allergies, you should avoid cigarette smoke and other air pollutants. If your allergies inflame your nasal passages, you are more likely to have a strong reaction to all irritants.

If you suspect that your sinus inflammation may be related to house dust mites, mold, pollen, or food—or any of the hundreds of allergens that can trigger an upper respiratory reaction—you should consult your health care provider who can use various tests to find out whether you have an allergy and if so, its cause. This will help you and your health care provider take the right steps to reduce or limit your allergy symptoms.

Other activities that can cause sinus problems include:

- drinking alcohol, which causes nasal and sinus membranes to swell;

- swimming in pools treated with chlorine, which irritates the lining of the nose and sinuses; and

- diving, which forces water into the sinuses from the nasal passages.

You may find that air travel poses a problem if you are suffering from acute or chronic sinusitis. As air pressure in a plane is reduced, pressure can build up in your head blocking your sinuses or eustachian tubes in your ears. Therefore, you might feel discomfort in your sinus or middle ear during the plane's ascent or descent. Some health experts recommend using decongestant nose drops or inhalers before a flight to avoid this problem.

Research

At least two thirds of sinusitis cases caused by bacteria are due to two germs that can also cause otitis media (middle ear infection) in children as well as pneumonia and acute worsening of chronic bronchitis. The National Institute of Allergy and Infectious Diseases (NIAID) is supporting multiple studies to better understand the basis for infectivity of these organisms as well as identifying potential candidates for future vaccine strategies that could eliminate these diseases.

A project supported by NIAID is developing an advanced sinuscope that will permit improved airway evaluation during a medical examination especially when surgical intervention is contemplated.

Scientific studies have shown a close relationship between having asthma and sinusitis. As many as 75 percent of people with asthma also get sinusitis. Some studies state that up to 80 percent of adults with chronic sinusitis also had allergic rhinitis. NIAID conducts and supports research on allergic diseases as well as bacteria and fungi that can cause sinusitis. This research is focused on developing better treatments and ways to prevent these diseases.

93

Scientists supported by NIAID and other institutions are investigating whether chronic sinusitis has genetic causes. They have found that certain alterations in the gene that causes cystic fibrosis may also increase the likelihood of developing chronic sinusitis. This research will give scientists new insights into the cause of the disease in some people and points to new strategies for diagnosis and treatment.

Another NIAID-supported research study has recently demonstrated that blood cells from people with chronic sinusitis make chemicals that produce inflammation when exposed to fungal antigens, suggesting that fungi may play a role in many cases of chronic sinusitis. Further research, including clinical trials of antifungal drugs, will help determine whether, and for whom, this new treatment strategy holds promise.

Section 9.2

Sinusitis and Headaches

"Headache," Copyright © 1999 American College of Allergy, Asthma and Immunology. Reprinted with permission. Reviewed and revised by David A. Cooke, M.D., January 5, 2007.

Headache is one of the top health complaints of Americans. We're bombarded with advertisements and we pay many millions of dollars for pain relievers. Headache also is one of the most common reasons people see physicians.

Everybody gets headaches. How do you know when you should see your doctor about them?

Because each of us is different in how we handle pain, you must decide yourself. However, here are some conditions that might call for a visit with your physician:

- The recent onset of frequent, moderate to severe headaches, associated with other symptoms such as nausea or vomiting

- Headaches that occur on a daily or weekly basis

- Headaches that make it impossible for you to think, do your work, go to school, or enjoy life

- Headaches that respond only to a great deal of over-the-counter pain-relief medication

- Headaches with fever that last more than a day or two

How are headaches diagnosed?

Your doctor will ask you to describe how severe your pain is, where it's strongest, how you obtain relief, if other symptoms accompany your headaches, and if you've found that some things make your headache worse. A physical examination will reveal the causes of some headaches. If necessary, your doctor will order laboratory tests, x-rays, and brain-wave tests. Often these tests are ordered after consultation with a neurologist, a physician who specializes in nerve and brain problems.

Some types of headaches have an allergic basis, but most do not. Before you see an allergist/immunologist for evaluation and treatment of your headaches, you should first visit your primary care physician to rule out the other more common causes of your headaches.

In some cases, a careful allergy evaluation may pinpoint the allergen (allergy-causing substance) causing a headache.

What kinds of headaches may be caused by allergies?

Three types of headaches may possibly be related to allergic disease—sinus headaches (facial pain), migraines, and cluster headaches.

What are the symptoms of sinus headache?

The four groups of sinus cavities in the head are hollow air spaces with openings into the nose for exchange of air and mucus. They're located inside each cheekbone, behind the eyes, behind the bridge of the nose, and in the forehead. Secretions from the sinus cavities normally drain into the nose.

Sinus headaches and pain occur when the sinuses are swollen and their openings into the nasal passages are obstructed, stopping normal drainage and causing pressure to build up. Often the pain is localized over the affected sinus, perhaps causing facial pain rather than a headache. For example, if the maxillary sinus in the cheeks is obstructed, your cheeks may be tender to the touch and pain may radiate to your jaw and teeth. Other sinuses can cause pain on the top of

95

your head or elsewhere. Sinus pain can be dull to intense, often begins in the morning, and becomes less intense after you move from a lying down to an upright position.

Similar pain can also be caused by severe nasal congestion, particularly if you have a septal deviation or septal "spur" from a previous nasal injury. Such headaches or facial pain can involve one side only.

Oral or nasal spray decongestants often help relieve symptoms of facial pain or headaches due to nasal or sinus blockage. Nasal steroid sprays are usually helpful because they reduce swelling that may cause sinuses to become blocked. Antihistamines are generally less helpful. Obstructed sinuses can get infected, requiring more intensive treatment, including antibiotics.

One hint that allergy might play a role in your sinus headaches or facial pain is if you have other upper airway symptoms such as the itching, sneezing, and runny nose of seasonal allergic rhinitis (hay fever). Allergy is not usually a direct cause of these types of headaches when the other allergic rhinitis symptoms are not present. Allergic reactions to things like airborne pollens, dust, animal dander, molds, as well as foods, can lead to sinus obstruction. Treatment of the underlying allergic cause of sinus pain can result in long-term relief. Medications used to treat allergies include antihistamines, decongestants, intranasal steroids, and cromolyn. In some cases, allergen immunotherapy (allergy shots) may be recommended. When possible, of course, avoid the allergen if an avoidable substance causes your allergy.

What are migraines?

Migraine headaches vary from very intense and disabling to mild. Migraines tend to be throbbing, usually one-sided headaches, that often are aggravated by sunlight and are frequently accompanied by nausea. Migraine headaches can run in families. There are two general types of migraine: classic and common (plus many variations). If you are having these types of headaches, you should schedule an appointment with your doctor for evaluation, because certain new medications are very effective in preventing and stopping migraines in their tracks.

Classic migraine attacks tend to be severe and of long duration. They are preceded by aura, a sensation that signals the start of a headache. The aura may be a funny smell, partial vision loss, or a strange sound.

Common migraine is more prevalent than classic migraine. Attacks are generally milder and shorter. There is no aura. However, because the attacks may occur more frequently, common migraine also can be quite disabling.

What is the role of allergy in these types of headaches?

Years of published data and clinical experience suggest that food allergy may be a trigger of recurrent, persistent migraine headaches in a few, but by no means all patients. In such cases, only a few foods trigger migraines and, by limiting or avoiding them, you can experience complete or marked relief without medication. If you have a firm diagnosis of migraine made by a physician expert in the diagnosis and treatment of migraine headaches, you may want to keep a diary of foods eaten and their relation to your headaches, and then request consultation with an allergist for evaluation and possible allergy testing. On a nonallergic basis, some migraines are provoked by food additives or naturally occurring food chemicals such as monosodium glutamate (often added to oriental food and packaged foods), tyramine (found in many cheeses), phenylethylamine (found in chocolate), or alcohol. The artificial sweetener aspartame has also been reported as a trigger migraine in some people.

If you have more questions, your allergist/immunologist will be happy to answer them. For more medical information, please contact an allergist in your area.

97

Section 9.3

Fungal Sinusitis: An Allergic Reaction to Environmental Fungi

Is there a fungus among us? In short, yes.

Fungi as a group are found nearly everywhere on the planet, including the human body. Of the approximately 50,000 kinds of fungi, only a few dozen have been implicated in human illness. In most cases, these various fungi coexist in a natural balance with other microorganisms that colonize our bodies. However, in certain circumstances, fungi can cause infection ranging from minor to life threatening in severity. Inflammation or infection of the sinuses by fungi is termed fungal sinusitis. Fungal sinusitis can be classified into four types:

- fungal ball;
- allergic fungal sinusitis;
- chronic invasive sinusitis; and
- acute invasive sinusitis.

Fungal Ball

A fungal ball is an overgrowth of fungal elements which typically occurs in the maxillary (or cheek) sinus. The organism involved is most often from the common bread mold family, *Aspergillus*. Patients with this condition may have a history of recurrent sinus infections, and the symptoms may be similar to bacterial sinusitis. A radiologic study (x-ray, CT [computed tomography], MRI [magnetic resonance imaging]) ordered to investigate this will show blockage of the involved sinus or sinuses, without any damage to the surrounding bone. Treatment consists of removal of the fungal ball. In most cases, this is possible with a minimally invasive procedure termed endoscopic sinus surgery, with excellent cure rates.

Allergic Fungal Sinusitis

The most common type of fungal infection is termed allergic fungal sinusitis. The fungi involved are mainly from the *Dematiaceous* family, including *Bipolaris, Curvularia*, and *Alternaria*, which are common in the environment. As in fungal ball, the symptoms can be similar to bacterial sinusitis. Nasal polyps and thick drainage are usually found on examination of the nose. Radiologic studies will show blockage of the affected sinuses and can show impressive bony thinning and occasionally bony destruction. Treatment consists of removal of the fungal elements, with re-establishment of sinus drainage. As in fungal ball, endoscopic sinus surgery is possible in most cases. Recurrence rates are higher than in fungal ball, due to the allergic component, inflammation, and nasal polyps associated with this condition. In many cases, lifelong medical and intermittent surgical management is necessary. Although the treatment of this condition is controversial, typical adjuncts to surgical removal may include systemic and/or topical steroids, antihistamines, antibiotics, antifungal medications, allergy immunotherapy, and irrigations.

Invasive Fungal Sinusitis

Acute and chronic invasive sinusitis are the most serious types of fungal sinusitis, and fortunately the least common. Acute invasive fungal sinusitis is a quickly advancing process that grows deeply into the sinus tissues and bones. Chronic invasive fungal sinusitis is a similar, but much slower, infection. Patients who are affected with acute invasive sinusitis typically have a compromised immune system, such as after chemotherapy or in patients with uncontrolled diabetes. In contrast, most patients with chronic invasive sinusitis have a normal immune system. Common environmental fungi from the families *Rhizopus, Mucor,* and *Aspergillus* are frequently found in this type of infection. Symptoms of this condition, like all types of fungal sinusitis, can be similar to bacterial sinusitis. On examination of the nose, mold spores and areas of dying tissue can be seen. The area involved in the infection can extend far beyond the confines of the nasal cavity and sinuses. Radiologic studies will show blockage of the involved sinuses, destruction of bone, and swelling in the affected areas of the facial tissues. A combination of surgery and antifungal medications are required in this often-fatal infection.

Final Comments

Indeed, as in humans' interaction with other microorganisms, our interaction with fungi varies from benign coexistence to deadly infection. Fungal sinusitis has been felt to be uncommon, however, recently published data contradicts previous reports. A topic of much debate, the diagnosis and treatment of fungal sinusitis continues to frustrate physicians and their patients.

For more information regarding sinus infections, fungal or otherwise, contact your local otorhinolaryngology specialist.

Section 9.4

Nasal Polyps and Sinusitis

Do you have a blocked nose? Does food seem less tasty? Do you have thick, discolored nasal drainage? You might be suffering from nasal polyps—a treatable nasal problem.

Nasal polyps are noncancerous growths occurring in the nose or sinuses. Other types of polyps occur in the bowel or urinary bladder, but have no relationship to those in the nose and sinuses. Polyps in the bowel or bladder have a chance of being cancerous; polyps in the nose and sinuses are rarely malignant.

Polyps can cause nasal blockage, making it hard to breathe, but most nasal polyp problems can be helped.

While some polyps are a result of swelling from an infection, most of the time, the cause for the nasal polyps is never known. A few individuals may have a combination of asthma, aspirin sensitivity, and nasal polyps. If aspirin is taken, the asthma and nasal polyps may worsen.

Because polyps block the nose, patients often notice a decrease in the sense of smell. Since much of our sense of taste is related to our sense of smell, patients with nasal polyps may describe a loss of both taste and smell.

Nasal polyps also cause nasal obstruction and may also block the pathways where the sinuses drain into the nose. This blockage by the polyps causes the mucus (which normally forms and drains through the nose) to remain in the sinuses. When this mucus stays in the sinuses too long, it can become infected. It is this infected mucus that the patient experiences as a thick, discolored drainage in the nose and down the throat. This type of nasal obstruction and infection may also cause pressure over the forehead and face.

Many people with nasal polyps have no symptoms and therefore require no treatment. For those patients whose polyps are causing symptoms, medical or surgical management is available.

Medical management to reduce the size of the polyps often requires a series of steroid pills and nasal steroid sprays. Since the nasal steroid sprays have very little absorption into the bloodstream, there are few, if any, side effects. For those patients whose polyps cannot be managed medically or choose not to manage them medically, surgery is usually effective.

Surgery for nasal polyps is usually done as an outpatient in an ambulatory surgery center where patients go home the same day as surgery. The polyps are removed from the nose and sinuses using small nasal telescopes, which not only removes the diseased tissue but also preserves the normal structures and reconstructs the normal inflow, outflow, and function of the sinuses.

While most patients with nasal polyps and asthma or nasal polyps, asthma, and aspirin sensitivity have the same 90% improvement, eighteen months after surgery 40% of patients with asthma and nasal polyps report continued improvement, and 35% of patients with the combination of aspirin sensitivity, asthma, and nasal polyps report still feeling well.

The asthmatic patient with nasal polyps is the most difficult to cure, but by using the endoscopic technique, as well as ongoing management with medication after surgery, we are able to help many patients breathe easier, regain their sense of smell, eliminate facial pressure, and have better controlled asthma.

Section 9.5

Postnasal Drip

"Nasal discharge," © 2006 A.D.A.M., Inc.
Reprinted with permission.

Definition

Nasal discharge is any mucus-like material that comes out of the nose.

Considerations

Nasal discharges are common, but rarely serious. Drainage from inflamed or infected sinuses may be thick or discolored.

Excess mucus production may run down the back of your throat (postnasal drip) or cause a cough that is usually worse at night. A sore throat may also result from excessive mucus drainage.

The mucus drainage may plug up the eustachian tube between the nose and the ear, causing an ear infection and pain. The mucus drip may also plug the sinus passages, causing sinus infection and pain.

Common Causes

- Colds
- Flu
- Hay fever—nasal discharge is usually clear and very thin
- Sinusitis—the nasal discharge may be thick and discolored yellow, brown, or green
- Head injury
- Bacterial infections
- Small objects in the nostril (especially in children)
- Nasal sprays—using drops containing vasoconstrictors for more than 3 days in a row may cause nasal discharge to come back

Home Care

Keep the mucus thin rather than thick and sticky. This helps prevent complications, such as ear and sinus infections and plugging of your nasal passages. To thin the mucus:

- use saline nasal sprays;
- drink extra fluids; and
- increase the humidity in the air with a vaporizer or humidifier.

Antihistamines may reduce the amount of mucus. Be careful because some antihistamines may make you drowsy. Don't use over-the-counter nasal sprays more frequently than 3 days on and 3 days off, unless ordered by the doctor.

Overuse of Antibiotics

Many people think that a green or yellow nasal discharge means a bacterial infection, which requires antibiotics. This is not true. Colds will often begin with a clear nasal discharge, but after several days it usually turns creamy yellow or green. Colds are caused by viruses, and antibiotics will not help. A green or yellow nasal discharge is not a sign you need antibiotics.

Call Your Health Care Provider

Call your health care provider if:

- a nasal discharge follows a head injury;
- the drainage is foul smelling, one-sided, or a color other than white or yellow;
- symptoms persist beyond 3 weeks; or
- there is fever along with nasal discharge.

What to Expect at Your Health Care Provider's Office

Your doctor may perform a physical examination, including an examination of the ears, nose, and throat.

Your doctor may ask medical history questions, such as:

- Is the discharge thin and watery or is it thick?

- Is it bloody?
- What color is it?
- How long has the nasal discharge been present?
- Is it present all the time?
- What other symptoms are also present?
- Is your nose stuffy or congested?
- Do you have a cough or headache?
- Do you have a sore throat?
- Do you have a fever?

Diagnostic tests that may be performed for persistent problems include:

- CT scan of the head
- X-rays of the skull and sinuses

For allergic rhinitis, antihistamines may be prescribed. Antibiotics should only be prescribed for bacterial infections.

Chapter 10

Treating Sinusitis

Chapter Contents

Section 10.1

Remedies for Sinus Headaches

Headache is a common complaint that is often associated with sinusitis. However, the true cause for a headache may be difficult to determine because headaches have many causes. The United States Centers for Disease Control and Prevention report that sinusitis affects over 30 million people and is the most common chronic disease in this country. Thus, many sinus sufferers will also suffer headaches. While headaches and sinusitis are common problems sometimes headaches occur with sinusitis and sometimes they do not.

The Nasal Sinus Problem

Typically, a nasal and/or sinus problem will include congestion and stuffiness, often with nasal drainage. If an infection is present there will be discolored, thick drainage in the front of the nose and down the back of the throat. If a headache is present, it is usually a pressure sensation varying in intensity from almost non-existent to somewhat severe.

Generally, a sinus headache will be located over the sinuses (forehead, corners of the eye, and cheek areas). On occasion, the pain will be felt behind the eyes, in the back of the neck, or may extend into the upper teeth. Head movement usually worsens this headache.

The true cause for headache may be difficult to determine; sometimes headaches occur with sinusitis and sometimes not.

Non-Sinus Headaches

Non-sinus headaches may give these same symptoms, thus making it difficult to determine if the headache is truly from a sinus problem. For example, tension headaches will occur in the forehead and neck; migraine headaches often occur in and around the eyes.

It is unusual for a person with a sinus or nasal problem to only have a headache. A sinus headache is nearly always accompanied by nasal stuffiness, congestion, obstruction, or drainage. When headache is the only symptom, it is rarely sinus related.

Sinus Headaches

The main cause of nasal and sinus headaches is the nasal turbinates—nasal structures that swell and contract throughout the day giving the feeling of nasal congestion and occasionally pressure. Worsened by irritants such as perfume, cigarette smoke, or allergens, the internal swelling causes facial pressure. When the turbinates swell, not only is the breathing passage blocked, but also normal sinus draining passages are blocked creating a backup situation.

Drainage remains trapped in the sinus cavity, causing the pain and pressure you feel over the sinuses. It may also cause an infection.

Oral decongestants (for example, pseudoephedrine) or a nasal spray (for example, Neo-Synephrine, oxymetazoline) will often give relief. However, these sprays should not be used for more than a few days since they can cause even more congestion when their effect wears off.

Caution is needed when using decongestant pills, especially is a person has a history of heart disease or high blood pressure. These adrenaline-like medications can cause a rapid heart rate or increased blood pressure.

If over-the-counter medical management for nasal congestion is not effective, a physician may choose to prescribe a steroid nasal spray.

If medical management fails or cannot be tolerated, surgery to reduce the turbinates is extremely successful.

Another cause for a sinus headache is the common cold, which may seem to be a sinus infection. If over-the-counter cold remedies fail and the symptoms continue beyond several days or if there are other debilitating medical problems, a physician should be called.

Section 10.2

Antibiotics and Sinusitis

An antibiotic is a soluble substance derived from a mold or bacterium that inhibits the growth of other microorganisms.

The first antibiotic was penicillin, discovered by Alexander Fleming in 1929, but it was not until World War II that the effectiveness of antibiotics was acknowledged, and large-scale fermentation processes were developed for their production.

Acute sinusitis is one of many medical disorders that can be caused by a bacterial infection. However, it is important to remember that colds, allergies, and environmental irritants, which are more common than bacterial sinusitis, can also cause sinus problems. Antibiotics are effective only against sinus problems caused by a bacterial infection.

The following symptoms may indicate the presence of a bacterial infection in your sinuses:

- pain in your cheeks or upper back teeth;

- a lot of bright yellow or green drainage from your nose for more than 10 days;

- no relief from decongestants; and/or

- symptoms that get worse instead of better after your cold is gone.

Most patients with a clinical diagnosis of acute sinusitis caused by a bacterial infection improve without antibiotic treatment. The specialist will initially offer appropriate doses of analgesics (pain relievers), antipyretics (fever reducers), and decongestants. However if symptoms persist, a treatment consisting of antibiotics may be recommended.

Antibiotic Treatment for Sinusitis

Antibiotics are labeled as narrow-spectrum drugs when they work against only a few types of bacteria. On the other hand, broad-spectrum antibiotics are more effective by attacking a wide range of bacteria, but are more likely to promote antibiotic resistance. For that reason, your ear, nose, and throat specialist will most likely prescribe narrow-spectrum antibiotics, which often cost less. He or she may recommend broad-spectrum antibiotics for infections that do not respond to treatment with narrow-spectrum drugs.

Acute Sinusitis

In most cases, antibiotics are prescribed for patients with specific findings of persistent purulent nasal discharge and facial pain or tenderness who are not improving after seven days or those with severe symptoms of rhinosinusitis, regardless of duration. On the basis of clinical trials, amoxicillin, doxycycline, or trimethoprim-sulfamethoxazole are preferred antibiotics.

Chronic Sinusitis

Even with a long regimen of antibiotics, chronic sinusitis symptoms can be difficult to treat. In general, however, treating chronic sinusitis, such as with antibiotics and decongestants, is similar to treating acute sinusitis. When antibiotic treatment fails, allergy testing, desensitization, and/or surgery may be recommended as the most effective means for treating chronic sinusitis. Research studies suggest that the vast majority of people who undergo surgery have fewer symptoms and better quality of life.

Pediatric Sinusitis

Antibiotics that are unlikely to be effective in children who do not improve with amoxicillin include trimethoprim-sulfamethoxazole (Bactrim) and erythromycin-sulfisoxazole (Pediazole), because many bacteria are resistant to these older antibiotics. For children who do not respond to two courses of traditional antibiotics, the dose and length of antibiotic treatment is often expanded or treatment with intravenous cefotaxime or ceftriaxone and/or a referral to an ENT [ear, nose, and throat] specialist is recommended.

Section 10.3

Sinus Surgery

Sinus surgery has truly evolved in the last several years. This procedure was once performed through external incisions, required extensive packing, and caused significant patient discomfort and a lengthy recovery. With recent advances in technology including the nasal endoscope, this procedure is now incisionless and can often be performed with minimal packing, pain, and recovery.

The most common indication for endoscopic sinus surgery is a chronic sinus infection refractory to medical management. Less common indications include (but are not limited to): recurrent infections (rather than a single chronic infection), complications of sinus infections, nasal polyps or mucoceles, chronic sinus headaches, impaired sense of smell, tumors of the nasal and sinus cavities, cerebrospinal fluid leaks, nasolacrimal duct obstruction, choanal atresia, and the need to decompress the orbit. Prior to undergoing endoscopic sinus surgery, patients should talk with their physicians to make sure that all reasonable medical options have been exhausted. In addition, patients should avoid any medications that may exacerbate bleeding, such as aspirin and ibuprofen products, as well as certain vitamins and herbal remedies.

Endoscopic sinus surgery may be performed under local or general anesthesia. The procedure involves the use of a small telescope (nasal endoscope) placed into the nasal cavity to visualize the surgery. The goal of the surgery is to identify the narrow channels that connect the paranasal sinuses to the nasal cavity and to enlarge these areas, thereby improving drainage from the sinuses to the nose. Sometimes sinus surgery may require simultaneous repair of the nasal septum, which divides the two sides of the nose, or the turbinates, which filter and humidify air inside of the nose. The use of nasal packing will depend on the extent of surgery and physician preference. The recovery period will also vary depending on the extent of surgery but postoperative discomfort, congestion, and drainage should significantly improve after the first few postoperative days, with mild symptoms sometimes lingering several weeks after the surgery.

Endoscopic sinus surgery generally yields excellent results, and significant symptomatic improvement is achieved in the majority of patients. Adverse events are rare but may include postoperative bleeding, orbital complications, complications from the general anesthetic, cerebrospinal fluid leaks, and intracranial complications such as meningitis.

However, it is important to realize that chronic sinus infections are located directly beneath the skull base and adjacent to the eye; the failure to treat this problem without surgery may lead to dire consequences such as intraorbital or intracranial spread of the infection.

Section 10.4

Complications of Sinus Surgery

Surgery on the nasal septum, turbinates, and sinuses is recommended only after it has been determined that medical management has been unsuccessful. While these procedures are generally very successful, patients must be aware of certain risks before electing to proceed. These risks include, but are not necessarily limited to, the following:

- **Postoperative bleeding:** Aspirin, ibuprofen, and certain non-prescription supplements (vitamin E, garlic, etc.) can increase the propensity to bleed, so patients should consult with their physicians before using these agents before or after surgery. Intranasal packing is utilized by many sinus surgeons to help avoid this complication but occasionally postoperative bleeding is encountered despite all precautions.

111

- **Anesthesia complications:** Adverse reactions to local or general anesthesia may occur, including cardiac and pulmonary complications. Fortunately, these risks are quite rare in this era of modern anesthesia.

- **Intracranial complications:** The base of the skull forms the roof of the ethmoid and sphenoid sinuses. If this layer is violated, a leak of cerebrospinal fluid (the fluid that bathes the brain and spinal cord) may occur. This can usually be repaired at the time of the initial surgery, although in rare cases further complications such as meningitis may ensue.

- **Intraorbital complications:** The orbit is situated immediately adjacent to several of the paranasal sinuses but is separated by a layer of bone. Because of this close proximity, in rare cases bleeding may occur into the orbit requiring repair at the time of the initial surgery. Visual loss and blindness have been reported but are extremely rare.

- **Smell:** The sense of smell usually improves, although it may occasionally worsen, depending on the extent of infection, allergy, or polyps.

- **Voice changes:** One of the functions of the sinuses is to affect resonance, so vocal professionals should be aware of potential changes in their voice after sinus surgery.

- **Infection:** The most common reason to undergo sinus surgery is a chronic infection that does not resolve with medications. The patient with sinusitis is therefore at risk of developing certain other infections in this area (abscesses, meningitis, etc.) regardless of whether they manage the sinusitis with or without surgery.

- **Nasal obstruction:** Much of the nasal septum is made of cartilage, which has "memory"—the propensity to move back to its original position. Despite certain measures performed by the surgeon at the time of septoplasty this may still occur and require a secondary procedure. Small scar bands may also occur in the nose and require removal by the surgeon at postoperative visits.

- **Numbness:** A transient numbness of the front upper teeth, lip, or nose may occur after surgery but is usually self-limiting.

While surgery may entail these complications, it is also crucial to remember that the failure to intervene surgically may also place the patient at risk for certain complications. When left untreated, the infection may rarely spread to adjacent structures such as the eye or brain and lead to abscesses in these areas, meningitis, visual loss, or even death. Fortunately, the rare patient suffers from complications of the infection or sinus surgery.

Section 10.5

What to Expect after Sinus Surgery

Many studies have demonstrated that the vast majority of patients who undergo endoscopic sinus surgery are ultimately very satisfied with their results. As with all surgeries, there is a convalescent period after this procedure, although it is usually much milder now than in years past with the advent of endoscopes, minimally invasive procedures, and smaller or absorbable packs. This recovery period can vary greatly depending on the extent of surgery, the use of nasal packing, and the individual patient.

Patients will often experience blood-tinged discharge during the first day or two after surgery. This is normal, and by keeping the head elevated above the heart (a recliner works very well), this symptom will be minimized. Discomfort is generally well managed with pain medications prescribed by the surgeon. All patients will experience some degree of congestion or nasal obstruction, and this will be significantly improved once any nasal packing or splints are removed. In addition, patients may notice postnasal drainage, headaches, and fatigue that is most noticeable the first few days after the surgery and gradually resolves completely over the ensuing weeks. Many of these symptoms will mimic those of a sinus infection until this healing process is complete.

Patients should avoid strenuous activities and medications that predispose them to bleeding (such as aspirin, ibuprofen, and certain herbal remedies) for at least two weeks after surgery or until the healing process is complete. Time off work varies from several days to even weeks depending on the patient's occupation and the extent of surgery. This should be discussed with the physician.

The postoperative care may be as important as the surgery itself. Sinus surgeons usually schedule frequent postoperative visits to clean the sinus cavities and ensure that they are patent [unobstructed], healing well, and are without scarring. In addition, the surgeon will often have patients on a regimen to clean the sinus cavities at home, although this varies greatly from physician to physician. For most patients, following the routine set forth by the sinus surgeon leads to excellent long-term results and patient satisfaction.

Chapter 11

Allergic Conjunctivitis

Believe your eyes, and see what they may be telling you. If your eyes itch, are red, tearing or burning, pay attention to what they may be telling you. You may have eye allergies, or allergic conjunctivitis, a condition that affects millions of Americans. It is a condition that can occur alone, but often accompanies nasal allergy symptoms, such as sneezing, sniffling, and a stuffy nose. And, while most people treat nasal allergy symptoms, they often ignore their itchy, red, watery eyes. This text answers questions about eye allergies and suggests effective ways for you to recognize and treat the symptoms.

What causes eye allergies?

Just like hay fever and skin rashes, eye allergies develop when the body's immune system becomes sensitized and overreacts to something that is ordinarily harmless. An allergic reaction can occur whenever that something—called an allergen—comes into contact with your eyes. The allergen causes certain cells in the eye (called mast cells) to release histamine and other substances or chemicals that cause blood vessels in the eyes to swell, and the eyes to become itchy, red, and watery.

115

What allergens trigger eye allergies?

Allergens that may be present indoors or outdoors can cause eye allergies. The most common outdoor airborne allergens are grass, tree, and weed pollens. People who are sensitive to these allergens suffer from seasonal allergic conjunctivitis, the most common type of eye allergy.

Pet hair or dander, dust mites, and molds are the most common indoor allergens. These indoor allergens can trigger symptoms for some people throughout the year, resulting in perennial allergic conjunctivitis.

Although cigarette smoke, perfume and diesel exhaust may inflame your eyes, they act as irritants rather than triggering an allergic response. They can, however, make your allergy symptoms worse.

Can eye allergies harm my eyesight?

No. Eye allergies can be extremely annoying and uncomfortable, and they may disrupt your day-to-day activities, but they cannot harm your eyes.

How are eye allergies treated?

As with any allergy, the first approach for successful management should be prevention or avoidance of the allergens that trigger your symptoms. Here are some avoidance tips to reduce exposure to allergens that affect your eyes.

- Stay indoors as much as possible when pollen counts are at their peak, usually during the mid-morning and early evening, and when wind is blowing pollens around.

- Keep windows closed and use air conditioning in your car and home. Air conditioning units should be kept clean. Avoid using window fans that can draw pollens and molds into the house.

- Wear glasses or sunglasses when outdoors to minimize pollen getting into your eyes.

- Avoid rubbing eyes, which will only irritate them or make your condition worse.

- Reduce dust mite exposure in your home, especially the bedroom. Bedding, particularly pillows, should be encased in "mite-proof" covers. Wash bedding often in hot water (at least 130 degrees Fahrenheit). Keep humidity in your home low (between 30 percent and 50 percent).

- Clean floors with a damp rag or mop rather than dry dusting or sweeping.

- Wash your hands immediately after petting any animals. Remove and wash clothing after visiting friends with pets.

- If you have a pet to which you are allergic, keep it out of your house as much as possible. If the pet must be in the house, keep it out of the bedroom so you are not exposed to animal allergens while you sleep. Close the air ducts to your bedroom if you have forced-air or central heating/cooling. Replace carpeting with hardwood, tile, or linoleum, which are easier to keep dander free.

- Reduce indoor molds caused by high humidity by cleaning bathrooms, kitchens, and basements regularly. A dehumidifier can be used to reduce molds, especially in damp, humid places like basements. Make sure the dehumidifier is cleaned often. To clean moldy areas in the home, use a 1-to-10 parts diluted mixture of chlorine bleach and water.

Because many of the allergens that trigger eye allergies are airborne, avoidance is not always possible. You should discuss your eye allergy symptoms with an allergy specialist or your personal physician to determine which of several treatment options is right for you. A list follows of the kinds of over-the-counter (OTC) and prescription eyedrops and oral medications that are available for the treatment of eye allergies.

Are the OTC and prescription eyedrops and medications safe for children?

There are eyedrops and oral medications available to treat eye allergies in children. Artificial tears are extremely safe and can be used at any age. Some eyedrops, such as antihistamines and antihistamines/mast cell stabilizers, can be used in children who are 3 and older. Any treatment should be discussed with your child's physician.

Do allergy shots treat eye allergies?

If avoidance, oral medication, and eyedrops do not control your symptoms, allergy shots or immunotherapy is another option for relieving eye allergies. Tiny amounts of the allergen are injected with gradually increasing doses over time. The shots can actually keep your body from reacting to the allergens. The treatment takes several months to achieve maximum results and some continuing medication may still be required.

What medications are used for the treatment of eye allergies?

Over-the-counter eyedrops and oral medications are commonly used for short-term relief of some eye allergy symptoms. However, they may not relieve all symptoms, and prolonged use of some OTC eyedrops may actually cause your condition to become worse.

Prescription eyedrops and oral medications also are used to treat eye allergies. Prescription eyedrops provide both short- and long-term targeted relief of eye allergy symptoms, and they can be used to manage eye allergy symptoms in conjunction with an oral antihistamine that might be taken to manage nasal allergy symptoms.

What OTC eyedrops and medications are used?

- **Tear Substitutes:** Artificial tears can temporarily wash allergens from the eye and also moisten the eyes, which often become dry when red and irritated. These drops, which can be refrigerated to provide additional soothing and comfort, are safe and can be used as often as necessary.

- **Decongestants/Antihistamines:** Decongestants or vasoconstrictors are available as over-the-counter eyedrops to reduce the redness associated with eye allergies. (Eyedrops containing vasoconstrictors should not be used by anyone with glaucoma.) The decongestant drops are available alone or in conjunction with an antihistamine, which provides additional relief of itching. The drops are weak and must be used frequently (four to six times a day). It is very important not to use these OTC eyedrops for more than two to three days. Prolonged use can actually lead to increased swelling and redness that may last even after discontinuing the drops. You may be familiar with this "rebound effect" that occurs when you use decongestant nasal sprays for more than three days, and your nose becomes even more congested than before.

- **Oral Antihistamines:** Oral antihistamines can be mildly effective in relieving the itching associated with eye allergies, however, these medications may cause dry eyes and potentially worsen eye allergy symptoms. Also, some OTC versions of these medications can cause side effects such as sedation, excitability, dizziness, or disturbed coordination.

What prescription eyedrops and medications are used?

- **Antihistamines:** Eyedrops that contain antihistamines can reduce the itching, redness, and swelling associated with eye allergies. Although antihistamine eyedrops provide quick relief, the effect may last only a few hours, and some of these drops need to be used four times a day.

- **Mast Cell Stabilizers:** Mast cell stabilizers are eyedrops that prevent the release of histamine and other substances that cause allergy symptoms. The drops must be taken before exposure to an allergen to prevent itching.

- **Antihistamine/Mast Cell Stabilizers:** Some of the newest eyedrops have both an antihistamine and a mast cell stabilizing action to treat and prevent eye allergies. They are used twice a day and provide quick and long-lasting relief of itching, redness, tearing, and burning.

- **NSAIDs:** Nonsteroidal anti-inflammatory drug (NSAID) eyedrops also are available to relieve itching. These drops may cause stinging or burning when applied and may need to be used four times a day.

- **Corticosteroids:** Steroid eyedrops can help treat chronic and severe eye allergy symptoms such as itching, redness, and swelling, but continued use of the drops can have side effects, such as a risk of secondary infection, glaucoma, and cataracts. These drops should only be used short-term and under the supervision of an ophthalmologist.

- **Nonsedating Oral Antihistamines:** Like OTC oral antihistamines, prescription antihistamines can be mildly effective in relieving the itching associated with eye allergies. They do not have the same sedating side effects as OTC antihistamines, but they still can cause dry eyes and worsen symptoms.

Your allergist or personal physician can help determine which treatments are best for you.

Chapter 12

Allergic Urticaria (Hives) and Angioedema

Definitions

Urticaria is a skin rash, also called hives, or nettle rash, which is often accompanied by swelling and itching of the skin.

Angioedema (in the past this was called giant urticaria or angioneurotic edema) is a condition involving swelling in the deeper layers of the skin, caused by a buildup of fluid leaking from thin-walled blood vessels. It can accompany hives or occur alone.

Symptoms

Hives are itchy and have a central, raised white wheal surrounded by an area of redness. Hives whiten if pressure is applied to the rash. The rash generally disappears within 24 hours.

Swelling of deeper layers of the skin, angioedema, is often seen with hives. The redness that accompanies hives isn't seen, but the swelling is very obvious. The swelling generally occurs on the fingers and toes, as well as areas of the head, neck, face, and, in men, the reproductive organs, and is often described as painful or burning.

"Urticaria and Angioedema" is reprinted with permission from the Allergic Diseases Resource Center at http://www.worldallergy.org. © 2006 World Allergy Organization. All rights reserved.

Classification

Hives and angioedema are described by the length of time that symptoms last. A rash and/or swelling lasting less than six weeks is called acute hives/angioedema. Episodes that last more than six weeks are described as chronic hives/angioedema. The causes and the body's reactions that lead to development of hives are different in acute and chronic hives/angioedema and so treatment is also different.

Acute Hives

Acute hives can be divided into two general types, depending on the rate at which hives develop and the length of time the rash lasts. In one type, the rash lasts 1 to 2 hours; this is usually the type found in physically induced hives (see the section titled Physical hives). The second type can last as long as 36 hours; this is the type commonly seen in food or drug reactions.

Chronic Hives and Angioedema

Chronic hives and angioedema are diagnosed when hives and swelling are present for more than six weeks. Before the diagnosis is made, it is important to make sure that what seems to be a long-lasting attack of hives is not really a series of short attacks occurring close together.

Chronic Idiopathic Hives and Idiopathic Angioedema

This is a common disorder, and the diagnosis of idiopathic hives and angioedema is made when no cause can be found. The skin symptoms may vary from severe to mild or may intermittently subside, and routine blood tests show no obvious abnormalities. Chronic hives does not appear to be a true allergic reaction, because IgE antibody is not involved, and no contact with an allergen is needed to bring on the symptoms.

Causes

Allergic Hives

Acute hives caused by an allergic reaction is a common condition in children and adults. When an allergen (for example, a food or insect sting) to which the person is allergic enters the bloodstream, it starts a series of reactions in the body's immune system. These reactions lead to the release of histamine and other chemicals into the blood and can result in hives and/or other allergic symptoms. Common allergens that can cause acute hives include foods, drugs (particularly antibiotics such as penicillin), and venoms from the stings of insects such as bee, wasp, yellow jacket, hornet, or fire ant, but virtually any allergen has the potential to cause hives.

In general, if an allergen causes hives or swelling, it is usually eaten (food, drug taken by mouth) or injected (drugs, stings). Allergens that are inhaled tend to cause asthma or rhinitis and may contribute to the development of eczema in children.

If an allergen can penetrate the skin, hives will develop at the site of exposure. For example, contact hives may occur following exposure to latex gloves if sufficient latex penetrates through the skin.

Non-Specific Causes

Acute hives can result from causes other than true (IgE-mediated) allergies. An example is exposure to certain dyes used in x-ray procedures, which can cause a whole-body reaction called anaphylaxis which includes hives. Acute viral illnesses in children can be associated with hives which last a few weeks and then spontaneously subside. This usually occurs in association with the symptoms of a common cold, sore throat, or bronchitis. If these patients are given an antibiotic, the cause of the hives becomes confused, because a reaction to the antibiotics may be causing the hives. If penicillin or related antibiotics have been taken, the doctor may perform an allergy skin test, or blood tests for IgE antibodies against the antibiotic, because it is important to know whether the patient has had an allergic reaction to the antibiotic. Hepatitis B, glandular fever, and intestinal parasites may all be associated with the development of hives.

Hives and angioedema can also result from drug treatments. These include codeine and opiate-derived medications, as well as aspirin and other non-steroidal anti-inflammatory drugs (NSAIDs). The responses to NSAIDs can be life-threatening because the angioedema can lead to serious swelling of the tongue and/or throat. Drugs used to treat high blood pressure, known as ACE [angiotensin-converting enzyme] inhibitors, can cause recurrent episodes of angioedema.

If chronic hives do not appear to be associated with any other disease, and are not due to a type of physically induced urticaria described, they are called idiopathic, that is, of unknown origin. Research suggests that in 35% to 45% of patients with idiopathic hives the cause may be autoimmunity—that is, the patient's immune system working against itself. These autoimmune types of hives are not serious and usually respond to treatment with antihistamines.

Physical Hives

Hives and/or angioedema can be caused by environmental factors, such as a change in temperature or pressure on the skin. Two rare causes of hives are exposure to sunlight or contact with water.

Cold-Dependent Disorders: Cold urticaria is the rapid onset of itching, redness, and swelling of the skin after exposure to cold. The symptoms of cold urticaria may occur for the first time some weeks after a viral infection and only affect those parts of the body that have been exposed to cold. To test for this, an ice-cube can be placed on the forearm for 4 to 5 minutes. A positive reaction leads to a hive in the shape of the ice cube within 10 minutes after the source of cold has been removed.

Cold urticaria can be restricted to certain areas of the body, for example, where there has been a cold injury, or at the sites of allergen immunotherapy (desensitization) injections or insect bites. Another skin condition that is related to cold is cold-dependent dermatographism, in which hives form if the skin is scratched and then chilled.

Exercise-Induced Disorders: Cholinergic or generalized heat urticaria is the onset of small wheals surrounded by a large area of redness, associated with exercise, hot showers, sweating and anxiety. The rash first appears on the neck and upper chest, giving a flushed appearance. This is accompanied by intense itching. The rash spreads gradually to the face, back, and extremities, and the wheals increase in size. In some people the hives join up and resemble angioedema. Watering eyes, increased saliva production, and diarrhea can occur at the same time. Cholinergic urticaria is the only form of hives that can be caused by emotional responses.

Exercise-induced anaphylaxis was first described in a series of people who experienced combinations of itching, skin rash, swelling, wheezing, and low blood pressure as a result of exercise. The hives seen with exercise-induced anaphylaxis are large, in contrast to the small hives seen in cholinergic urticaria. A type of exercise-induced anaphylaxis has been described that is related to food and occurs only if exercise takes place 5 to 24 hours after eating a food to which the individual is allergic.

Pressure-Induced Hives/Angioedema: Pressure-induced hives/ angioedema occurs 4 to 6 hours after pressure has been applied to the skin. There may be either a rash or swelling, or both, occurring around tight clothing; the hands may swell with activity such as hammering; foot swelling is common after walking; and buttock swelling may occur after sitting for a few hours.

Solar Urticaria: Solar urticaria is a rare disorder in which brief exposure to light causes the development of hives within 1 to 3 minutes. It starts with itching about 30 seconds after exposure to sunlight, and is followed by swelling and redness of the light-exposed area. The symptoms usually disappear within 1 to 3 hours.

Aquagenic Urticaria: Individuals develop small wheals after contact with water, regardless of its temperature.

Association with Autoimmune Thyroid Disease: Patients with chronic hives have an increased frequency of Hashimoto disease (thyroiditis), and tests of thyroid function and thyroid antibody levels can be performed to see if this is responsible for the skin symptoms.

Treatment

Treatment of Acute Hives and Angioedema

Acute episodes of hives and/or swelling can be treated with antihistamines, and 1% menthol in aqueous cream may help control itching. If the allergens causing hives and/or swelling have been identified, either from the description of the attacks, or by blood testing for specific IgE antibodies, allergen avoidance will help to prevent further attacks. If the hives or swelling has resulted from taking medications, the patient's physician will be able to identify different types of medications for future treatment. Tightly fitting clothes should be avoided, as wheals often occur in areas of pressure. As the itching associated with hives can be more severe in warm conditions, it may help to keep the home cool, and to ensure that the bedroom is not too hot. Urticaria and angioedema can be symptoms of a systemic reaction called anaphylaxis and may require urgent administration of intramuscular epinephrine (adrenaline).

Treatment of Chronic Hives

Antihistamines are valuable in the treatment of chronic hives and are more effective on the itching than the wheals. If the symptoms continue when the maximum recommended amount of antihistamines has been given, a short course of corticosteroid tablets may be helpful.

Epidemiology: Who Develops Urticaria and Angioedema and Why?

Urticaria and angioedema are thought to affect 20% of the population at some time during their lifetimes. Hives alone or associated with the swelling of angioedema are more common in women, whereas angioedema alone, in the absence of hives, is more common in men.

Less than 10% of hives develop into a chronic problem. Very often an attack of hives occurs without anyone understanding why it has happened, with little or no risk of the symptoms recurring.

Chapter 13

Contact Dermatitis: Skin Reactions to Allergens or Irritants

Chapter Contents

Section 13.1

Understanding Contact Dermatitis

Definition

Contact dermatitis (CD) is an inflammation of the skin characterized by redness, itching, blistering and, in chronic cases, flaking of scales
of skin, resulting from exposure of the skin to substances in the environment. The site and shape of the affected areas of skin are directly
related to the area that has been exposed to the causative substance.

Classification

Irritant Contact Dermatitis

Irritant CD develops following prolonged and repeated exposure
to irritants such as caustic agents or detergents. This is not an IgE-
mediated, allergic condition, and prior contact and sensitization to the
causative substance is not necessary for the development of symptoms.
Susceptibility to irritants varies, but, given sufficient exposure, most
people would develop irritant CD.

Phototoxic reactions are the result of exposure to sunlight in combination with certain chemicals. All individuals with sufficient skin
exposure to chemical photosensitizers such as psoralens (naturally occurring substances found in some plants) together with ultraviolet light
(UV) would develop a phototoxic skin reaction. This reaction resembles
sunburn and is not caused by a reaction of the immune system.

Allergic Contact Dermatitis (Allergic CD)

Allergic CD results from inflammation caused by a group of blood cells
called allergen specific T lymphocytes. Prior exposure, which results in
an allergic reaction, i.e., sensitization, is essential. Rapid development
of skin inflammation, i.e., dermatitis, occurs following re-exposure to low

concentrations of allergen, which would not cause a reaction in non-sensitized non-allergic individuals.

Photoallergic reactions result from new allergens created by the photochemical reaction of UV on certain chemicals and body proteins. The new allergens stimulate an allergic "immune" response, which causes a skin reaction similar to that of allergic CD.

Epidemiology

Eighty-five to 95% of all occupational-related skin disease in the working population of industrialized countries is due to contact dermatitis. In these countries hand dermatitis affects between 2% and 6% of the population.

Symptoms and Characteristics

The fundamental characteristic of contact dermatitis is the relationship to environmental exposure, which determines the site and shape of the skin reaction. A sharp edge to an otherwise shapeless rash, or an abrupt cutoff, is a characteristic of contact dermatitis.

Irritant CD

- Irritant CD most frequently affects the hands.

- Phototoxic and photoallergic CD can occur due to a combination of drugs taken by mouth, a sensitizing agent (such as fragrance) applied to the skin, and subsequent exposure to sunlight. Patches of CD will appear only on the areas of skin exposed to the sun.

Allergic CD

- Nickel allergy involves ears, skin under knuckles, and often the hands; accidental spread from the hands can affect the face.

- Hair products—dyes and sprays—affect the face, neck, and ears.

- Dyes in socks and shoes affect the feet.

- Medications for the treatment of leg ulcers can cause dermatitis of the legs.

- In the case of an allergy, an itchy, red rash develops at the site of re-exposure to the causative substance within 6 to 12 hours.

- The reaction is worse after 48 to 72 hours, and, if exposure continues, the skin becomes scaly, weepy, and flaky.

- Strongly allergic people require very little contact with the causative agent for severe acute weeping eczematous reactions to occur.

- Contact with the allergen can occur even through several layers of clothing. For example, nickel can be leached from keys, money, or earring studs by perspiration.

Differential Diagnosis

It is important to obtain a correct diagnosis of either allergic or irritant CD, particularly when the dermatitis is caused by contact with a substance encountered at work, because the correct diagnosis of an irritant cause may allow the patient to continue at work with appropriate skin protection. A detailed history of all substances with which the individual comes into contact during domestic, occupational, sporting and leisure activities, together with the results of patch testing, is required.

Contact dermatitis can be similar in appearance to most inflammatory skin diseases. However the majority of skin diseases that are not related to contact have a symmetrical distribution, as is the case with IgE-mediated eczema, drug rashes, psoriasis, and connective tissue diseases.

Fixed drug eruptions (a rash occurring repeatedly at the same place following ingestion of a medicine to which the individual is sensitized) can be single and round, and skin cells can be examined to ensure the eruption is not a symptom of a lymphoma (a form of cancer).

Allergens Causing Allergic CD

Nickel

Nickel is the most common cause of allergic CD in most countries. It is present in most metal alloys including 14-karat gold. Most nickel-allergic individuals can avoid problems by wearing 18-karat gold and testing other suspect alloys with a dimethylglyoxime test. The role of dietary nickel in skin eruptions is controversial.

Rubber Accelerators: Thiurams, Carbamates, Mercaptobenzothiazole

Allergic CD to rubber usually results from sensitization to these compounds and occurs where rubber is worn next to or close to the skin.

Examples are elastic bands in underclothes and rubber in gloves, shoes, and barrier contraceptives. Carbamates are found not only in rubber products but also in garden fungicides. Allergy to black rubber may also be the result of sensitization to paraphenylenediamine dye.

Latex rubber can also cause so called allergic contact urticaria (hives), which is an IgE-mediated reaction to protein allergens from the latex. Patients with a history of contact urticaria should not undergo patch testing because there is a risk of anaphylaxis.

Paraphenylenediamine

Paraphenylenediamine is a black dye used in permanent oxidative hair dyes and is used with cross-linkers to produce all hair dye colors. It is a major cause of allergic CD in hairdressers. Paraphenylenediamine is also used as an antioxidant in oils and greases, as a component in color film developers and as a dye for leather and rubber. It is an important cause of occupational dermatitis in a wide variety of trades.

Fragrances: Balsam of Peru and Cinnamic Aldehyde

Fragrances containing balsam of Peru and cinnamic aldehyde are present in many topical preparations, cosmetics, soaps, perfumes, and toothpastes. Allergic patients must use "fragrance free" products— unscented products are not suitable because they may contain masking fragrances.

Adhesives and Varnishes

P-Tertiary-butyl phenol formaldehyde resin (PTBP) is a phenolic contact adhesive used in the manufacture of plastics, plywood, cardboard boxes, varnish, rubber cements, leather products, and lacquers. PTBT is a factor in dermatitis caused by some shoes, and in allergic CD caused by plastic products and oils.

Epoxy resins are widely used as adhesives in electronics, the construction industry, and in marine paints and varnishes and are an important cause of allergic CD.

Formaldehyde and Formaldehyde Releasers

Formaldehyde is one of the most widespread allergens in the environment and is present in fixatives, adhesives, preservatives and disinfectants. Many cosmetics and disinfectants contain either formaldehyde or the formaldehyde releasers imidazolidinyl urea and quaternium-15. Formaldehyde is also used as a fabric treatment particularly in the "care-free" type of garments, which retain their shape. Many formaldehyde allergic patients can, however, tolerate garments that have been washed many times.

Chromates

Exposure to potassium chromate is common in tanning of leather and in the construction industry due to cement. Allergic CD to chromate in leather shoes may be seasonal as a result of the allergen being leached out by perspiration.

Medications

Benzocaine is a sensitizer and is present in many nonprescription medications such as preparations for the treatment of hemorrhoids and burns and as a topical anesthetic. Cross-reactions with procaine occur. The antibacterial agent neomycin is a common cause of allergic CD. Bacitracin may also cause sensitization.

Tests

Patch Testing

Patch testing requires three visits. On the first day, the allergens are applied to the back in a dermatitis-free area. These are applied by taping to the skin a number of small chambers containing the substances to be tested. Forty-eight hours later, the patches are removed and the skin is examined. The patient returns the following day for a final assessment of any skin reactions. Topical corticosteroids must not be applied to the test site, and oral corticosteroids should not be taken by the patient for at least 2 weeks prior to patch testing. Standardized allergens are used for patch testing whenever possible, because these are extensively tested and should not induce skin irritation or sensitization. It may be necessary on occasion to use non-standardized materials such as clippings of shoes and clothing. Non-standardized compounds that are generally safe for patch testing are cosmetics, moisturizers, and medications that are applied directly to the skin.

Interpretation of Patch Test Reactions

All patch test results will be interpreted in the light of the patient's clinical history and the size, shape, and location of the affected areas of skin. Positive patch tests may not be relevant to the patient's present condition and may simply represent allergies that have occurred in the past. Perspiration and moisture are important factors in the development of allergic CD, because they may be necessary to leach out the allergen from the article of clothing that is in contact with the skin. For this reason in some patients, the skin may only be affected during hot weather.

Standardized Patch Test Allergen Series

The standardized patch test allergen series consists of 20 commonly encountered contact sensitizers. The frequency with which these or indeed other contact allergens are encountered will vary between countries worldwide.

False-Positive Patch Test Reactions

Sometimes a false positive test can occur because:

- the petrolatum used to apply the allergens may cause a mild occasional skin reaction around hair follicles, some reddening, or a pus-filled spot;

- allergic or irritant reactions to the tape used to hold the allergen chambers in place are recognized by their relation to the site of the tape rather than to the area of the patch test; or

- a large skin reaction may overrun into the area of the next test, and, if any doubt exists about the allergen responsible for the skin reaction, the tests need to be repeated a greater distance apart.

Treatment

Allergen/Irritant Avoidance

Contact dermatitis resolves spontaneously when the causative agent is identified by clinical history, site, appearance, and patch testing and is removed.

Antihistamines

Neither the itching nor the inflammation of contact dermatitis responds to antihistamine therapy. However, sedating antihistamines, such as diphenhydramine and hydroxyzine, are often administered at night to aid sleep.

Topical Corticosteroids

If allergen avoidance is not possible or on rare occasions not helpful, topical corticosteroids are the mainstay of therapy. Depending on the type of skin reaction, either a gel, ointment or cream may be recommended.

Potent corticosteroid preparations should not be used on the face because they can cause thinning of the skin.

Systemic Corticosteroid Treatment

This treatment may be prescribed if contact dermatitis involves a large area of the body, and interferes with essential aspects of daily life. Treatment is given for 14 days, at which time the corticosteroids are discontinued.

Patients should be informed of the possible unwanted effects of systemic corticosteroid treatment, because it can affect the immune system and lead to infection of the affected areas of skin. Blood pressure and glucose levels may be monitored while the patient is taking corticosteroid treatment.

Section 13.2

Facial Contact Dermatitis

The irony of facial contact dermatitis is that, in search of a cause, patients often overlook what was once literally right in front of them. Since allergic reactions can take several days to develop after initial exposure, the substance responsible for the dermatitis on the face has plenty of time for a clean getaway.

Speaking at the 62nd Annual Meeting of the American Academy of Dermatology Academy, dermatologist Susan T. Nedorost, M.D., Director, Contact Dermatitis Program and Patch Test Clinic, Department of Dermatology, Case Western Reserve University, Cleveland, Ohio, discussed some of the common causes of facial contact dermatitis.

Dermatitis by Allergy

Contact dermatitis is characterized by redness, swelling, itching, and scaling caused by an allergic substance that makes direct contact with the skin. The condition can develop at any age, although the facial version of the disorder is most often seen in young and middle-aged adults.

"Facial contact dermatitis often stems from fragrances or preservatives in cosmetics and other personal care products; hence, more women are affected because they use a greater number of personal care products," said Dr. Nedorost. "Facial contact dermatitis is also common in patients who also have hand dermatitis, signaling that the cause is a substance the patient touches that is transferred from the hands to the face."

Allergens: Common and Covert

Dermatologists rely on patch testing to identify contact allergens. Small concentrations of suspected allergens are applied to the skin on the back and held in place with tape for 48 hours. If small, red spots, that may also itch, appear within three to five days, this indicates that the patient is allergic to the substance.

Patch testing for facial contact dermatitis may reveal an allergen that the patient or dermatologist had not previously considered because it was not intentionally or directly applied to the face. There are a variety of sources of allergens that patients may not recognize as likely causes of dermatitis and include the following.

Rubber

Rubber contains several allergenic chemicals in addition to latex. "Rubber allergy may cause dermatitis where applicators used to apply eye shadow contact the skin, or where foam rubber sponges are used to apply and remove cosmetics," said Dr. Nedorost.

Metals

Metal allergy is the most common form of contact dermatitis, and nickel is the most common of all metal allergens. Nickel may be present in costume jewelry, such as earrings, and in eyelash curlers or tweezers used on the face. Gold is also a common allergen and may be transferred to the face from gold rings on the hands.

Acrylates

Acrylates are used in the application of artificial nails and in both home and salon nail repair kits. "Ironically, nail products can cause dermatitis on the face without causing it on the nail itself, as the nail plate is composed of dead tissue and cannot exhibit dermatitis," commented Dr. Nedorost. "Instead, patients may notice itching or burning of the skin following a nail salon service or the application of nail cosmetics at home." Acrylates are also found in eyeglass frames and dental resins, as well as in adhesives used in industrial work.

Pine Resin

Colophony, or pine resin, is a sticky material that may cause allergy. "In addition to being used in mascara, pine resin may also be transferred from the fingers due to exposure in hobbies such as bowling, baseball, or playing stringed instruments," stated Dr. Nedorost.

Sunscreen Ingredients

The sunscreen ingredient benzophenone, which blocks both types of harmful ultraviolet (UV) radiation, can also cause allergy. "Photo contact dermatitis is common on areas of the face and neck where sunscreen has been applied and is most often noticed after UV exposure because UV light activates the sunscreen," stated Dr. Nedorost.

Hair Products

Benzophenone can also be found in hair care products but a more common ingredient in these products that may cause facial contact dermatitis is cocamidopropyl betaine, which is found in baby shampoos and many adult shampoos. "Ingredients in hair care products can cause facial or neck dermatitis, even if they don't cause scalp dermatitis," said Dr. Nedorost. "The face and neck are more sensitive than the scalp and may react where hair products run off of the scalp or are not completely rinsed."

Vital Diagnosis

It is common for patients to self-treat facial contact dermatitis with topical corticosteroids, which are available over-the-counter. "Unfortunately, long-term use of these medications on the face can cause thinning of the skin with visible blood vessels, rosacea, or even cataracts and glaucoma if used near the eye," stated Dr. Nedorost.

Individuals who suspect they may have contact dermatitis should seek evaluation and treatment from a dermatologist. The dermatologist will take a thorough history from the patient, including asking for information about the type and brands of personal care products used, occupation, hobbies, and prior treatments for the rash.

"By working with the dermatologist to identify the allergens, successful treatment for even longstanding facial dermatitis is possible for patients," stated Dr. Nedorost. "After allergens are identified, dermatologists can advise patients how to avoid the substances, as well as substitute products that do not cause reactions."

Section 13.3

Metal Allergy: A Form of Allergic Contact Dermatitis

That itchy rash you get when you wear earrings might not be because you bought them from the sales rack, and the redness on your finger when you wear your wedding ring is not a sign that your marriage is in trouble. You may be one of the million of individuals who have allergic contact dermatitis. Look around you and at what you're wearing. You may find the cause of your discomfort: you may have a metal allergy.

Speaking at the American Academy of Dermatology's 2003 Annual Meeting in San Francisco, dermatologist Joseph F. Fowler, Jr., M.D., spoke about allergic contact dermatitis and the various metals that can trigger it.

"Allergic contact dermatitis accounts for a significant number of visits to a dermatologist's office and is usually caused by substances that come into contact with the skin," said Dr. Fowler, Clinical Professor, Division of Dermatology at the University of Louisville, Louisville, Kentucky. "Metal is one of the most common culprits of allergic contact dermatitis especially due to the popular trend of body piercing, which can lead to irritation and rashes in not only the earlobes, but upper portions of the ears, lips, nose, tongue, navel, breasts, and genitalia as well."

After poison ivy, metal allergy is the most common form of allergic contact dermatitis. In the past, women have been more susceptible to metal allergy than men due to the amount of jewelry worn, but the numbers of males wearing jewelry is increasing and so is the incidence of metal allergy in this population.

Symptoms of metal allergy usually occur between six to 24 hours following exposure and will dissipate if exposure to the allergen is eliminated. The affected skin may become red, swollen, and blisters often appear, which may break, leaving crusts and scales. Later the skin

138

may darken and become leathery and cracked. The rash is generally confined to the site of contact, although severe cases may extend outside the contact area, especially if the allergen is on your fingers and then transmitted to the face, eyelids, or genitals.

"It's important to note that allergic contact dermatitis, such as metal allergy, can be difficult to distinguish from other rashes," stated Dr. Fowler. "However, dermatologists can determine clues about the nature of a rash based on its location on the body and the patient's lifestyle and work habits."

Another way dermatologists can discover the source of an allergy is through patch testing. During patch testing, small amounts of possible allergens are applied to the skin on strips of tape and then removed after two days. An allergy shows up as a small red spot at the site of the patch and a dermatologist notes what the patient is most sensitive to.

Nickel

The most common of all metal allergens is nickel, which is found in costume jewelry, clothing ornamentation, such as zippers, buttons and snaps, and virtually all common metal objects. Approximately 16 percent of all individuals who are patch tested for allergies turn out to be allergic to nickel. Because sweat allows the metal ions to be better absorbed into the skin, areas on the body where nickel is present and where sweating may occur can see an increase in the severity of the dermatitis.

The most common location of nickel dermatitis is on the earlobes from earrings containing the metal. This reaction may start with the needle used to pierce the ears and continue as individuals begin to change their earrings daily. Dermatologists suggest that individuals with an allergy to nickel wear only nickel-free or plastic earrings.

Trace amounts of metal are found in food and people with sensitivity to metal can experience dermatitis. In particular, beans, lettuce, and whole-grain foods are high in nickel, but most people do not ingest enough of them to develop a serious rash.

"While nickel dermatitis is associated most often with costume jewelry or watchbands, which have a high concentration of nickel, it can occur with finer jewelry which is usually worn for prolonged periods, for example a wedding ring," said Dr. Fowler. "If sentimental reasons prevent you from not wearing an item on a daily basis, the best way to prevent the reaction is to have it plated in a non-allergic metal, such as platinum."

Cobalt

Cobalt is also a common allergen that is found in many of the same items that contain nickel thereby making this allergen difficult to pinpoint. It is also found naturally in soil, dust, and seawater. In the home, it is most often found in the blue pigments in porcelain, glass, pottery, or ceramics, as well as blue and green water color paints and crayons. In the workplace, cobalt is found in cement, bricks, and mortars.

"Combined allergic reactions are not uncommon and represent simultaneous specific sensations to each individual metals as opposed to being reactions to the combination," stated Dr. Fowler. "Whenever possible, patients are encouraged to avoid the allergen, use plastic or wooden items, such as kitchen utensils or scissors, and wear protective clothing and a face mask at their workplace."

Chromate

Chromate is another dermatitis-causing metal, which is also found in cement, but more commonly used as a leather tanning agent. "Shoe dermatitis" may result from leather containing chromates and patients should change their shoes and socks throughout the day especially if they are allergic or if there is excess perspiration.

In addition, some matches contain chromates and touching unlit matches can contaminate fingers. The fumes from a lit match and the charred match head also contain small amounts of chromate.

"When a metal allergy is suspected, it's important for people to seek the medical advice of a dermatologist especially since nickel, cobalt, and chromate can all be found in some common metal objects that people may touch every day," said Dr. Fowler. "If avoidance of an item isn't possible, your dermatologist can recommend some other treatment options and lifestyle changes that can help patients live and work without the itchy rash of allergic contact dermatitis."

Section 13.4

Poison Ivy, Oak, and Sumac Allergy

"Outsmarting Poison Ivy and Its Cousins," by Isadora B. Stehlin, is from *FDA Consumer* magazine (www.fda.gov/fdac), published by the U.S. Food and Drug Administration, September 1996. Reviewed by David A. Cooke, M.D., October 27, 2006.

Pamela Lillian Isley can manipulate plants in unexplained ways. They bend to her will, growing and threatening the environment and society—at least in Gotham City. In the world of Batman, the fictional Isley is better known as the beautiful criminal Poison Ivy. Her alias is fitting. Just as she is the bane of Batman's existence, in the real world the poison ivy plant—along with its cousins poison oak and poison sumac—is the bane of millions of campers, hikers, gardeners, and others who enjoy the great outdoors.

Approximately 85 percent of the population will develop an allergic reaction if exposed to poison ivy, oak, or sumac, according to the American Academy of Dermatology. Nearly one third of forestry workers and firefighters who battle forest fires in California, Oregon, and Washington develop rashes or lung irritations from contact with poison oak, which is the most common of the three in those states.

Usually, people develop a sensitivity to poison ivy, oak, or sumac only after several encounters with the plants, sometimes over many years. However, sensitivity may occur after only one exposure.

The cause of the rash, blisters, and infamous itch is urushiol, a chemical in the sap of poison ivy, oak, and sumac plants. Because urushiol is inside the plant, brushing against an intact plant will not cause a reaction. But undamaged plants are rare.

"Poison oak, ivy, and sumac are very fragile plants," says William L. Epstein, M.D., professor of dermatology, University of California, San Francisco. Stems or leaves broken by the wind or animals, and even the tiny holes made by chewing insects, can release urushiol.

Reactions, treatments, and preventive measures are the same for all three poison plants. Avoiding direct contact with the plants reduces the risk but doesn't guarantee against a reaction. Urushiol can stick to pets, garden tools, balls, or anything it comes in contact with. If the urushiol isn't washed off those objects or animals, just touching them—for example, picking up a ball or petting a dog—could cause a reaction in a susceptible person. (Animals, except for a few higher primates, are not sensitive to urushiol.)

Urushiol that's rubbed off the plants onto other things can remain potent for years, depending on the environment. If the contaminated object is in a dry environment, the potency of the urushiol can last for decades, says Epstein. Even if the environment is warm and moist, the urushiol could still cause a reaction a year later.

"One of the stories I tell people is of the hunter who gets poison oak on his hunting coat," says Epstein. "He puts it on a year later to go hunting and gets a rash [from the urushiol still on the coat]."

Almost all parts of the body are vulnerable to the sticky urushiol, producing the characteristic linear (in a line) rash. Because the urushiol must penetrate the skin to cause a reaction, places where the skin is thick, such as the soles of the feet and the palms of the hands, are less sensitive to the sap than areas where the skin is thinner. The severity of the reaction may also depend on how big a dose of urushiol the person got.

Quick Action Needed

Because urushiol can penetrate the skin within minutes, there's no time to waste if you know you've been exposed. "The earlier you cleanse the skin, the greater the chance that you can remove the urushiol before it gets attached to the skin," says Hon-Sum Ko, M.D., an allergist and immunologist with the U.S. Food and Drug Administration (FDA)'s Center for Drug Evaluation and Research. Cleansing may not stop the initial outbreak of the rash if more than 10 minutes has elapsed, but it can help prevent further spread.

If you've been exposed to poison ivy, oak, or sumac, if possible, stay outdoors until you complete the first two steps:

- First, Epstein says, cleanse exposed skin with generous amounts of isopropyl (rubbing) alcohol. (Don't return to the woods or yard the same day. Alcohol removes your skin's protection along with the urushiol and any new contact will cause the urushiol to penetrate twice as fast.)

- Second, wash skin with water. (Water temperature does not matter; if you're outside, it's likely only cold water will be available.)

- Third, take a regular shower with soap and warm water. Do not use soap before this point because "soap will tend to pick up some of the urushiol from the surface of the skin and move it around," says Epstein.

- Clothes, shoes, tools, and anything else that may have been in contact with the urushiol should be wiped off with alcohol and water. Be sure to wear gloves or otherwise cover your hands while doing this and then discard the hand covering.

Dealing with the Rash

If you don't cleanse quickly enough, or your skin is so sensitive that cleansing didn't help, redness and swelling will appear in about 12 to 48 hours. Blisters and itching will follow. For those rare people who react after their very first exposure, the rash appears after seven to 10 days.

Because they don't contain urushiol, the oozing blisters are not contagious nor can the fluid cause further spread on the affected person's body. Nevertheless, Epstein advises against scratching the blisters because fingernails may carry germs that could cause an infection.

The rash will only occur where urushiol has touched the skin; it doesn't spread throughout the body. However, the rash may seem to spread if it appears over time instead of all at once. This is either because the urushiol is absorbed at different rates in different parts of the body or because of repeated exposure to contaminated objects or urushiol trapped under the fingernails.

The rash, blisters, and itch normally disappear in 14 to 20 days without any treatment. But few can handle the itch without some relief. For mild cases, wet compresses or soaking in cool water may be effective. Oral antihistamines can also relieve itching.

FDA also considers over-the-counter topical corticosteroids (commonly called hydrocortisones under brand names such as Cortaid and Lanacort) safe and effective for temporary relief of itching associated with poison ivy.

For severe cases, prescription topical corticosteroid drugs can halt the reaction, but only if treatment begins within a few hours of exposure. "After the blisters form, the [topical] steroid isn't going to do much," says Epstein. The American Academy of Dermatology recommends that people who have had severe reactions in the past should contact a dermatologist as soon as possible after a new exposure.

Severe reactions can be treated with prescription oral corticosteroids. Phillip M. Williford, M.D., assistant professor of dermatology, Wake Forest University, prescribes oral corticosteroids if the rash is on the face, genitals, or covers more than 30 percent of the body. The drug must be taken for at least 14 days, and preferably over a three-week period, says FDA's Ko. Shorter courses of treatment, he warns, will cause a rebound with an even more severe rash.

There are a number of over-the-counter products to help dry up the oozing blisters, including:

- aluminum acetate (Burrows solution)
- baking soda
- Aveeno (oatmeal bath)
- aluminum hydroxide gel
- calamine
- kaolin
- zinc acetate
- zinc carbonate
- zinc oxide

Desensitization, vaccines, and barrier creams have been studied over the last several decades for their potential to protect against poison ivy reactions, but none have been approved by FDA for this purpose.

Right now, prevention seems the best treatment, unless you plan to take lessons from Batman's bane with Poison Ivy's name.

Getting Rid of the Plants

Poison ivy, oak, and sumac are most dangerous in the spring and summer, when there is plenty of sap, the urushiol content is high, and the plants are easily bruised. However, the danger doesn't disappear over the winter. Dormant plants can still cause reactions, and cases have been reported in people who used the twigs of the plant for firewood or the vines for Christmas wreaths. Even dead plants can cause a reaction, because urushiol remains active for several years after the plant dies.

If poison ivy invades your yard, "there's really no good news for you," says David Yost, a horticulturist (specialist in fruits, vegetables, flowers, and general gardening) with the state of Virginia. The two herbicides most commonly used for poison ivy—Roundup and Ortho Poison Ivy Killer—will kill other plants as well. Spraying Roundup (active ingredient glyphosate) on the foliage of young plants will kill the poison ivy, but if the poison ivy vine is growing up your prize rhododendron or azalea, for example, the Roundup will kill them, too, he says.

Ortho Poison Ivy Killer (active ingredient triclopyr), if used sparingly, will kill poison ivy but not trees it grows around, says Joseph Neal, Ph.D., associate professor of weed science, Cornell University. "But don't use it around shrubs, broadleaf ground cover, or herbaceous garden plants," he says. Neal explains it is possible to spray the poison ivy without killing other plants if you pull the poison ivy vines away from the desirable plants and wipe the ivy foliage with the herbicide, or use a shield on the sprayer to direct the chemical.

If you don't want to use chemicals, "manual removal will get rid of the ivy if you're diligent," says Neal. You must get every bit of the plant—leaves, vines, and roots—or it will sprout again.

The plants should be thrown away according to your municipality's regulations, says Neal. Although urushiol will break down with composting, Neal doesn't recommend that because the plants must be chopped into small pieces first, which just adds to the time you're exposed to the plant and risk of a rash. "It's a health issue," he says.

Never burn the plants. The urushiol can spread in the smoke and cause serious lung irritation.

The American Academy of Dermatology recommends that whenever you're going to be around poison ivy—trying to clear it from your yard or hiking in the woods—you wear long pants and long sleeves and, if possible, gloves and boots. Neal recommends wearing plastic gloves over cotton gloves when pulling the plants. Plastic alone isn't enough because the plastic rips, and cotton alone won't work because after a while the urushiol will soak through.

Identification Please

Unfortunately, poison ivy, oak, and sumac don't grow with little picture ID badges around their stems, so you have to know what to look for. The famous rule "leaves of three, let it be" is good to follow, except that some of the plants don't always play by the rules and have leaves in groups of five to nine. To avoid these plants and their itchy consequences, here's what to look for.

Poison Ivy

- grows around lakes and streams in the Midwest and the East
- woody, rope-like vine, a trailing shrub on the ground, or a free-standing shrub

- normally three leaflets (groups of leaves all on the same small stem coming off the larger main stem), but may vary from groups of three to nine
- leaves are green in the summer and red in the fall
- yellow or green flowers and white berries

Poison Oak

- eastern (from New Jersey to Texas) grows as a low shrub; western (along the Pacific coast) grows to 6-foot-tall clumps or vines up to 30 feet long
- oak-like leaves, usually in clusters of three
- clusters of yellow berries

Poison Sumac

- grows in boggy areas, especially in the Southeast
- rangy shrub up to 15 feet tall
- seven to 13 smooth-edged leaflets
- glossy pale yellow or cream-colored berries

Isadora B. Stehlin is a member of FDA's public affairs staff.

Chapter 14

Eczema (Atopic Dermatitis)

Chapter Contents

Section 14.1

All about Eczema

"Handout on Health: Atopic Dermatitis" is excerpted from a booklet by the National Institute of Arthritis and Musculoskeletal and Skin Diseases (NIAMS, www.niams.nih.gov), part of the National Institutes of Health, revised April 2003.

Defining Atopic Dermatitis

Atopic dermatitis is a chronic (long-lasting) disease that affects the skin. It is not contagious; it cannot be passed from one person to another. The word dermatitis means inflammation of the skin. Atopic refers to a group of diseases where there is often an inherited tendency to develop other allergic conditions, such as asthma and hay fever. In atopic dermatitis, the skin becomes extremely itchy. Scratching leads to redness, swelling, cracking, weeping clear fluid, and finally, crusting and scaling. In most cases, there are periods of time when the disease is worse (called exacerbations or flares) followed by periods when the skin improves or clears up entirely (called remissions). As some children with atopic dermatitis grow older, their skin disease improves or disappears altogether, although their skin often remains dry and easily irritated. In others, atopic dermatitis continues to be a significant problem in adulthood.

Atopic dermatitis is often referred to as eczema, which is a general term for the several types of inflammation of the skin. Atopic dermatitis is the most common of the many types of eczema. Several have very similar symptoms.

Incidence and Prevalence of Atopic Dermatitis

Atopic dermatitis is very common. It affects males and females and accounts for 10 to 20 percent of all visits to dermatologists (doctors who specialize in the care and treatment of skin diseases). Although atopic dermatitis may occur at any age, it most often begins in infancy and childhood. Scientists estimate that 65 percent of patients develop symptoms in the first year of life, and 90 percent develop symptoms before the age of 5. Onset after age 30 is less common and is often due to exposure of the skin to harsh or wet conditions. Atopic dermatitis is a common cause of workplace disability. People who live in cities and in dry climates appear more likely to develop this condition.

Although it is difficult to identify exactly how many people are affected by atopic dermatitis, an estimated 20 percent of infants and young children experience symptoms of the disease. Roughly 60 percent of these infants continue to have one or more symptoms of atopic dermatitis in adulthood. This means that more than 15 million people in the United States have symptoms of the disease.

Types of Eczema (Dermatitis)

- **Allergic contact eczema (dermatitis):** a red, itchy, weepy reaction where the skin has come into contact with a substance that the immune system recognizes as foreign, such as poison ivy or certain preservatives in creams and lotions

- **Atopic dermatitis:** a chronic skin disease characterized by itchy, inflamed skin

- **Contact eczema:** a localized reaction that includes redness, itching, and burning where the skin has come into contact with an allergen (an allergy-causing substance) or with an irritant such as an acid, a cleaning agent, or other chemical

- **Dyshidrotic eczema:** irritation of the skin on the palms of hands and soles of the feet characterized by clear, deep blisters that itch and burn

- **Neurodermatitis:** scaly patches of the skin on the head, lower legs, wrists, or forearms caused by a localized itch (such as an insect bite) that become intensely irritated when scratched

- **Nummular eczema:** coin-shaped patches of irritated skin—most common on the arms, back, buttocks, and lower legs—that may be crusted, scaling, and extremely itchy

- **Seborrheic eczema:** yellowish, oily, scaly patches of skin on the scalp, face, and occasionally other parts of the body

- **Stasis dermatitis:** a skin irritation on the lower legs, generally related to circulatory problems

Cost of Atopic Dermatitis

In a recent analysis of the health insurance records of 5 million Americans under age 65, medical researchers found that approximately

2.5 percent had atopic dermatitis. Annual insurance payments for medical care of atopic dermatitis ranged from $580 to $1,250 per patient. More than one quarter of each patient's total health care costs were for atopic dermatitis and related conditions. The researchers project that U.S. health insurance companies spend more than $1 billion per year on atopic dermatitis.

Causes of Atopic Dermatitis

The cause of atopic dermatitis is not known, but the disease seems to result from a combination of genetic (hereditary) and environmental factors.

Children are more likely to develop this disorder if one or both parents have had it or have had allergic conditions like asthma or hay fever. While some people outgrow skin symptoms, approximately three fourths of children with atopic dermatitis go on to develop hay fever or asthma. Environmental factors can bring on symptoms of atopic dermatitis at any time in individuals who have inherited the atopic disease trait.

Atopic dermatitis is also associated with malfunction of the body's immune system: the system that recognizes and helps fight bacteria and viruses that invade the body. Scientists have found that people with atopic dermatitis have a low level of a cytokine (a protein) that is essential to the healthy function of the body's immune system and a high level of other cytokines that lead to allergic reactions. The immune system can become misguided and create inflammation in the skin even in the absence of a major infection. This can be viewed as a form of autoimmunity, where a body reacts against its own tissues.

In the past, doctors thought that atopic dermatitis was caused by an emotional disorder. We now know that emotional factors, such as stress, can make the condition worse, but they do not cause the disease.

Skin Features of Atopic Dermatitis

- Atopic pleat (Dennie-Morgan fold): an extra fold of skin that develops under the eye
- Cheilitis: inflammation of the skin on and around the lips
- Hyperlinear palms: increased number of skin creases on the palms
- Hyperpigmented eyelids: eyelids that have become darker in color from inflammation or hay fever

- Ichthyosis: dry, rectangular scales on the skin

- Keratosis pilaris: small, rough bumps, generally on the face, upper arms, and thighs

- Lichenification: thick, leathery skin resulting from constant scratching and rubbing

- Papules: small raised bumps that may open when scratched and become crusty and infected

- Urticaria: hives (red, raised bumps) that may occur after exposure to an allergen, at the beginning of flares, or after exercise or a hot bath

Symptoms of Atopic Dermatitis

Symptoms (signs) vary from person to person. The most common symptoms are dry, itchy skin and rashes on the face, inside the elbows and behind the knees, and on the hands and feet. Itching is the most important symptom of atopic dermatitis. Scratching and rubbing in response to itching irritates the skin, increases inflammation, and actually increases itchiness. Itching is a particular problem during sleep when conscious control of scratching is lost.

The appearance of the skin that is affected by atopic dermatitis depends on the amount of scratching and the presence of secondary skin infections. The skin may be red and scaly, be thick and leathery, contain small raised bumps, or leak fluid and become crusty and infected. The portion of text titled "Skin Features of Atopic Dermatitis" lists common skin features of the disease. These features can also be found in people who do not have atopic dermatitis or who have other types of skin disorders.

Atopic dermatitis may also affect the skin around the eyes, the eyelids, and the eyebrows and lashes. Scratching and rubbing the eye area can cause the skin to redden and swell. Some people with atopic dermatitis develop an extra fold of skin under their eyes. Patchy loss of eyebrows and eyelashes may also result from scratching or rubbing.

Researchers have noted differences in the skin of people with atopic dermatitis that may contribute to the symptoms of the disease. The outer layer of skin, called the epidermis, is divided into two parts: an inner part containing moist, living cells, and an outer part, known as the horny layer or stratum corneum, containing dry, flattened, dead cells. Under normal conditions the stratum corneum acts as a barrier, keeping the rest of the skin from drying out and protecting other

151

layers of skin from damage caused by irritants and infections. When this barrier is damaged, irritants act more intensely on the skin.

The skin of a person with atopic dermatitis loses moisture from the epidermal layer, allowing the skin to become very dry and reducing its protective abilities. Thus, when combined with the abnormal skin immune system, the person's skin is more likely to become infected by bacteria (for example, *Staphylococcus* and *Streptococcus*) or viruses, such as those that cause warts and cold sores.

Stages of Atopic Dermatitis

When atopic dermatitis occurs during infancy and childhood, it affects each child differently in terms of both onset and severity of symptoms. In infants, atopic dermatitis typically begins around 6 to 12 weeks of age. It may first appear around the cheeks and chin as a patchy facial rash, which can progress to red, scaling, oozing skin. The skin may become infected. Once the infant becomes more mobile and begins crawling, exposed areas, such as the inner and outer parts of the arms and legs, may also be affected. An infant with atopic dermatitis may be restless and irritable because of the itching and discomfort of the disease. The skin may improve by 18 months of age, although the infant has a greater than normal risk of developing dry skin or hand eczema later in life.

In childhood, the rash tends to occur behind the knees and inside the elbows; on the sides of the neck; around the mouth; and on the wrists, ankles, and hands. Often, the rash begins with papules that become hard and scaly when scratched. The skin around the lips may be inflamed, and constant licking of the area may lead to small, painful cracks in the skin around the mouth.

In some children, the disease goes into remission for a long time, only to come back at the onset of puberty when hormones, stress, and the use of irritating skin care products or cosmetics may cause the disease to flare.

Although a number of people who developed atopic dermatitis as children also experience symptoms as adults, it is also possible for the disease to show up first in adulthood. The pattern in adults is similar to that seen in children; that is, the disease may be widespread or limited to only a few parts of the body. For example, only the hands or feet may be affected and become dry, itchy, red, and cracked. Sleep patterns and work performance may be affected, and long-term use of medications to treat the atopic dermatitis may cause complications. Adults with atopic dermatitis also have a predisposition toward irritant contact dermatitis, where the skin becomes red and inflamed from contact with detergents, wool, friction from clothing, or other potential irritants. It is more likely to occur in occupations involving frequent hand washing or exposure to chemicals. Some people develop a rash around their nipples. These localized symptoms are difficult to treat. Because adults may also develop cataracts, the doctor may recommend regular eye exams.

Diagnosing Atopic Dermatitis

Each person experiences a unique combination of symptoms, which may vary in severity over time. The doctor will base a diagnosis on the symptoms the patient experiences and may need to see the patient several times to make an accurate diagnosis and to rule out other diseases and conditions that might cause skin irritation. In some cases, the family doctor or pediatrician may refer the patient to a dermatologist (doctor specializing in skin disorders) or allergist (allergy specialist) for further evaluation.

A medical history may help the doctor better understand the nature of a patient's symptoms, when they occur, and their possible causes. The doctor may ask about family history of allergic disease; whether the patient also has diseases such as hay fever or asthma; and about exposure to irritants, sleep disturbances, any foods that seem to be related to skin flares, previous treatments for skin-related symptoms, and use of steroids or other medications. A preliminary diagnosis of atopic dermatitis can be made if the patient has three or more features from each of two categories: major features and minor features.

Currently, there is no single test to diagnose atopic dermatitis. However, there are some tests that can give the doctor an indication of allergic sensitivity.

Pricking the skin with a needle that contains a small amount of a suspected allergen may be helpful in identifying factors that trigger flares of atopic dermatitis. Negative results on skin tests may help rule out the possibility that certain substances cause skin inflammation. Positive skin prick test results are difficult to interpret in people with atopic dermatitis because the skin is very sensitive to many substances, and there can be many positive test sites that are not meaningful to a person's disease at the time. Positive results simply indicate that the individual has IgE (allergic) antibodies to the substance tested. IgE (immunoglobulin E) controls the immune system's allergic response and is often high in atopic dermatitis.

Recently, it was shown that if the quantity of IgE antibodies to a food in the blood is above a certain level, it is diagnostic of a food allergy. If the level of IgE to a specific food does not exceed the level needed for diagnosis but a food allergy is suspected, a person might be asked to record everything eaten and note any reactions. Physician-supervised food challenges (that is, the introduction of a food) following a period of food elimination may be necessary to determine if symptomatic food allergy is present. Identifying the food allergen may be difficult when a person is also being exposed to other possible allergens at the same time or symptoms may be triggered by other factors, such as infection, heat, and humidity.

Factors That Make Atopic Dermatitis Worse

Many factors or conditions can make symptoms of atopic dermatitis worse, further triggering the already overactive immune system, aggravating the itch-scratch cycle, and increasing damage to the skin. These factors can be broken down into two main categories: irritants and allergens.

Irritants are substances that directly affect the skin and, when present in high enough concentrations with long enough contact, cause the skin to become red and itchy or to burn. Specific irritants affect people with atopic dermatitis to different degrees. Over time, many patients and their family members learn to identify the irritants causing the most trouble. For example, frequent wetting and drying of the skin may affect the skin barrier function. Also, wool or synthetic fibers and rough or poorly fitting clothing can rub the skin, trigger inflammation, and cause the itch-scratch cycle to begin. Soaps and detergents may have a drying effect and worsen itching, and some perfumes and cosmetics may irritate the skin. Exposure to certain substances, such as solvents, dust, or sand, may also make the condition worse. Cigarette smoke may irritate the eyelids. Because the effects of irritants vary from one person to another, each person can best determine what substances or circumstances cause the disease to flare.

Allergens are substances from foods, plants, animals, or the air that inflame the skin because the immune system overreacts to the substance. Inflammation occurs even when the person is exposed to small amounts of the substance for a limited time. Although it is known that allergens in the air, such as dust mites, pollens, molds, and dander from animal hair or skin, may worsen the symptoms of atopic dermatitis in some people, scientists aren't certain whether inhaling these allergens or their actual penetration of the skin causes the problems. When people with atopic dermatitis come into contact with an irritant or allergen they are sensitive to, inflammation-producing cells become active. These cells release chemicals that cause itching and redness. As the person responds by scratching and rubbing the skin, further damage occurs.

Common Irritants

- Wool or synthetic fibers
- Soaps and detergents
- Some perfumes and cosmetics
- Substances such as chlorine, mineral oil, or solvents
- Dust or sand
- Cigarette smoke

A number of studies have shown that foods may trigger or worsen atopic dermatitis in some people, particularly infants and children. In general, the worse the atopic dermatitis and the younger the child, the more likely food allergy is present. An allergic reaction to food can cause skin inflammation (generally an itchy red rash), gastrointestinal symptoms (abdominal pain, vomiting, diarrhea), and/or upper respiratory tract symptoms (congestion, sneezing, and wheezing). The most common allergenic (allergy-causing) foods are eggs, milk, peanuts, wheat, soy, and fish. A recent analysis of a large number of studies on allergies and breastfeeding indicated that breastfeeding an infant for at least 4 months may protect the child from developing allergies. However, some studies suggest that mothers with a family history of atopic diseases should avoid eating common allergenic foods during late pregnancy and breastfeeding.

In addition to irritants and allergens, emotional factors, skin infections, and temperature and climate play a role in atopic dermatitis. Although the disease itself is not caused by emotional factors, it can be made worse by stress, anger, and frustration. Interpersonal problems or major life changes, such as divorce, job changes, or the death of a loved one, can also make the disease worse.

Bathing without proper moisturizing afterward is a common factor that triggers a flare of atopic dermatitis. The low humidity of winter or the dry year-round climate of some geographic areas can make the disease worse, as can overheated indoor areas and long or hot baths and showers. Alternately sweating and chilling can trigger a flare in some people. Bacterial infections can also trigger or increase the severity of atopic dermatitis. If a patient experiences a sudden flare of illness, the doctor may check for infection.

Treatment of Atopic Dermatitis

Treatment is more effective when a partnership develops that includes the patient, family members, and doctor. The doctor will suggest a treatment plan based on the patient's age, symptoms, and general health. The patient or family member providing care plays a large role in the success of the treatment plan by carefully following the doctor's instructions and paying attention to what is or is not helpful. Most patients will notice improvement with proper skin care and lifestyle changes.

The doctor has two main goals in treating atopic dermatitis: healing the skin and preventing flares. These may be assisted by developing skin care routines and avoiding substances that lead to skin irritation and trigger the immune system and the itch-scratch cycle. It is important for the patient and family members to note any changes in the skin's condition in response to treatment, and to be persistent in identifying the treatment that seems to work best.

Medications

New medications known as immunomodulators have been developed that help control inflammation and reduce immune system reactions when applied to the skin. Examples of these medications are tacrolimus ointment (Protopic) and pimecrolimus cream (Elidel). They can be used in patients older than 2 years of age and have few side effects (burning or itching the first few days of application). They not only reduce flares, but also maintain skin texture and reduce the need for long-term use of corticosteroids.

Corticosteroid creams and ointments have been used for many years to treat atopic dermatitis and other autoimmune diseases affecting the skin. Sometimes over-the-counter preparations are used, but in many cases the doctor will prescribe a stronger corticosteroid cream or ointment. When prescribing a medication, the doctor will take into account the patient's age, location of the skin to be treated, severity of the symptoms, and type of preparation (cream or ointment) that will be most effective. Sometimes the base used in certain brands of corticosteroid creams and ointments irritates the skin of a particular patient. Side effects of repeated or long-term use of topical corticosteroids can include thinning of the skin, infections, growth suppression (in children), and stretch marks on the skin.

When topical corticosteroids are not effective, the doctor may prescribe a systemic corticosteroid, which is taken by mouth or injected instead of being applied directly to the skin. An example of a commonly prescribed corticosteroid is prednisone. Typically, these medications are used only in resistant cases and only given for short periods of time. The side effects of systemic corticosteroids can include skin damage, thinned or weakened bones, high blood pressure, high blood sugar, infections, and cataracts. It can be dangerous to suddenly stop taking corticosteroids, so it is very important that the doctor and patient work together in changing the corticosteroid dose.

Antibiotics to treat skin infections may be applied directly to the skin in an ointment, but are usually more effective when taken by mouth. If viral or fungal infections are present, the doctor may also prescribe specific medications to treat those infections.

Certain antihistamines that cause drowsiness can reduce nighttime scratching and allow more restful sleep when taken at bedtime. This effect can be particularly helpful for patients whose nighttime scratching makes the disease worse.

In adults, drugs that suppress the immune system, such as cyclosporine, methotrexate, or azathioprine, may be prescribed to treat severe cases of atopic dermatitis that have failed to respond to other forms of therapy. These drugs block the production of some immune cells and curb the action of others. The side effects of drugs like cyclosporine can include high blood pressure, nausea, vomiting, kidney problems, headaches, tingling or numbness, and a possible increased risk of cancer and infections. There is also a risk of relapse after the drug is stopped. Because of their toxic side effects, systemic corticosteroids and immunosuppressive drugs are used only in severe cases and then for as short a period of time as possible. Patients requiring systemic corticosteroids should be referred to dermatologists or allergists specializing in the care of atopic dermatitis to help identify trigger factors and alternative therapies.

In rare cases, when home-based treatments have been unsuccessful, a patient may need a few days in the hospital for intense treatment.

Phototherapy

Use of ultraviolet A or B light waves, alone or combined, can be an effective treatment for mild to moderate dermatitis in older children (over 12 years old) and adults. A combination of ultraviolet light therapy and a drug called psoralen can also be used in cases that are resistant to ultraviolet light alone. Possible long-term side effects of this treatment include premature skin aging and skin cancer. If the doctor thinks that phototherapy may be useful to treat the symptoms of atopic dermatitis, he or she will use the minimum exposure necessary and monitor the skin carefully.

Skin Care

Healing the skin and keeping it healthy are important to prevent further damage and enhance quality of life. Developing and sticking with a daily skin care routine is critical to preventing flares.

A lukewarm bath helps to cleanse and moisturize the skin without drying it excessively. Because soaps can be drying to the skin, the doctor may recommend use of a mild bar soap or nonsoap cleanser. Bath oils are not usually helpful.

After bathing, a person should air-dry the skin, or pat it dry gently (avoiding rubbing or brisk drying), and then apply a lubricant to seal in the water that has been absorbed into the skin during bathing. In addition to restoring the skin's moisture, lubrication increases the rate of healing and establishes a barrier against further drying and irritation. Lotions that have a high water or alcohol content evaporate more quickly, and alcohol may cause stinging. Therefore, they generally are not the best choice. Creams and ointments work better at healing the skin.

Another key to protecting and restoring the skin is taking steps to avoid repeated skin infections. Signs of skin infection include tiny pustules (pus-filled bumps), oozing cracks or sores, or crusty yellow blisters. If symptoms of a skin infection develop, the doctor should be consulted and treatment should begin as soon as possible.

Protection from Allergen Exposure

The doctor may suggest reducing exposure to a suspected allergen. For example, the presence of the house dust mite can be limited by encasing mattresses and pillows in special dust-proof covers, frequently washing bedding in hot water, and removing carpeting. However, there is no way to completely rid the environment of airborne allergens.

Changing the diet may not always relieve symptoms of atopic dermatitis. A change may be helpful, however, when the medical history, laboratory studies, and specific symptoms strongly suggest a food allergy. It is up to the patient and his or her family and physician to decide whether the dietary restrictions are appropriate. Unless properly monitored by a physician or dietitian, diets with many restrictions can contribute to serious nutritional problems, especially in children.

Treating Atopic Dermatitis in Infants and Children

- Give lukewarm baths.
- Apply lubricant immediately following the bath.
- Keep child's fingernails filed short.
- Select soft cotton fabrics when choosing clothing.
- Consider using sedating antihistamines to promote sleep and reduce scratching at night.
- Keep the child cool; avoid situations where overheating occurs.
- Learn to recognize skin infections and seek treatment promptly.
- Attempt to distract the child with activities to keep him or her from scratching.
- Identify and remove irritants and allergens.

Atopic Dermatitis and Quality of Life

Despite the symptoms caused by atopic dermatitis, it is possible for people with the disorder to maintain a good quality of life. The keys to quality of life lie in being well-informed; awareness of symptoms and their possible cause; and developing a partnership involving the patient or caregiving family member, medical doctor, and other health professionals. Good communication is essential.

When a child has atopic dermatitis, the entire family may be affected. It is helpful if families have additional support to help them cope with the stress and frustration associated with the disease. A child may be fussy and difficult and unable to keep from scratching and rubbing the skin. Distracting the child and providing activities that keep the hands busy are helpful but require much effort on the part of the parents or caregivers. Another issue families face is the social and emotional stress associated with changes in appearance caused by atopic dermatitis. The child may face difficulty in school or with social relationships and may need additional support and encouragement from family members.

Adults with atopic dermatitis can enhance their quality of life by caring regularly for their skin and being mindful of the effects of the disease and how to treat them. Adults should develop a skin care regimen as part of their daily routine, which can be adapted as circumstances and skin conditions change. Stress management and relaxation techniques may help decrease the likelihood of flares. Developing a network of support that includes family, friends, health professionals, and support groups or organizations can be beneficial. Chronic anxiety and depression may be relieved by short-term psychological therapy.

Recognizing the situations when scratching is most likely to occur may also help. For example, many patients find that they scratch more when they are idle, and they do better when engaged in activities that keep the hands occupied. Counseling also may be helpful to identify or change career goals if a job involves contact with irritants or involves frequent hand washing, such as kitchen work or auto mechanics.

Atopic Dermatitis and Vaccination against Smallpox

Although scientists are working to develop safer vaccines, persons diagnosed with atopic dermatitis (or eczema) should not receive the current smallpox vaccine. According to the Centers for Disease Control and Prevention (CDC), a U.S. Government organization, persons who have ever been diagnosed with atopic dermatitis, even if the condition is mild or not presently active, are more likely to develop a serious complication if they are exposed to the virus from the smallpox vaccine.

People with atopic dermatitis should exercise caution when coming into close physical contact with a person who has been recently vaccinated, and make certain the vaccinated person has covered the vaccination site or taken other precautions until the scab falls off (about 3 weeks). Those who have had physical contact with a vaccinated person's unhealed vaccination site or to their bedding or other items that might have touched that site should notify their doctor, particularly if they develop a new or unusual rash.

During a smallpox outbreak, these vaccination recommendations may change. Persons with atopic dermatitis who have been exposed to smallpox should consult their doctor about vaccination.

Tips for Working with Your Doctor

- Provide complete, accurate medical information.
- Make a list of your questions and concerns in advance.

- Be honest and share your point of view with the doctor.
- Ask for clarification or further explanation if you need it.
- Talk to other members of the health care team, such as nurses, therapists, or pharmacists.
- Don't hesitate to discuss sensitive subjects with your doctor.
- Discuss changes to any medical treatment or medications with your doctor.

Current Research

Researchers supported by the National Institute of Arthritis and Musculoskeletal and Skin Diseases and other institutes of the National Institutes of Health are gaining a better understanding of what causes atopic dermatitis and how it can be managed, treated, and, ultimately, prevented. Some promising avenues of research are described in the following text.

Genetics

Although atopic dermatitis runs in families, the role of genetics (inheritance) remains unclear. It does appear that more than one gene is involved in the disease.

Research has helped shed light on the way atopic dermatitis is inherited. Studies show that children are at increased risk for developing the disorder if there is a family history of other atopic disease, such as hay fever or asthma. The risk is significantly higher if both parents have an atopic disease. In addition, studies of identical twins, who have the same genes, show that in an estimated 80 to 90 percent of cases, atopic disease appears in both twins. Fraternal (nonidentical) twins, who have only some genes in common, are no more likely than two other people in the general population to both have an atopic disease. These findings suggest that genes play an important role in determining who gets the disease.

Biochemical Abnormalities

Scientists suspect that changes in the skin's protective barrier make people with atopic dermatitis more sensitive to irritants. Such people have lower levels of fatty acids (substances that provide moisture and elasticity) in their skin, which causes dryness and reduces the skin's ability to control inflammation.

Other research points to a possible defect in a type of white blood cell called a monocyte. In people with atopic dermatitis, monocytes appear to play a role in the decreased production of an immune system hormone called interferon gamma, which helps regulate allergic reactions. This defect may cause exaggerated immune and inflammatory responses in the blood and tissues of people with atopic dermatitis.

Faulty Regulation of Immunoglobulin E (IgE)

As already described in the section on diagnosis, IgE is a type of antibody that controls the immune system's allergic response. An antibody is a special protein produced by the immune system that recognizes and helps fight and destroy viruses, bacteria, and other foreign substances that invade the body. Normally, IgE is present in very small amounts, but levels are high in 80 to 90 percent of people with atopic dermatitis.

In allergic diseases, IgE antibodies are produced in response to different allergens. When an allergen comes into contact with IgE on specialized immune cells, the cells release various chemicals, including histamine. These chemicals cause the symptoms of an allergic reaction, such as wheezing, sneezing, runny eyes, and itching. The release of histamine and other chemicals alone cannot explain the typical long-term symptoms of the disease. Research is underway to identify factors that may explain why too much IgE is produced and how it plays a role in the disease.

Immune System Imbalance

Researchers also think that an imbalance in the immune system may contribute to the development of atopic dermatitis. It appears that the part of the immune system responsible for stimulating IgE is overactive, and the part that handles skin viral and fungal infections is underactive. Indeed, the skin of people with atopic dermatitis shows increased susceptibility to skin infections. This imbalance appears to result in the skin's inability to prevent inflammation, even in areas of skin that appear normal. In one project, scientists are studying the role of the infectious bacterium *Staphylococcus aureus* (*S. aureus*) in atopic dermatitis. Researchers also think that an imbalance in the immune system may contribute to the development of atopic dermatitis.

Researchers believe that one type of immune cell in the skin, called a Langerhans cell, may be involved in atopic dermatitis. Langerhans cells pick up viruses, bacteria, allergens, and other foreign substances that invade the body and deliver them to other cells in the immune defense system. Langerhans cells appear to be hyperactive in the skin of people with atopic diseases. Certain Langerhans cells are particularly potent at activating white blood cells called T cells in atopic skin, which produce proteins that promote allergic response. This function results in an exaggerated response of the skin to tiny amounts of allergens.

Scientists have also developed mouse models to study step-by-step changes in the immune system in atopic dermatitis, which may eventually lead to a treatment that effectively targets the immune system.

Drug Research

Some researchers are focusing on new treatments for atopic dermatitis, including biologic agents, fatty acid supplements, and new forms of phototherapy. For example, they are studying how ultraviolet light affects the skin's immune system in healthy and diseased skin. They are also investigating biologic agents, including several aimed at modifying the response of the immune system. A biologic agent is a new type of drug based on molecules that occur naturally in the body. One promising treatment is the use of thymopentin to reestablish balance in the immune system.

Researchers also continue to look for drugs that suppress the immune system. In this regard, they are studying the effectiveness of cyclosporine A. Clinical trials are underway with another drug called FK506, which is applied to the skin rather than taken orally. Also, anti-inflammatory drugs have been developed that affect multiple cells and cell functions, and may prove to be an effective alternative to corticosteroids in the treatment of atopic dermatitis.

Several experimental treatments are being evaluated that attempt to replace substances that are deficient in people with atopic dermatitis. Evening primrose oil is a substance rich in gamma-linolenic acid, one of the fatty acids that is decreased in the skin of people with atopic dermatitis. Studies to date using evening primrose oil have yielded contradictory results. In addition, dietary fatty acid supplements have not proven highly effective. There is also a great deal of interest in the use of Chinese herbs and herbal teas to treat the disease. Studies to date show some benefit, but not without concerns about toxicity and the risks involved in suppressing the immune system without close medical supervision.

Hope for the Future

Although the symptoms of atopic dermatitis can be difficult and uncomfortable, the disease can be successfully managed. People with atopic dermatitis can lead healthy, productive lives. As scientists learn more about atopic dermatitis and what causes it, they continue to move closer to effective treatments, and perhaps, ultimately, a cure.

Additional Resources

National Institute of Arthritis and Musculoskeletal and Skin Diseases

NIAMS/National Institutes of Health
1 AMS Circle
Bethesda, MD 20892-3675
Toll-Free: 877-22-NIAMS (226-4267)
Phone: 301-495-4484
TTY: 301-565-2966
Fax: 301-718-6366
Website: www.niams.nih.gov
E-mail: niamsinfo@mail.nih.gov

NIAMS provides information about various forms of skin diseases; arthritis and rheumatic diseases; and bone, muscle, and joint diseases. It distributes patient and professional education materials and refers people to other sources of information. Additional information and updates can be found on the NIAMS website. Listings of clinical trials recruiting patients who have or are at risk of developing a skin disease can be found at www.ClinicalTrials.gov.

Section 14.2

Caring for a Child with Eczema

"Eczema" was provided by KidsHealth, one of the largest resources online for medically reviewed health information written for parents, kids, and teens. For more articles like this one, visit www.KidsHealth.org, or www. TeensHealth.org. © 2005 The Nemours Foundation. This document was reviewed by Barbara P. Homeier, M.D., May 2005.

Most kids get itchy rashes at one time or another. But eczema can be a nuisance that may prompt scratching that can only make the problem worse.

The term eczema refers to a number of different skin conditions in which the skin is red and irritated and occasionally results in small, fluid-filled bumps that become moist and ooze. The most common cause of eczema is atopic dermatitis, sometimes called infantile eczema although it occurs in infants and older children.

The word "atopic" describes conditions that occur when someone is overly sensitive to allergens in their environment such as pollens, molds, dust, animal dander, and certain foods. Dermatitis means that the skin is inflamed, or red and sore.

Kids who get eczema often have family members with hay fever, asthma, or other allergies. Some scientists think these children may be genetically predisposed to get eczema, which means characteristics have been passed on from parents through genes that make a child more likely to get it.

About half of the kids who get eczema will also someday develop hay fever or asthma themselves. Eczema is not an allergy itself, but allergies can trigger eczema. Some environmental factors (such as excessive heat or emotional stress) can also trigger the condition.

About one out of every 10 kids develops eczema. Typically, symptoms appear within the first few months of life, and almost always before a child turns 5. But the good news is that more than half of the kids who have eczema today will be over it by the time they're teenagers.

What are the signs and symptoms?

Signs and symptoms of eczema can vary widely during the early phases. Between 2 and 6 months of age (and almost always before the age of 5 years), children with eczema usually develop itchy, dry, red skin and small bumps on their cheeks, forehead, or scalp. The rash may spread to the extremities (the arms and legs) and the trunk, and red, crusted, or open lesions may appear on any area affected.

Kids with eczema may also experience circular, slightly raised, itchy, and scaly rashes in the bends of the elbows, behind the knees, or on the backs of the wrists and ankles.

As children get older, the rash is usually less oozy and scalier than it was when the eczema first began, and the skin is extremely itchy and dry. These symptoms also tend to worsen and improve over time, with flare-ups occurring periodically.

Children often try to relieve the itching by rubbing the affected areas with a hand or anything within reach. But scratching can make the rash worse and can eventually lead to thickened, brownish areas on the skin. This is why eczema is often called the "itch that rashes" rather than the "rash that itches."

How long does it last?

In many cases, eczema goes into remission and symptoms may disappear altogether for months or even years.

For many children, the condition begins to improve by the age of 5 or 6, but others may experience flare-ups throughout adolescence and early adulthood.

In some kids, the condition may improve and then resurface at the onset of puberty when hormones, stress, and irritating skin products or cosmetics are introduced (or due to other factors that scientists don't yet understand). And some people will experience some degree of dermatitis into adulthood, experiencing areas of itching and a dry, scaly appearance.

Is it contagious?

Eczema is not contagious, so there's no need to keep a baby or child who has it away from siblings, other children, or anyone else.

Can it be prevented?

Scientists believe that eczema is inherited, so there's no way to prevent the condition. However, because specific triggers may tend to make it worse, flare-ups can be prevented or improved by avoiding possible triggers such as:

- pollen;
- mold;
- dust;
- animal dander;
- dry winter air with little moisture;
- allowing the skin to become too dry;
- certain harsh soaps and detergents;
- certain fabrics (such as wool or coarsely woven materials);
- certain skin care products, perfumes, and colognes (particularly those that contain alcohol);
- tobacco smoke;
- some foods (which foods may be eczema triggers depends on the person, but dairy products and acidic foods like tomatoes seem to be common culprits);
- emotional stress;
- excessive heat; and
- sweating.

Also, curbing the tendency to scratch the rash can prevent the condition from worsening and progressing to cause more severe skin damage or secondary infection.

How is it diagnosed?

Diagnosing eczema can be challenging because:

- each child experiences a unique combination of symptoms that also tend to vary in severity;
- it's sometimes confused with other skin conditions, such as seborrheic dermatitis (better known as cradle cap), psoriasis (a genetic disease that causes the skin to become scaly and inflamed), and contact dermatitis (caused by direct skin contact with an irritating substance, such as a metal, medicine, or soap); and
- there's no test available to diagnose it definitively.

If your child's doctor suspects eczema, a thorough medical history is likely to be the most valuable diagnostic tool. A personal or family history of hay fever, other allergies, or asthma is often an important clue.

In addition to doing a physical examination, the doctor will likely ask you and your child about any concerns and symptoms your child has, your child's past health, your family's health, any medications your child is taking, any allergies your child may have, and other issues.

The doctor will also help you identify things in your child's environment that may be contributing to the skin irritation. For example, if your child started using a new soap or lotion before the symptoms appeared, mention this to the doctor because a substance in the soap might be irritating your child's skin.

Your child's doctor may also ask you and your child about any stress he or she might be feeling at home, school, or work (for older kids), because stress can lead to eczema flare-ups.

Your child's doctor will also probably:

- examine the distribution and appearance of the rash;
- ask about how long the rash has been there; and
- look for evidence of thickening of the skin from itching or rubbing (this is called lichenification).

The doctor will also want to rule out other diseases and conditions that can cause skin inflammation, which means that your child may have to be seen more than once before a diagnosis is made. The doctor may also recommend sending your child to a dermatologist or an allergist.

Sometimes, the doctor may refer your child to an allergist to perform allergy testing to find out if the rash is an allergic reaction to a certain substance.

Allergy testing can involve one or more of the following:

- a blood test;
- a patch test (which involves placing a patch of suspected allergen, such as dyes or fragrances, on the skin); or
- scratch/prick tests (which involve placing suspected allergens on the skin or injecting them into the skin).

Your child's doctor may also ask you to eliminate certain foods (such as eggs, milk, soy, or nuts) from your child's diet, switch detergents or soaps, or make other changes for a certain period of time to find out whether your child has a reaction to a particular substance.

How is it treated?

Topical corticosteroids, also called cortisone or steroid creams or ointments, are commonly used to treat eczema and are not the same as the steroids used by some athletes. These medicines are usually applied directly to the affected areas twice a day.

Continue to apply the corticosteroids for as long as your child's doctor suggests. It's also important not to use a topical steroid prescribed for someone else. These creams and ointments vary in strength, and using the wrong strength in sensitive areas can damage the skin, especially in infants.

Nonsteroid medications are also available now in creams or ointments that can be used instead of—or in conjunction with—topical steroids.

Other prescription treatments your child's doctor may recommend could include:

- antihistamines (to help to control itching), or

- oral or topical antibiotics (to prevent or treat secondary infections, which are common in children with eczema).

Some older children with severe eczema may also be treated with ultraviolet light under the supervision of a dermatologist to help clear up their condition and make them more comfortable. In some cases, newer medications that change the way the skin's immune system reacts are also prescribed.

What can I do to help my child?

You can help prevent or treat your child's eczema by keeping your child's skin from becoming dry or itchy and avoiding known triggers that cause flare-ups. It may help to follow these suggestions:

- Avoid giving your child frequent hot baths, which tend to dry the skin.

- Use warm water with mild soaps or nonsoap cleansers when bathing your child.

- Avoid using scented soaps.

- Ask your child's doctor if it's OK to use oatmeal soaking products in the bath to help control the itching.

- Avoid excessive scrubbing and toweling after bathing your child. Instead, gently pat your child's skin dry.

169

- Avoid dressing your child in harsh or irritating clothing, such as wool or coarsely woven materials. Dress your child in soft clothes that "breathe," such as those made from cotton.

- Apply moisturizing ointments (such as petroleum jelly), lotions, or creams to your child's skin regularly and always within a few minutes of bathing, after a very light towel dry. Even if your child is using a corticosteroid cream prescribed by the doctor, apply moisturizers or lotions frequently (ideally, two to three times a day). But be sure to avoid alcohol-containing lotions and moisturizers, which can make your child's skin drier. Some baby products can also contribute to children's dry skin.

- Apply cool compresses (such as a wet, cool washcloth) on the irritated areas of your child's skin to ease itching.

- Keep your child's fingernails short to minimize any skin damage caused by scratching.

- Try having your child wear comfortable, light gloves to bed if scratching at night is a problem.

- Help your child avoid becoming overheated, which can lead to flare-ups.

- Eliminate any known allergens such as certain foods, dust, or pet dander from your household. (This has been shown to help the condition in some young children.)

- Have your child drink plenty of water, which adds moisture to the skin.

Although eczema can be annoying and uncomfortable for children, its emotional impact can become the most significant problem as your child gets older—especially during the preteen and teen years. And your child will need to take responsibility for following the strategies described above.

You can help by teaching your preteen or teen to:

- establish a skin care routine. Brief, lukewarm showers or baths and moisturizing regularly will help to avoid or alleviate flare-ups.

- use only hypoallergenic makeup and sunscreens and facial moisturizers labeled noncomedogenic and oil free.

- recognize stressful situations (such as taking tests at school or sports competitions) and how to manage them (such as by breathing, focusing on an enjoyable activity, or taking a break).

• be aware of scratching and minimize it as much as possible.

When should you call your child's doctor?

Children and teens with eczema are prone to skin infections, especially with *Staph* [*Staphylococcal*] bacteria and herpesvirus. Call your child's doctor immediately if you notice any of the early signs of skin infection, which may include:

• increased fever;

• redness and warmth on or around affected areas;

• pus-filled bumps on or around affected areas; and

• areas on the skin that look like cold sores or fever blisters.

Also, call your child's doctor if you notice a sudden change or worsening of your child's condition or if your child's eczema isn't responding to the doctor's recommendations.

Even though eczema can certainly be bothersome for kids and parents alike, taking some preventative precautions and following the doctor's orders can help to keep your child's eczema under control.

Section 14.3

Information for Teenagers with Eczema

"All About Eczema" was provided by TeensHealth, one of the largest resources online for medically reviewed health information written for parents, kids, and teens. For more articles like this one, visit www.TeensHealth.org, or www.KidsHealth.org. © 2006 The Nemours Foundation. Reviewed by Patrice Hyde, M.D., August 2006.

Rick was exhausted. Increased stress at school, home, and work had made him extremely tired. It also made his skin act up. Not again, he thought—not another eczema flare-up!

Eczema is a common skin problem. If you have eczema or think you might have it, here's how to deal with it.

Some Skin Facts

Your skin, which protects your organs, muscles, and bones and regulates your body temperature, can run into plenty of trouble. Acne occurs when your pores become clogged. But zits aren't the only skin problem you may encounter. Have you ever tried a new type of soap and developed an itchy rash? That reaction may just be eczema in action.

What Is Eczema?

Eczema (pronounced: ek-zeh-ma) is a group of skin conditions that cause skin to become red, irritated, itchy, and sometimes develop small, fluid-filled bumps that become moist and ooze.

There are many forms of eczema, but atopic (pronounced: ay-tah-pik) eczema is one of the most common and severe. Doctors don't know exactly what causes atopic eczema, also called atopic dermatitis (pronounced: der-muh-tie-tis), but they think it could be a difference in the way a person's immune system reacts to things. Skin allergies may be involved in some forms of eczema.

If you have eczema, you're probably not the only person you know who has it. Eczema isn't contagious like a cold, but most people with eczema have family members with the condition. Researchers think

172

it's inherited or passed through the genes. In general, eczema is fairly common—approximately 1 in 10 people in the world will be affected by it at some point in their lives.

People with eczema also may have asthma and certain allergies, such as hay fever. For some, food allergies (such as allergies to cow's milk, soy, eggs, fish, or wheat) may bring on or worsen eczema. Allergies to animal dander, rough fabrics, and dust may also trigger the condition in some people.

Signs and Symptoms

It can be difficult to avoid all the triggers, or irritants, that may cause or worsen eczema flare-ups. In many people, the itchy patches of eczema usually appear where the elbow bends; on the backs of the knees, ankles, and wrists; and on the face, neck, and upper chest— although any part of the body can be affected.

In an eczema flare-up, skin may feel hot and itchy at first. Then, if the person scratches, the skin may become red, inflamed, or blistered. Some people who have eczema scratch their skin so much it becomes almost leathery in texture. Others find that their skin becomes extremely dry and scaly. Even though many people have eczema, the symptoms can vary quite a bit from person to person.

What Do Doctors Do?

If you think you have eczema, your best bet is to visit your doctor, who may refer you to a dermatologist (a doctor who specializes in treating skin). Diagnosing atopic eczema can be difficult because it may be confused with other skin conditions. For example, eczema can easily be confused with a skin condition called contact dermatitis, which happens when the skin comes in contact with an irritating substance like the perfume in a certain detergent.

In addition to a physical examination, a doctor will take your medical history by asking about any concerns and symptoms you have, your past health, your family's health, any medications you're taking, any allergies you may have, and other issues. Your doctor can also help identify things in your environment that may be contributing to your skin irritation. For example, if you started using a new shower gel or body lotion before the symptoms appeared, mention this to your doctor because a substance in the cream or lotion might be irritating your skin.

Emotional stress can also lead to eczema flare-ups, so your doctor might also ask you about any stress you're feeling at home, school, or work.

If you're diagnosed with eczema, your doctor might:

- prescribe medications to soothe the redness and irritation, such as creams or ointments that contain corticosteroids, or antihistamine pills; or

- recommend other medications to take internally if the eczema is really bad or you get it a lot.

For some people with severe eczema, ultraviolet light therapy can help clear up the condition. Newer medications that change the way the skin's immune system reacts may also help.

If eczema doesn't respond to normal treatment, your doctor may do allergy testing to see if something else is triggering the condition, especially if you have asthma or seasonal allergies.

If you're tested for food allergies, you may be given certain foods (such as eggs, milk, soy, or nuts) and observed to see if the food causes an eczema flare-up. Food allergy testing can also be done by pricking the skin with an extract of the food substance and observing the reaction. But sometimes allergy testing can be misleading because someone may have an allergic reaction to a food that is not responsible for the eczema flare-up.

If you're tested for allergy to dyes or fragrances, a patch of the substance will be placed against the skin and you'll be monitored to see if skin irritation develops.

Can I Prevent Eczema?

Eczema can't be cured, but there are plenty of things you can do to prevent a flare-up. For facial eczema, wash gently with a nondrying facial cleanser or soap substitute, use a facial moisturizer that says noncomedogenic/oil-free, and apply only hypoallergenic makeup and sunscreens.

In addition, these tips may help:

- **Avoid substances that stress your skin.** Besides your known triggers, some things you may want to avoid include household cleaners, drying soaps, detergents, and fragranced lotions.

- **H_2O is a no-no.** Too much exposure to water can dry out your skin, so take short warm—not hot—showers and baths and wear gloves if your hands will be in water for long periods of time. Be sure to gently and thoroughly pat your skin dry, as rubbing with a coarse towel will irritate the eczema. Also, it isn't the water that causes your skin to react; it's the water evaporating if not dried soon enough.

- **Say yes to cotton.** Clothes made of scratchy fabric like wool can irritate your skin. Cotton clothes are a better bet.

- **Moisturize!** A fragrance-free moisturizer such as petroleum jelly will prevent your skin from becoming irritated and cracked.

- **Don't scratch that itch.** Even though it's difficult to resist, scratching your itch can worsen eczema and make it more difficult for the skin to heal because you can break the skin and bacteria can get in, causing an infection.

- **Keep your cool.** Sudden changes in temperature, sweating, and becoming overheated may cause your eczema to kick in.

- **Take your meds.** Follow your doctor's or dermatologist's directions and take your medication as directed.

- **Unwind.** Stress can aggravate eczema, so try to relax.

Dealing with Eczema

There's good news if you have eczema—it usually clears up before the age of 25. Until then, you can learn to tune in to what triggers eczema and manage the condition. For example, if you have eczema and can't wear certain types of makeup, find brands that are free of fragrances and dyes. Your dermatologist may be able to recommend some brands that are less likely to irritate your skin.

Your self-esteem doesn't have to suffer just because you have eczema, and neither does your social life. Getting involved in your school and extracurricular activities can be a great way to get your mind off the itch. If certain activities aggravate your eczema, such as swimming in a heavily chlorinated pool, suggest activities to your friends that won't harm your skin.

Even if sweat tends to aggravate your skin, it's still a good idea to exercise. Exercise is a great way to blow off stress—just try walking, bike riding, or another sport that keeps your skin cool and dry while you work out.

Chapter 15

Medications Used to Treat Eczema

Chapter Contents

177

Section 15.1

Overview of New Treatments for Eczema

For the millions of Americans with psoriasis and eczema, searching for a treatment to alleviate their red, itchy, and scaly skin is a top priority. While current therapies provide some relief for these bothersome symptoms, they also can produce serious side effects and lifestyle sacrifices. Now, thanks to the development of new targeted therapies that address the causes of these common skin conditions, these medications are revolutionizing treatment and improving patients' quality of life.

Speaking at the American Academy of Dermatology's Derm Update 2002, dermatologist Mark Lebwohl, M.D., Professor and Chairman, Department of Dermatology, Mount Sinai School of Medicine, New York, explained the science behind these emerging treatments as well as their benefits to patients.

"These new medications, which are injected or applied on the skin, more effectively clear the skin conditions rather than only treating the symptoms," stated Dr. Lebwohl. "Since they target the diseased area and do not affect surrounding, healthy tissue, these medications are not associated with dangerous side effects, some of which can affect the kidney, liver, and bone marrow."

Topical Immunomodulators

For over a decade, potent systemic immunomodulators have been used for the treatment of psoriasis and eczema. But in the past two years, these medications have been incorporated into topical preparations. When applied topically, these therapies exert their powerful anti-inflammatory effects on the skin without hampering the immune system's ability to defend itself from bacteria, viruses, and other diseases.

Two topical immunomodulators (TIMs), tacrolimus ointment and pimecrolimus cream, have been approved for the treatment of eczema, a chronic skin condition characterized by itchy, inflamed skin—typically on the insides of the elbows, backs of the knees, and the face. These steroid-free treatments are effective in treating eczema without the side effects found with using corticosteroids, medications tradition-ally used to treat eczema that can cause thinning of the skin, forma-tion of dilated blood vessels, stretch marks, and infection.

"By reducing our reliance on topical corticosteroids, TIMs are spar-ing patients significant side effects," stated Dr. Lebwohl. "Not only have these therapies been shown to be effective for eczema, but they are profoundly changing the way that we treat a number of inflam-matory skin diseases, including psoriasis."

By specifically interfering with the activation of T-cells, a type of white blood cell in the body responsible for triggering immune re-sponses which contribute to the development of psoriasis, TIMs have been shown to effectively treat this common skin disorder. Studies have also shown that the side effects of topical corticosteroids on the face and other areas in patients with psoriasis can be avoided by treat-ing those areas with TIMs. In addition, the use of TIMs on the eyelids has dramatically reduced the need for topical corticosteroids, which can cause glaucoma and cataracts.

Another breakthrough has been in the use of TIMs to treat actinic keratoses, or AKs, which are known as the early beginnings of skin cancer. Imiquimod, which is approved for the treatment of genital warts, has been shown in recent studies to dramatically improve the treatment of AKs as well as some skin cancers.

Biologic Agents

New biologic agents are also showing promise in the treatment of psoriasis. Since these agents create molecules that target specific steps in the development of psoriasis, they have substantial advantages over previously used systemic therapies that could cause kidney and liver damage.

Two agents already approved for rheumatoid arthritis and Crohn disease, but not approved to treat psoriasis, are etanercept and inflix-imab. These medications are TNF blockers, which work by interfer-ing with specific immune responses that are responsible for psoriasis. Both have been shown to dramatically improve psoriatic arthritis and psoriasis. Patients can give themselves injections of etanercept at home and those taking infliximab can receive intravenous injections in the doctor's office, clinic, or hospital.

Two other biologic therapies that are not FDA approved but are show-ing promising results in clearing psoriasis are alefacept and efalizumab.

Both of these biologic agents work by blocking the over-activation of T-cells. Alefacept, which is given by injection, appears to keep the disease from flaring for long periods of time. Patients on alefacept are reporting that their psoriasis has cleared for a year or more without recurring. An advantage of efalizumab is that it works rapidly to treat psoriasis, allowing almost immediate relief in most cases. Another benefit is that patients can use the medication at home once they receive training on giving themselves injections.

"These biologic agents are leading the way in the development of innovative ways to treat common skin conditions," remarked Dr. Lebwohl. "As more and more research is conducted in this area, I am confident that dermatologists can help more patients than ever before find the best therapy available for their condition."

Traditional Treatments

"While these new therapies have been shown to have significant advantages for many patients with eczema and psoriasis, dermatologists will continue to use traditional treatments, especially those that have been shown to work well and are well tolerated by patients," said Dr. Lebwohl. "However, patients who have trouble complying with their treatment regimen may be the most likely candidates for these new medications. For example, patients who have difficulty fitting in ultraviolet light treatments, which can involve three treatments a week for months at a time, may benefit from TIMs and biologic agents."

"The introduction of topical immunomodulators and biologic agents is revolutionizing the way that we treat patients with psoriasis, eczema, and skin cancer," said Dr. Lebwohl. "They are making a tremendous impact in the quality of life of patients of all ages, including young children."

Section 15.2

Medications and Other Therapies Used to Treat Eczema

Topical (applied to the skin) medications play an integral role in controlling the signs and symptoms of eczema, and moisturizer is an essential part of most treatment plans. Systemic medication (medication that circulates throughout the body and is taken orally or given by injection or infusion) also may be prescribed.

Dermatologists use medication and other therapies to:

- control itching;
- reduce skin inflammation;
- clear infection;
- loosen and remove scaly lesions; and
- reduce formation of new lesions.

A patient (or parent) may be instructed to use one medication or a combination of therapies. Research is showing that combination therapy (use of two or more therapeutic agents) can, in some cases, increase effectiveness and reduce side effects. Medications and other therapies that dermatologists may use to treat eczema include the following.

Medications

Antibiotics

Skin affected by eczema frequently becomes infected. A topical or systemic antibiotic may be prescribed to clear the infection.

Research demonstrates that an oral antibiotic can be highly beneficial when the skin becomes infected or a secondary infection develops. Oral antibiotics are frequently prescribed when a patient has atopic dermatitis because individuals with this condition often have

181

Staphylococcus aureus, a bacterium that causes *Staph* infections, colonizing their skin. This bacterium is frequently the cause of secondary infection. Oral antibiotics should be taken exactly as prescribed.

What it does: Kills bacteria causing the infection.

Usage: This depends on the antibiotic prescribed and severity of the infection. It is especially important to use antibiotics as prescribed. Patients should not skip doses nor stop using the medication as soon as they feel better. Doing so may allow some of the bacteria to remain and possibly become resistant to the medication.

Antihistamines

When itching is severe, antihistamines may be prescribed. While there is little scientific evidence that either sedating or nonsedating antihistamines are effective in relieving itch and other symptoms, sedating antihistamines can be useful for patients experiencing significant sleep disruption due to a constant, unbearable itch and other symptoms. It is believed that the improvements associated with antihistamine use are due primarily to the patient getting a restful sleep.

What it does: These pills do not clear eczema. However, sedative antihistamines may promote a restful sleep, and this restful sleep is believed to decrease the severity and improve the patient's quality of life.

Usage: This depends on the antihistamine and severity of the eczema. Antihistamines should be taken exactly as prescribed. While research shows that antihistamines are safe and not associated with significant adverse effects, even in very young patients when taken as prescribed, taking a higher dose than prescribed can be dangerous, especially for young children.

Calcineurin Inhibitors

Pimecrolimus and tacrolimus belong to a class of drugs called calcineurin inhibitors, which effectively reduce the inflammation of atopic dermatitis. Available in topical form by prescription, these two steroid-free medications are the newest treatment option for atopic dermatitis and a much-welcomed addition because they do not produce the side effects, such as thinning skin and loss of effectiveness, associated with long-term use of topical corticosteroids. As such, calcineurin inhibitors can be used for longer periods.

Currently, pimecrolimus and tacrolimus are FDA [U.S. Food and Drug Administration]-approved for treating atopic dermatitis in patients who are two years of age or older and cannot use or have not responded to other treatments for eczema. Both medications can be used for short-term and intermittent long-term treatment. Tacrolimus received FDA approval for the treatment of moderate to severe atopic dermatitis in December 2000. Pimecrolimus received approval in December 2001 for treating mild to moderate atopic dermatitis.

In clinical trials, side effects were mild and temporary. Some patients using pimecrolimus experienced a mild to moderate temporary sensation of warmth or burning at the application site, headache, or cold-like symptoms. When applying tacrolimus, some patients also experienced stinging and burning upon application. The more severe the eczema, the more likely the patient was to experience these side effects. The burning sensation was usually confined to the area being treated and tended to subside after the first week.

What it does: Topical calcineurin inhibitors (TCIs) reduce inflammation. Scientists believe that these medications work by selectively modifying or suppressing the over-response that occurs in the immune system, which causes the inflammation.

Usage: The recommended dosage for both pimecrolimus and tacrolimus is to apply a thin layer twice a day to the affected areas until the skin clears.

Who should not use: Neither medication should be used by a patient with a weakened immune system.

Avoid sunlight and other UV exposure: Patients should avoid exposure to sunlight, tanning beds, sun lamps, and treatment with ultraviolet (UV) light while taking these medications. Sun protection is essential. Be sure to avoid the midday (between 10 a.m. and 4 p.m.) sun. Even when going outdoors for a few minutes sun-protection practices must be followed. Wear loose-fitting clothing that protects the treated area from sunlight, apply a sunscreen with an SPF [sun protection factor] of 15 or higher to all exposed skin 20 minutes before going outdoors, use a sunscreen for the lips that has an SPF of at least 15, and wear a wide-brimmed hat and sunglasses.

Pregnancy: Women who are pregnant, breastfeeding, or may become pregnant should discuss safety with their dermatologist. Research shows that the oral form of tacrolimus crosses the placenta and appears in breast milk, making it inappropriate for use by pregnant or breast-feeding women.

Coal Tar

Coal tar has a soothing effect on inflamed skin and has been used for many years to treat atopic dermatitis. Today, coal tar comes in numerous preparations, and some of these are available over the counter. Best results are typically seen when use is supervised by a dermatologist. While effective and free of serious side effects, patients often prefer other treatment options because coal tar has an unpleasant odor and stains just about everything it touches.

What it does: Reduces inflammation and itching.

Usage: Coal tar preparations are available in many forms, including lotion, shampoo, and a preparation that can be added to the bath. All forms should be used as directed by a dermatologist.

Corticosteroids

Available both over the counter and by prescription, topical corticosteroids have been used since the 1950s to treat eczema. Today, dermatologists use topical corticosteroids more than any other medication to alleviate the signs and symptoms of eczema. Also known as glucocorticoids and steroids, corticosteroids come in a variety of strengths, ranging from mild to extremely potent. The strength prescribed depends on the patient's age and medical history, severity of the eczema, where on the body the medication will be used, and the size of the areas to be treated. While many patients have concerns about using corticosteroids due to potential side effects, the likelihood of a side effect occurring is rare when corticosteroids are used as prescribed. Side effects, such as thinning skin, dilated blood vessels, stretch marks, and loss of effectiveness, tend to occur when high-potency corticosteroids are used over long periods of time.

In severe cases, intramuscular injections of a corticosteroid or short-term therapy with a corticosteroid in pill or liquid form may be prescribed to provide relief from chronic itching. These therapies also may be used to prevent major exacerbations of atopic dermatitis. However, systemic corticosteroids are used sparingly in adults and rarely in children due to the possibility of:

- potential side effects;
- diminished effectiveness with use; and
- rebound flare-ups that may occur when the medication is stopped.

Systemic treatment is not recommended for long-term use. Fortunately, significant improvement is usually seen within a few weeks, and the remaining signs and symptoms can be successfully treated with topical agents and lifestyle modifications.

What it does: Corticosteroids tend to rapidly and effectively reduce inflammation, which relieves itching.

Usage: Topical corticosteroids are applied in a thin layer to the skin as prescribed and used for limited periods of time. To prevent potential side effects, care should be taken when applying this medication around the eye, to skin that is diapered or bandaged, and to body folds. Systemic corticosteroids may be prescribed in a pill or liquid form or given as an injection.

Pregnancy: Pregnant and breastfeeding women should not take systemic corticosteroids because these medications cross the placenta. Children who may have been exposed to systemic corticosteroids before birth (or while being breastfed) should be monitored for suppression of adrenal and pituitary hormones. A woman who is pregnant or becomes pregnant during a course of systemic or high-potency topical corticosteroid therapy should discuss safety issues with her dermatologist or obstetrician.

Note: A corticosteroid should only be used as prescribed. This medication should not be used more frequently or for a longer period of time than directed, and a corticosteroid should never be shared. This last fact is especially important for parents to know. Since atopic dermatitis tends to run in families, a parent with atopic dermatitis may believe that using a corticosteroid already in the home will help a child. This should never be done without consulting a dermatologist.

Cyclosporine

Cyclosporine is a potent immunosuppressant used to prevent rejection of a transplanted heart, kidney, or liver. It also is used to treat severe cases of psoriasis and atopic dermatitis. In fact, oral cyclosporine has been used for many years to treat severe atopic dermatitis that does not respond to other treatment. In clinical trials, patients taking cyclo-sporine experienced prompt relief from the symptoms of eczema; how-ever, rapid relapse usually occurs soon after the patient stops taking the medication. Long-term maintenance therapy tends to gives patients satisfactory remission.

A number of side effects, including lowered immune response, limit the use of oral cyclosporine. Due to potential side effects, each patient's kidney function and blood pressure must be checked before the drug can be prescribed, and these need to be monitored regularly during therapy. Other side effects include increased risk of developing can-cers, headache, tingling or burning sensations in the arms or legs, fatigue, abdominal upset, and musculoskeletal or joint pain.

Topical preparations of cyclosporine are not available due to the medication's inability to effectively penetrate the skin.

What it does: Reduces skin inflammation by inhibiting T-cell (a type of white blood cell) activity.

Usage: Take only as prescribed.

Interferon Gamma

Not traditionally used to treat eczema, interferon gamma has been investigated in a small number of studies. Findings indicate that while injections can provide significant relief, a high overall rate of side ef-fects was demonstrated. Interferon gamma is a protein produced by the human body that is involved in the regulation of the immune sys-tem and inflammatory responses.

What it does: More research is needed to fully understand how interferon gamma works. It is believed that interferon gamma regu-lates immune responses; thereby, preventing the overactive immune response that leads to inflammation of the skin.

Usage: Take only as prescribed.

Mycophenolate Mofetil

Approved for preventing organ rejection in transplant patients, research suggests that the medication may effectively treat severe atopic dermatitis in adults. Potential side effects include increased risk of cancers and infections. In animal studies, mycophenolate mofetil has been shown to cause birth defects. Women are advised to use effective contraception before and during therapy and for six weeks after stopping therapy with mycophenolate mofetil.

What it does: Prevents the exaggerated, one-sided immune response that leads to inflammation.

Usage: Take only as prescribed.

Other Therapies

Cold Compresses

A cold compress is a cloth dipped in ice water that is wrung out and applied directly to the skin that itches. When first placed on the skin, the itching or pain may become more intense; however, this soon subsides.

What it does: Helps relieve inflammation and itching.

Usage: If your dermatologist believes cold compresses are beneficial, the parent or patient will be instructed in how to use and how often to use.

Moisturizers

Most eczema treatment plans include use of moisturizers, also called emollients, since one of the symptoms of eczema is an intense almost unbearable itching.

Contrary to popular belief, moisturizers do not add moisture to the skin. Rather moisturizers serve as a barrier that reduces water loss from the skin. This is why dermatologists recommend that a moisturizer be applied after bathing while the skin is still damp. This "locks in" the moisture from the bath or shower. Moisturizers come in many, many forms. Ointments are best for very dry skin. Creams and lotions are used to treat mild to moderate eczema. Most moisturizers are applied directly to the skin; however, some are added to a bath.

Since many moisturizers contain added preservatives and fragrances that can irritate the skin, people with eczema should consult a dermatologist to find appropriate products.

What it does: Acts as a protective barrier to prevent water loss from the skin, which prevents the dry skin that leads to itching.

Usage: Moisturizer should be applied to the skin or added to a bath.

References

1. AAD *Guidelines of Care for Atopic Dermatitis.* July 26, 2003.

2. MacReady, N. Hydrocortisone Cuts Irritation Associated with Tacrolimus, *Skin & Allergy News.* February 2004, p. 28.

Section 15.3

Pimecrolimus Cream

McEvoy GK, ed. Pimecrolimus Topical. Bethesda, MD: AHFS MedMaster Consumer Medication Information database; 2006 [cited 2006 Nov 7]. Available from http://www.nlm.nih.gov/medlineplus/druginfo/medmaster/a603027.html.

Important Warning Regarding Pimecrolimus Topical

A small number of patients who used pimecrolimus cream or another similar medication developed skin cancer or lymphoma (cancer in a part of the immune system). There is not enough information available to tell whether pimecrolimus cream caused these patients to develop cancer. Studies of transplant patients and laboratory animals and an understanding of the way pimecrolimus works suggest that there is possibility that people who use pimecrolimus cream have a greater risk of developing cancer. More study is needed to understand this risk. Follow these directions carefully to decrease the possible risk that you will develop cancer during your treatment with pimecrolimus cream:

- Use pimecrolimus cream only when you have symptoms of eczema. Stop using pimecrolimus cream when your symptoms go away or when your doctor tells you that you should stop.

- Do not use pimecrolimus cream continuously for a long time.

- Call your doctor if you have used pimecrolimus cream for 6 weeks and your eczema symptoms have not improved. A different medication may be needed.

- Call your doctor if your eczema symptoms come back after your treatment with pimecrolimus cream.

- Apply pimecrolimus cream only to skin that is affected by eczema.

- Use the smallest amount of cream that is needed to control your symptoms.

- Do not use pimecrolimus cream to treat eczema in children who are younger than 2 years old.

- Tell your doctor if you have or have ever had cancer, especially skin cancer, or any condition that affects your immune system.

- Ask your doctor if you are not sure if a condition that you have has affected your immune system. Pimecrolimus may not be right for you.

- Protect your skin from real and artificial sunlight during your treatment with pimecrolimus cream. Do not use sun lamps or tanning beds, and do not undergo ultraviolet light therapy. Stay out of the sunlight as much as possible during your treatment, even when the medication is not on your skin.

- If you need to be outside in the sun, wear loose-fitting clothing to protect the treated skin, and ask your doctor about other ways to protect your skin from the sun.

- Your doctor or pharmacist will give you the manufacturer's patient information sheet (Medication Guide) when you begin treatment with pimecrolimus and each time you refill your prescription. Read the information carefully and ask your doctor or pharmacist if you have any questions. You can also visit the Food and Drug Administration (FDA) website (http://www.fda.gov/cder) or the manufacturer's website to obtain the Medication Guide.

- Talk to your doctor about the risks of using pimecrolimus.

Why is this medication prescribed?

Pimecrolimus is used to control the symptoms of eczema (atopic dermatitis; a skin disease that causes the skin to be dry and itchy and to sometimes develop red, scaly rashes). Pimecrolimus is only used to treat patients who cannot use other medications for eczema, or whose symptoms were not controlled by other medications. Pimecrolimus is in a class of medications called topical calcineurin inhibitors. It works by stopping the immune system from producing substances that may cause eczema.

How should this medicine be used?

Pimecrolimus comes as a cream to apply to the skin. It is usually applied twice a day for up to 6 weeks at a time. Follow the directions on your prescription label carefully, and ask your doctor or pharmacist to explain any part you do not understand. Apply pimecrolimus cream exactly as directed. Do not apply more or less of it or apply it more often than prescribed by your doctor.

Pimecrolimus cream is only for use on the skin. Be careful not to get pimecrolimus cream in your eyes or mouth. If you get pimecrolimus cream in your eyes, rinse them with cold water. If you swallow pimecrolimus cream, call your doctor.

To use the cream, follow these steps:

- Wash your hands with soap and water.

- Be sure that the skin in the affected area is dry.

- Apply a thin layer of pimecrolimus cream to all affected areas of your skin. You can apply pimecrolimus to all affected skin surfaces including your head, face, and neck.

- Rub the cream into your skin gently and completely.

- Wash your hands with soap and water to remove any leftover pimecrolimus cream. Do not wash your hands if you are treating them with pimecrolimus cream.

- You may cover the treated areas with normal clothing, but do not use any bandages, dressings, or wraps.

- Be careful not to wash the cream off of affected areas of your skin. Do not swim, shower, or bathe immediately after applying pimecrolimus cream. Ask your doctor if you should apply more pimecrolimus cream after you swim, shower, or bathe.

- After you apply pimecrolimus cream and allow time for it be completely absorbed into your skin, you may apply moisturizers, sunscreen, or makeup to the affected area. Ask your doctor about the specific products you plan to use.

What are other uses for this medicine?

This medication may be prescribed for other uses; ask your doctor or pharmacist for more information.

What special precautions should I follow?

Before using pimecrolimus cream:

- tell your doctor and pharmacist if you are allergic to pimecrolimus or any other medications.

- tell your doctor and pharmacist what prescription and nonprescription medications, vitamins, nutritional supplements, and herbal products you are taking. Be sure to mention any of the following: antifungals such as fluconazole (Diflucan), itraconazole (Sporanox), and ketoconazole (Nizoral); calcium channel blockers such as diltiazem (Cardizem, Dilacor, Tiazac, others), and verapamil (Calan, Isoptin, Verelan); cimetidine (Tagamet); clarithromycin (Biaxin); cyclosporine (Neoral, Sandimmune); danazol (Danocrine); delavirdine (Rescriptor); erythromycin (E.E.S., E-Mycin, Erythrocin); fluoxetine (Prozac, Sarafem); fluvoxamine (Luvox); HIV protease inhibitors such as indinavir (Crixivan), and ritonavir (Norvir); isoniazid (INH, Nydrazid); metronidazole (Flagyl); nefazodone; oral contraceptives (birth control pills); other ointments, creams, or lotions; troleandomycin (TAO); and zafirlukast (Accolate). Your doctor may need to change the doses of your medications or monitor you carefully for side effects.

- tell your doctor if you have or have ever had Netherton syndrome (an inherited condition that causes the skin to be red, itchy, and scaly), redness and peeling of most of your skin, any other skin disease, or any type of skin infection, especially chickenpox, shingles (a skin infection in people who have had chickenpox in the past), herpes (cold sores), or eczema herpeticum (viral infection that causes fluid-filled blisters to form on the skin of people who have eczema). Also tell your doctor if your eczema rash has turned crusty or blistered or if you think that your eczema rash is infected.

- tell your doctor if you are pregnant, plan to become pregnant, or are breastfeeding. If you become pregnant while taking pimecrolimus, call your doctor.

- ask your doctor about the safe use of alcohol during your treatment with pimecrolimus cream. Your face may become flushed or red or feel hot if you drink alcohol during your treatment.

- avoid exposure to chickenpox, shingles and other viruses. If you are exposed to one of these viruses while using pimecrolimus, call your doctor immediately.

- you should know that good skin care and moisturizers may help relieve the dry skin caused by eczema. Talk to your doctor about the moisturizers you should use, and always apply them after applying pimecrolimus cream.

What special dietary instructions should I follow?

Talk to your doctor about eating grapefruit and drinking grape-fruit juice while taking this medicine.

What should I do if I forget a dose?

Apply the missed dose as soon as you remember it. However, if it is almost time for the next dose, skip the missed dose and continue your regular dosing schedule. Do not apply extra cream to make up for a missed dose.

What side effects can this medication cause?

Pimecrolimus may cause side effects. Tell your doctor if any of these symptoms are severe or do not go away:

- burning, warmth, stinging, soreness, or redness in the areas where you applied pimecrolimus (call your doctor if this lasts more than 1 week)
- warts, bumps, or other growths on skin
- eye irritation
- headache
- cough
- red, stuffy, or runny nose
- nosebleed
- diarrhea
- painful menstrual periods

Some side effects can be serious. If you experience any of the following symptoms, call your doctor immediately:

- sore or red throat
- fever
- flu-like symptoms
- ear pain, discharge, and other signs of infection
- hives
- new or worsening rash
- itching
- swelling of the face, throat, tongue, lips, eyes, hands, feet, ankles, or lower legs
- difficulty breathing or swallowing
- crusting, oozing, blistering, or other signs of skin infection
- cold sores
- chickenpox or other blisters
- swollen glands in the neck

Pimecrolimus may cause other side effects. Call your doctor if you have any unusual problems while taking this medication.

If you experience a serious side effect, you or your doctor may send a report to the Food and Drug Administration's (FDA) MedWatch Adverse Event Reporting program online [at http://www.fda.gov/MedWatch/report.htm] or by phone [1-800-332-1088].

What storage conditions are needed for this medicine?

Keep this medication in the container it came in, tightly closed, and out of reach of children. Store it at room temperature and away from excess heat and moisture (not in the bathroom). Throw away any medication that is outdated or no longer needed. Talk to your pharmacist about the proper disposal of your medication.

What other information should I know?

Keep all appointments with your doctor.

Do not let anyone else take your medication. Ask your pharmacist any questions you have about refilling your prescription.

What brand name is used?

Elidel®

Chapter 16

Facts about Anaphylaxis: Allergic Disorders Can Be Deadly

What is anaphylaxis?

Anaphylaxis is a severe allergic reaction—the extreme end of the allergic spectrum. The whole body is affected, often within minutes of exposure to the allergen but sometimes after hours. Peanut allergy and nut allergy are frequently severe and for that reason have received widespread publicity. Causes of anaphylaxis also include other foods, insect stings, latex, and drugs, but on rare occasions there may be no obvious trigger.

What are the symptoms?

Symptoms include:

- generalized flushing of the skin;
- nettle rash (hives) anywhere on the body;
- sense of impending doom;
- swelling of throat and mouth;
- difficulty in swallowing or speaking;
- alterations in heart rate;
- severe asthma;

- abdominal pain, nausea, and vomiting;
- sudden feeling of weakness (drop in blood pressure); and
- collapse and unconsciousness.

Nobody would necessarily experience all of these symptoms.

What are mild allergy symptoms?

Some people find that the allergy symptoms they experience are always mild. For example, there may be a tingling or itching in the mouth or a localized rash—nothing more. This is not serious in itself and may be treated with oral antihistamines. However, in some cases the allergy may become worse over time. It is wise in all cases to make an appointment with the doctor and seek a referral to a specialist allergy clinic.

If there is marked difficulty in breathing or swallowing and/or a sudden weakness or floppiness, regard these as serious symptoms requiring immediate treatment.

What is the treatment for a severe reaction?

Preloaded adrenaline injection kits are available on prescription for those believed to be at risk. These are available in two strengths—adult and junior.

The injection must be given, as directed, as soon as a serious reaction is suspected and an ambulance must be called. If there is no improvement in 5 to 10 minutes, give a second injection.

Why does anaphylaxis occur?

Any allergic reaction, including the most extreme form, anaphylactic shock, occurs because the body's immune system reacts inappropriately in response to the presence of a substance that it wrongly perceives as a threat.

What exactly is going on?

An anaphylactic reaction is caused by the sudden release of chemical substances, including histamine, from cells in the blood and tissues where they are stored. The release is triggered by the reaction between the allergic antibody (IgE) with the substance (allergen) causing the anaphylactic reaction. This mechanism is so sensitive that minute quantities of the allergen can cause a reaction. The released chemicals act on blood vessels to cause the swelling in the mouth and anywhere on the skin. There is a fall in blood pressure and, in asthmatics, the effect is mainly on the lungs.

Why does adrenaline work?

During anaphylaxis, blood vessels leak, bronchial tissues swell, and blood pressure drops, causing choking and collapse. Adrenaline (epinephrine) acts quickly to constrict blood vessels, relax smooth muscles in the lungs to improve breathing, stimulate the heartbeat, and help to stop swelling around the face and lips (angioedema).

How do I know if I am at risk from anaphylaxis?

If you have suffered a bad allergic reaction in the past—whatever the cause—then any future reaction is also likely to be severe. If you have suffered a significant reaction to a tiny dose, or have reacted on skin contact, this might also be a sign that a larger dose may trigger a severe reaction. If you have asthma as well as allergies, a referral is particularly important because asthma can put you in a higher risk category. Where foods such as nuts, seeds, shellfish, and fish are concerned, even mild symptoms should not be ignored because future reactions may be severe.

What are the most common causes of anaphylaxis?

Common causes include foods such as peanuts, tree nuts (e.g., almonds, walnuts, cashews, Brazils), sesame, fish, shellfish, dairy products, and eggs. Non-food causes include wasp or bee stings, natural latex (rubber), penicillin, or any other drug or injection. In some people, exercise can trigger a severe reaction—either on its own or in combination with other factors such as food or drugs (e.g., aspirin).

Fresh fruit allergy may occur in people who are allergic to pollen. This is frequently mild, but a doctor's advice should be sought.

What will an allergy specialist do?

There is no perfect way to measure an individual's potential for a severe allergic reaction, but, in making a diagnosis, an allergy consultant can do several things that will provide clues. Most importantly, the specialist will take a detailed history of previous reactions and other allergic conditions you may have. Valuable information can also be provided by means of skin prick tests and blood tests (RAST [radioallergosorbent test] or CAP [ImmunoCAP Specific IgE blood test] assay).

How can I avoid problems?

- Minimize the risk by taking great care and being vigilant. If you are food allergic, read labels like Sherlock Holmes: look for the "hidden" allergen. You can easily recognize a packet of peanuts but may miss the word "groundnuts" in tiny print on the side of a tin of curry sauce, or the Latin term *arachis* used to signify the presence of peanut in pharmaceutical products.

- If you are food-allergic, be assertive about asking for detailed information from manufacturers and supermarket staff.

- Be particularly careful in restaurants, where proprietors are under no obligation to list ingredients. Question staff very directly. It may be necessary to speak with a senior manager. Some restaurants have ingredient lists available for you to check. You may wish to telephone the restaurant in advance to ensure your allergy is taken seriously.

- Be alert to all symptoms and take them seriously. Reach for the adrenaline (epinephrine) if you think you are beginning to show signs of a severe reaction. Do not wait until you are sure. Even if adrenaline is administered, you will still need to get to hospital as soon as possible. Someone must call an ambulance.

- Make sure others in your family know how to administer the adrenaline kit—and when. Do not be frightened of adrenaline. It is a well-understood drug. The dose you will administer has very few side effects, which will pass quickly in any case. However, if you have heart difficulties, discuss these with your doctor.

- Develop a crisis plan for how to handle an emergency. Get your allergist or GP [general practitioner] to help. Have this written out for family and friends—put it on the bulletin board at home; carry one in your pocket. If a child is the person at risk, make sure his teachers and friends' parents have a copy—along with the adrenaline. Make sure everyone knows where the adrenaline is when you go out or when you are at home.

- Wear a Medic Alert talisman.

- Be open about your allergy problem with your family, friends, and colleagues. It's easy to avoid a Thai, Chinese, or Indian restaurant if everyone knows you are allergic to peanuts.

What should I do if I think I am having a serious reaction?

Follow your crisis plan. These are some key points:

- Is there a marked difficulty in breathing or swallowing? Is there sudden weakness or floppiness? Is there a steady deterioration? Any of these are signs of a serious reaction.

- Administer adrenaline (epinephrine) without delay if you believe the symptoms are serious or becoming serious.

- Dial 911 or get someone else to do it.

Part Three

Foods and Food Additives
That Trigger Allergic Reactions

Chapter 17

Understanding Food Allergy

Introduction

Food allergy affects up to 6 to 8 percent of children under the age of three and 2 percent of adults. If you have an unpleasant reaction to something you have eaten, you might wonder if you have a food allergy. One out of three people either believe they have a food allergy or modify their or their family's diet. Thus, while food allergy is commonly suspected, health care providers diagnose it less frequently than most people believe.

This text describes allergic reactions to foods and their possible causes as well as the best ways to diagnose and treat allergic reactions to food. It also describes other reactions to foods, known as food intolerances, which can be confused with food allergy, and describes some unproven and controversial food allergy theories.

What Is Food Allergy?

Food allergy is an abnormal response to a food triggered by the body's immune system.

Allergic reactions to food can cause serious illness and, in some cases, death. Therefore, if you have a food allergy, it is extremely important

From the pamphlet "Food Allergy: An Overview," by the National Institute of Allergy and Infectious Diseases (NIAID, www.niaid.nih.gov), part of the National Institutes of Health, NIH Publication No. 04-5518, July 2004.

for you to work with your health care provider to find out what food(s) causes your allergic reaction.

Sometimes, a reaction to food is not an allergy at all but another type of reaction called food intolerance.

Food intolerance is more common than food allergy. The immune system does not cause the symptoms of a food intolerance, though these symptoms can look and feel like those of a food allergy.

How Do Allergic Reactions Work?

An immediate allergic reaction involves two actions of your immune system.

- Your immune system produces immunoglobulin E (IgE), a type of protein that works against a specific food. This protein is called a food-specific antibody, and it circulates through the blood.

- The food-specific IgE then attaches to mast cells, cells found in all body tissues. They are more often found in areas of your body that are typical sites of allergic reactions. Those sites include your nose, throat, lungs, skin, and gastrointestinal (GI) tract.

Generally, your immune system will form IgE against a food if you come from a family in which allergies are common—not necessarily food allergies but perhaps other allergic diseases such as hay fever or asthma. If you have two allergic parents, you are more likely to develop food allergy than someone with one allergic parent.

If your immune system is inclined to form IgE to certain foods, you must be exposed to the food before you can have an allergic reaction.

- As this food is digested, it triggers certain cells in your body to produce a food-specific IgE in large amounts. The food-specific IgE is then released and attaches to the surfaces of mast cells.

- The next time you eat that food, it interacts with food-specific IgE on the surface of the mast cells and triggers the cells to release chemicals such as histamine.

- Depending upon the tissue in which they are released, these chemicals will cause you to have various symptoms of food allergy.

Food allergens are proteins within the food that enter your bloodstream after the food is digested. From there, they go to target organs, such as your skin or nose, and cause allergic reactions.

An allergic reaction to food can take place within a few minutes to an hour. The process of eating and digesting food affects the timing and the location of a reaction.

- If you are allergic to a particular food, you may first feel itching in your mouth as you start to eat the food.

- After the food is digested in your stomach, you may have GI symptoms such as vomiting, diarrhea, or pain.

- When the food allergens enter and travel through your bloodstream, they may cause your blood pressure to drop.

- As the allergens reach your skin, they can cause hives or eczema.

- When the allergens reach your lungs, they may cause asthma.

Cross-Reactivity

If you have a life-threatening reaction to a certain food, your health care provider will show you how to avoid similar foods that might trigger this reaction. For example, if you have a history of allergy to shrimp, testing will usually show that you are not only allergic to shrimp but also to crab, lobster, and crayfish. This is called cross-reactivity.

Another interesting example of cross-reactivity occurs in people who are highly sensitive to ragweed. During ragweed pollen season, they sometimes find that when they try to eat melons, particularly cantaloupe, they experience itching in their mouths and simply cannot eat the melon. Similarly, people who have severe birch pollen allergy also may react to apple peels. This is called the oral allergy syndrome.

Common Food Allergies

In adults, the foods that most often cause allergic reactions include:

- shellfish such as shrimp, crayfish, lobster, and crab;
- peanuts;
- tree nuts such as walnuts;
- fish; and
- eggs.

The most common foods that cause problems in children are:

- eggs;

205

- milk; and
- peanuts.

Tree nuts and peanuts are the leading causes of deadly food allergy reactions called anaphylaxis.

Adults usually keep their allergies for life, but children sometimes outgrow them. Children are more likely to outgrow allergies to milk or soy, however, than allergies to peanuts or shrimp. The foods to which adults or children usually react are those foods they eat often. In Japan, for example, rice allergy is more frequent. In Scandinavia, codfish allergy is more common.

Food Allergy or Food Intolerance?

If you go to your health care provider and say, "I think I have a food allergy," your provider has to consider other possibilities that may cause symptoms and could be confused with food allergy, such as food intolerance. To find out the difference between food allergy and food intolerance, your provider will go through a list of possible causes for your symptoms. This is called a differential diagnosis. This type of diagnosis helps confirm that you do indeed have a food allergy rather than a food intolerance or other illness.

Types of Food Intolerance

Food Poisoning

One possible cause of symptoms like those of food allergy is foods contaminated with microbes, such as bacteria, and bacterial products, such as toxins. Contaminated meat and dairy products sometimes cause symptoms, including GI discomfort, that resemble a food allergy when it is really a type of food poisoning.

Histamine Toxicity

There are substances, such as histamine present in certain foods, that cause a reaction like an allergic reaction. For example, histamine can reach high levels in cheese, some wines, and certain kinds of fish such as tuna and mackerel.

In fish, histamine is believed to come from contamination by bacteria, particularly in fish that are not refrigerated properly. If you eat one of these foods with a high level of histamine, you could have a reaction that strongly resembles an allergic reaction to food. This reaction is called histamine toxicity.

Lactose Intolerance

Another cause of food intolerance confused with a food allergy is lactose intolerance or lactase deficiency. This common food intolerance affects at least one out of ten people.

- Lactase is an enzyme that is in the lining of the gut.
- Lactase breaks down lactose, a sugar found in milk and most milk products.
- There is not enough lactase in the gut to digest lactose.
- Lactose, instead, is used by bacteria to form gas, which causes bloating, abdominal pain, and sometimes diarrhea. There are tests your health care provider can use to find out whether your body can digest lactose.

Food Additives

Another type of food intolerance is a reaction to certain products that are added to food to enhance taste, provide color, or protect against the growth of microbes. Several compounds, such as MSG (monosodium glutamate) and sulfites, are tied to reactions that can be confused with food allergy.

MSG: MSG is a flavor enhancer, and, when taken in large amounts, can cause some of the following signs:

- flushing;
- sensations of warmth;
- headache;
- chest discomfort; and
- feelings of detachment.

These passing reactions occur rapidly after eating large amounts of food to which MSG has been added.

Sulfites: Sulfites occur naturally in foods or may be added to increase crispness or prevent mold growth. Sulfites in high concentrations sometimes pose problems for people with severe asthma. Sulfites can give off a gas called sulfur dioxide that the asthmatic person inhales while eating the sulfited food. This irritates the lungs and can send an asthmatic person into severe bronchospasm, a tightening of the lungs.

The Food and Drug Administration (FDA) has banned sulfites as spray-on preservatives in fresh fruits and vegetables. Sulfites are still used in some foods, however, and occur naturally during the fermentation of wine.

Gluten Intolerance

Gluten intolerance is associated with the disease called gluten-sensitive enteropathy, or celiac disease. It happens if your immune system responds abnormally to gluten, which is a part of wheat and some other grains.

Psychological Causes

Some people may have a food intolerance that has a psychological trigger. If your food intolerance is caused by this type of trigger, a careful psychiatric evaluation may identify an unpleasant event in your life, often during childhood, tied to eating a particular food. Eating that food years later, even as an adult, is associated with a rush of unpleasant sensations.

Other Causes

There are several other conditions, including ulcers and cancers of the GI tract, that cause some of the same symptoms as food allergy. These problems include vomiting, diarrhea, and cramping and abdominal pain made worse by eating.

Diagnosis

After ruling out food intolerances and other health problems, your health care provider will use several steps to find out if you have an allergy to specific foods.

Detailed History

This technique is the most valuable. Your provider will ask you several questions and listen to your history of food reactions to decide if the facts go with a food allergy.

- What was the timing of your reaction?

- Did your reaction come on quickly, usually within an hour after eating the food?

- Did allergy medicines help? Antihistamines should relieve hives, for example.

- Is your reaction always associated with a certain food?

- Did anyone else who ate the same food get sick? For example, if you ate fish contaminated with histamine, everyone who ate the fish should be sick.

- How much did you eat before you had a reaction? The severity of a reaction is sometimes related to the amount of food eaten.

- How was the food prepared? Some people will have a violent allergic reaction only to raw or undercooked fish. Complete cooking of the fish may destroy the allergen, and they can then eat it with no allergic reaction.

- Did you eat other foods at the same time you had the reaction? Some foods may delay digestion and thus delay the start of the allergic reaction.

Diet Diary

Sometimes your health care provider can't make a diagnosis solely on the basis of your history. In that case, you may be asked to keep a record of the contents of each meal you eat and whether you have a reaction. This gives more detail from which you and your provider can see if there is a consistent pattern in your reactions.

Elimination Diet

The next step some health care providers use is an elimination diet. Under your provider's direction:

- You don't eat a food suspected of causing the allergy, such as eggs.

- You then substitute another food—in the case of eggs, another source of protein.

- Your provider can almost always make a diagnosis if the symptoms go away after you remove the food from your diet.

The diagnosis is confirmed if you then eat the food and the symptoms come back. You should do this only when the reactions are not significant and under health care provider direction.

209

Your provider can't use this technique, however, if your reactions are severe or don't happen often. If you have a severe reaction, you should not eat the food again.

Skin Test

If your history, diet diary, or elimination diet suggests a specific food allergy is likely, your health care provider will then use tests to confirm the diagnosis.

One of these is a scratch skin test, during which an extract of the food is placed on the skin of your lower arm. Your provider will then scratch this portion of your skin with a needle and look for swelling or redness, which would be a sign of a local allergic reaction. If the scratch test is positive, it means that there is IgE on the skin's mast cells that is specific to the food being tested. Skin tests are rapid, simple, and relatively safe.

You can have a positive skin test to a food allergen, however, without having an allergic reaction to that food. A health care provider diagnoses a food allergy only when someone has a positive skin test to a specific allergen and the history of reactions suggests an allergy to the same food.

Blood Test

If you are extremely allergic and have severe anaphylactic reactions, your health care provider cannot use skin testing because causing an allergic reaction could be dangerous. Skin testing also cannot be done if you have eczema over a large portion of your body.

In those cases, a health care provider may use blood tests such as the RAST (radioallergosorbent test) or the ELISA (enzyme-linked immunosorbent assay). These tests measure the presence of food-specific IgE in your blood. As with skin testing, positive tests do not necessarily mean you have a food allergy.

Double-Blind Food Challenge

The final method health care providers use to diagnose food allergy is double-blind food challenge. This testing has come to be the "gold standard" of allergy testing.

- Your health care provider will give you individual opaque capsules containing various foods, some of which are suspected of starting an allergic reaction.

- You swallow a capsule and are watched to see if a reaction occurs. This process is repeated until you have swallowed all the capsules.

In a true double-blind test, your health care provider is also "blinded" (the capsules having been made up by another medical person). In that case your provider does not know which capsule contains the allergen.

The advantage of such a challenge is that if you react only to suspected foods and not to other foods tested, it confirms the diagnosis. You cannot be tested this way if you have a history of severe allergic reactions.

In addition, this testing is difficult because it takes a lot of time to perform and many food allergies are difficult to evaluate with this procedure. Consequently, health care providers seldom do double-blind food challenges.

This type of testing is most commonly used if your health care provider thinks the reaction you describe is not due to a specific food and wishes to obtain evidence to support this. If your provider finds that your reaction is not due to a specific food, then additional efforts may be used to find the real cause of the reaction.

Treatment

Food allergy is treated by avoiding the foods that trigger the reaction. Once you and your health care provider have identified the food(s) to which you are sensitive, you must remove them from your diet. To do this, you must read the detailed ingredient lists on each food you are considering eating.

Many allergy-producing foods such as peanuts, eggs, and milk, appear in foods one normally would not associate them with. Peanuts, for example, are often used as a protein source, and eggs are used in some salad dressings.

FDA requires ingredients in a packaged food to appear on its label. You can avoid most of the things to which you are sensitive if you read food labels carefully and avoid restaurant-prepared foods that might have ingredients to which you are allergic.

If you are highly allergic, even the tiniest amounts of a food allergen (for example, a small portion of a peanut kernel) can prompt an allergic reaction.

If you have severe food allergies, you must be prepared to treat unintentional exposure. Even people who know a lot about what they are sensitive to occasionally make a mistake. To protect yourself if you have had allergic reactions to a food, you should:

- wear a medical alert bracelet or necklace stating that you have a food allergy and are subject to severe reactions;

- carry a syringe of adrenaline (epinephrine), obtained by pre- scription from your health care provider, and be prepared to give it to yourself if you think you are getting a food allergic reaction; and

- seek medical help immediately by either calling the rescue squad or by getting transported to an emergency room.

Anaphylactic allergic reactions can be fatal even when they start off with mild symptoms such as a tingling in the mouth and throat or GI discomfort.

Schools and day care centers must have plans in place to address any food allergy emergency. Parents and caregivers should take spe- cial care with children and learn how to:

- protect children from foods to which they are allergic;

- manage children if they eat a food to which they are allergic; and

- give children epinephrine.

There are several medicines that you can take to relieve food al- lergy symptoms that are not part of an anaphylactic reaction. These include:

- antihistamines to relieve GI symptoms, hives, or sneezing and a runny nose and

- bronchodilators to relieve asthma symptoms.

You should take these medicines if you have accidentally eaten a food to which you are allergic. They do not prevent an allergic reac- tion when taken before eating the food. No medicine in any form will reliably prevent an allergic reaction to that food before eating it.

Exercise-Induced Food Allergy

At least one situation may require more than simply eating food with allergens to start a reaction: exercise-induced food allergy. People who have this reaction only experience it after eating a specific food before exercising. As exercise increases and body temperature rises, itching and lightheadedness start and allergic reactions such as hives may appear and even anaphylaxis may develop.

The cure for exercised-induced food allergy is simple—avoid eating for a couple of hours before exercising.

Food Allergy in Infants and Children

Allergy to cow's milk is particularly common in infants and young children. In addition to causing hives and asthma, it can lead to colic and sleeplessness, and perhaps blood in the stool or poor growth. Infants are thought to be particularly susceptible to this allergic syndrome because their immune and digestive systems are immature. Milk allergy can develop within days to months of birth.

If your baby is on cow's milk formula, your provider may suggest a change to soy formula or an elemental formula if possible. Elemental formulas are produced from processed proteins with supplements added (basically sugars and amino acids). There are few if any allergens within these materials.

Health care providers sometimes prescribe glucocorticosteroid drugs to treat infants with very severe GI reactions to milk formulas. Fortunately, this food allergy tends to go away within the first few years of life.

Breastfeeding often helps babies avoid feeding problems related to allergic reactions. Therefore, health experts often suggest that mothers feed their babies only breast milk for the first 6 to 12 months of life to avoid milk allergy from developing within that time frame.

Some babies are very sensitive to a certain food. If you are nursing and eat that food, sufficient amounts can enter your breast milk to cause a food reaction in your baby. To keep possible food allergens out of your breast milk, you might try not eating those foods that could cause an allergic reaction in your baby, such as peanuts.

There is no conclusive evidence that breastfeeding prevents allergies from developing later in your child's life. It does, however, delay the start of food allergies by delaying your infant's exposure to those foods that can prompt allergies. Plus, it may avoid altogether food allergy problems sometimes seen in infants.

By delaying the introduction of solid foods until your baby is 6 months old or older, you can also prolong your baby's allergy-free period. In addition, the American Academy of Pediatrics recommends you delay adding eggs to your child's diet until he or she is 2 years old and peanuts, tree nuts, and fish until he or she is 3 years old.

Some Controversial and Unproven Theories

There are several disorders that are popularly thought by some to be caused by food allergies. There is not enough scientific evidence or evidence that does exist goes against such claims.

Migraine Headaches

There is controversy about whether migraine headaches can be caused by food allergy. Studies show people who are prone to migraines can have their headaches brought on by histamines and other substances in foods. The more difficult issue is whether food allergies actually cause migraines in such people.

Arthritis

There is virtually no evidence that most rheumatoid arthritis or osteoarthritis can be made worse by foods, despite claims to the contrary.

Allergic Tension Fatigue Syndrome

There is no evidence that food allergies can cause a disorder called the allergic tension fatigue syndrome, in which people are tired, nervous, and may have problems concentrating, or have headaches.

Cerebral Allergy

Cerebral allergy is a term that has been given to people who have trouble concentrating and have headaches as well as other complaints. These symptoms are sometimes blamed on mast cells activated in the brain but no other place in the body. Researchers have found no evidence that such a scenario can happen. Most health experts do not recognize cerebral allergy as a disorder.

Environmental Illness

In a seemingly pristine environment, some people have many non-specific complaints such as problems concentrating or depression. Sometimes this is blamed on small amounts of allergens or toxins in the environment. There is no evidence that such problems are due to food allergies.

Childhood Hyperactivity

Some people believe hyperactivity in children is caused by food allergies. But researchers have found that this behavioral disorder in children is only occasionally associated with food additives, and then only when such additives are consumed in large amounts. There is no evidence that a true food allergy can affect a child's activity except for the possibility that if a child itches and sneezes and wheezes a lot, the child may be uncomfortable and therefore more difficult to guide. Also, children who are on antiallergy medicines that cause drowsiness may get sleepy in school or at home.

Controversial and Unproven Diagnostic Methods

Cytotoxicity Testing: One controversial diagnostic technique is cytotoxicity testing, in which a food allergen is added to your blood sample. A technician then examines the sample under the microscope to see if white cells in the blood "die." Scientists have evaluated this technique in several studies and have found it does not effectively diagnose food allergy.

Provocative Challenge: Another controversial approach is called sublingual (placed under the tongue) or subcutaneous (injected under the skin) provocative challenge. In this procedure, diluted food allergen is put under your tongue if you feel that your arthritis, for instance, is due to foods. The technician then asks you if the food allergen has made your arthritis symptoms worse. In clinical studies, researchers have not shown that this procedure can effectively diagnose food allergy.

Immune Complex Assay: An immune complex assay is sometimes done on people suspected of having food allergies to see if groups, or complexes, of certain antibodies connect to the food allergen in the bloodstream. Some think that these immune groups link with food allergies. But the formation of such immune complexes is a normal offshoot of food digestion, and everyone, if tested with a sensitive enough measurement, has them. To date, no one has conclusively shown that this test links with allergies to foods.

IgG Subclass Assay: Another test is the IgG subclass assay, which looks specifically for certain kinds of IgG antibody. Again, there is no evidence that this diagnoses food allergy.

Controversial and Unproven Treatments

Controversial treatments include putting a diluted solution of a particular food under your tongue about a half hour before you eat the food suspected of causing an allergic reaction. This is an attempt to "neutralize" the subsequent exposure to the food that you believe is harmful. The results of a carefully conducted clinical study show this procedure does not prevent an allergic reaction.

Allergy Shots: Another unproven treatment involves getting shots (immunotherapy) containing small quantities of the food extracts to which you are allergic. These shots are given regularly for a long period of time with the aim of "desensitizing" you to the food allergen. Researchers have not yet proven that allergy shots reliably relieve food allergies.

Research

The National Institute of Allergy and Infectious Diseases does research on food allergy and other allergic diseases. This research is focused on understanding what happens to the body during the allergic process—the sequence of events leading to the allergic response and the factors responsible for allergic diseases. This understanding will lead to better methods of diagnosing, preventing, and treating allergic diseases. Researchers also are looking at better ways to study allergic reactions to foods.

One study by the Johns Hopkins Children's Center showed that simply washing your hands with soap and water will remove peanut allergens. Also, most household cleaners will remove them from surfaces such as food preparation areas at home as well as day care facilities and schools. These easy-to-do measures will help prevent peanut allergy reactions in children and adults.

Educating people, including patients, health care providers, school teachers, and day care workers, about the importance of food allergy is also an important research focus. The more people know about the disorder, the better equipped they will be to control food allergies.

Chapter 18

Food Allergy Myths and Facts

Do you, or someone you know, shun certain foods because you are "allergic?" Surveys show that nearly one third of all adults believe they have a food allergy. The following text seeks to shed light on such frequently asked questions as: What is a food allergy? How do you know if you have one? What should you do if you have a food allergy? And, if it is not a food allergy, what might it be?

Myth: Lots of people have food allergies.

Reality: "From talking with the public, you might think almost everyone has a food allergy," said Daryl Altman, M.D., Fellow of the American College of Allergy, Asthma and Immunology and researcher at Allergy Information Services in Long Island, New York. "In surveys, nearly one in three American adults indicated he or she was allergic to some food." But in reality, the most conservative estimates indicate two percent of the population in the United States are food allergic. Children are more susceptible than adults to food allergy—up to five percent have some type of food allergy. However, common allergens such as eggs and milk are typically outgrown by age five.

The eight most common food allergens in people are: Peanuts, tree nuts (for example, almonds, pecans, and walnuts), dairy, soy, wheat, eggs, fish, and shellfish (for example, shrimp and crab). Nevertheless, allergies to nearly 175 different types of food have been documented. "These foods are responsible for over 90 percent of serious allergic reactions to food," stated Susan L. Hefle, Ph.D., co-director of the Food Allergy Research and Resource Program at the University of Nebraska-Lincoln.

Myth: A food allergy means I'll just get a runny nose, right?

Reality: No—although food allergy is rare, it is a serious condition and should be diagnosed by a board-certified allergist. Food allergy is a reaction of the body's immune system to a certain component, usually a protein, in a food or ingredient. The reactions can be uncomfortable and mild including vomiting, diarrhea, skin rashes or runny nose, sneezing, coughing, and wheezing, and may occur within hours or days after eating. However, anaphylaxis, a more serious and life-threatening reaction, may occur. Anaphylaxis is a rapidly occurring reaction that often involves hives and swelling, enlarging of the larynx with a choking sensation, wheezing, severe vomiting, diarrhea, and even shock. These symptoms can also occur within minutes, hours, or days. "Food allergic patients should have an anaphylaxis reaction plan worked out ahead of time with their allergist," according to Anne Muñoz-Furlong, president and founder of the Food Allergy & Anaphylaxis Network. "The plan should be practiced with family and friends in case of an emergency."

Allergic Reactions: An allergic reaction occurs when a susceptible person is exposed to a specific protein. Because the body perceives this protein (an allergen) as being a threat, it produces a special material—a substance that recognizes allergens—known as immunoglobulin E (IgE) antibody. A person who has a tendency to develop allergies tends to produce increased amounts of IgE. After the initial exposure to a specific allergen (such as cat or dog protein) the body reacts to future exposures by creating millions of IgE antibodies. These newly produced IgE antibodies then connect to special blood cells called basophils, and special tissue cells called mast cells. These cells are then "stimulated" to release histamine that causes the allergy symptoms: Itchy watery eyes and nose, scratchy throat, rashes, hives, eczema, and even life-threatening anaphylaxis.

Myth: Any negative reaction to a food is a food allergy.

Reality: Adverse reactions to food can have many causes. If something does not agree with you, it does not necessarily mean you are allergic to it. Food allergy is a very specific reaction involving the immune system of the body, and it is important to distinguish food allergy from other food sensitivities. Whereas food allergies are rare, food intolerances, which are the other classification of food sensitivities, are more common. Intolerances are reactions to foods or ingredients that do not involve the body's immune system. Intolerance reactions are generally localized, transient, and rarely life threatening with one possible exception—sulfite sensitivity. "A good example of a food intolerance is lactose intolerance. And, it is extremely important to know the difference between it and a milk allergy," said Robert K. Bush, M.D., University of Wisconsin. He emphasized that, "Whereas lactose intolerance may result in a bloated feeling or flatulence after consuming milk or dairy products, milk allergy can have life-threatening consequences. The milk allergic patient must avoid all milk proteins."

Myth: I think I'm allergic to a food—I just won't eat it, so I don't need to be seen by a doctor.

Reality: Just thinking you are allergic to a food does not mean you have an allergy. To properly diagnose a food allergy or sensitivity, the offending substance must be accurately identified. Avoiding a food may deprive you of food choices and important nutrients, and could be dangerous if the allergen is actually different. Diagnosis of a food allergy can be complex, with three major components. The first and most important involves a board-certified allergist, preferably a food allergy specialist. Second, a history of a specific food causing an allergic reaction is necessary; a food diary can help. Third, an IgE antibodies test is only useful when combined with the former components, but it does not always pinpoint a food allergy. Hugh Sampson, M.D., director, Food Allergy Clinic, Mt. Sinai Medical Center, and chair of the American Academy of Allergy, Asthma and Immunology's Adverse Reactions to Foods Committee, emphasized an examination by a board-certified allergist: "Due to many people claiming to have food allergies, many physicians have become 'desensitized' to taking their symptoms seriously."

Double-Blind Placebo-Controlled Food Challenge: This test, considered the gold standard for food allergy testing, is performed by a board-certified allergist. The suspected allergen is placed in a capsule or hidden in food, and fed to the patient under strict supervision. Neither the allergist, nor the patient, is aware of which capsule, or food, contains the suspected allergen—hence the name double-blind.

In order for the test to be effective, the patient must also be fed capsules or food which do not contain the allergen to make sure the reaction, if any, being observed is to the allergen and not some other factor—hence the name placebo-controlled. It is tests of this kind that have enabled allergists to identify the most common allergens, and also to determine what foods, ingredients, and additives do not cause allergic reactions.

Myth: I don't frequently eat food I'm allergic to, so I can eat a little bit for a special occasion.

Reality: Because food allergy can be life threatening, the allergen must be completely avoided—even the most minute amounts. Although an extreme case, a man allergic to shellfish died of anaphylaxis shock after encountering simply the steam from shrimp. It can be fatal to assume a given food environment is safe and not be cautious. A board-certified allergist can help the food allergic patient manage diet issues without sacrificing nutrition or pleasure when eating at and away from home. Since most life-threatening, and sometimes fatal, allergic reactions to foods occur when eating away from home, it is imperative that the food-allergic individual or responsible guardian clearly explain the risks of exposure to a certain food or ingredient to food service workers, family, and friends—and always ask before eating.

Myth: With all the ingredients in processed food I can never completely avoid my allergen.

Reality: When purchasing groceries, labels should be read for every product purchased—every time. Although food and beverage manufacturers are often improving and changing their products, changes in ingredients must be listed on ingredient labels.

According to Fred Shank, Ph.D., director of the Center for Food Safety and Applied Nutrition, Food and Drug Administration (FDA), "Foods which contain allergenic substances must be properly labeled or be subject to recall. The FDA supports the activities of independent organizations to inform consumers of these recall activities." The FDA includes on its list of recall substances all eight of the major allergens, so if these substances are present in a food, but not listed on the label, they must be recalled. Additionally, substances which cause non-allergic-based reactions, such as the additives sulfites and tartrazine (FD&C Yellow #5), are on this list. Some individuals have unique sensitivities to these food components which are not allergenic or allergy-causing in nature, but may cause comparably severe reactions.

Sulfite Sensitivity: Sulfiting agents are commonly used to preserve the color of foods, such as dried fruits and vegetables, and to inhibit the growth of microorganisms in fermented foods, like wine. Sulfites can also be found in beer, some fruit drinks, shrimp, and some prepared foods. Although sulfites are safe for the majority of people, for some, they have been found to cause a reaction. For this reason, the FDA requires that when sulfites are added to foods in greater than 10 parts/million (or, 10 sulfite molecules per million molecules) they must be indicated on the label.

Myth: Since I'm allergic to peanuts, I can't eat anything with peanut oil.

Reality: There are many misunderstandings regarding exactly what might stimulate the food allergic reaction. "Virtually all food allergens are proteins," explained Steve L. Taylor, Ph.D., co-director of the Food Allergy Research and Resource Program at the University of Nebraska-Lincoln. "And, the process of refining oil removes the protein which would trigger an allergic reaction." Oils used in processed foods and in cosmetics are highly refined and should pose no problem for the food allergic individual. Yet, caution should be taken with natural, cold pressed, or flavored oils. These oils, as well as oil that has been used to cook peanuts (or another food to which an individual might have an allergy), might contain the protein of the allergen and should be avoided. For example, an individual with a fish allergy should ensure that the oil used to cook his or her food was not first used to fry fish.

Myth: I'm allergic to food additives.

Reality: Other common misconceptions regarding food allergy are additives and preservatives. Although some—sulfites and tartrazine— have been shown to trigger asthma or hives in certain people, these reactions do not follow the same pathway observed with food. There are other food additives that have historically been associated with adverse reactions, but because they do not contain proteins or involve the immune system, true allergic pathways cannot be used to explain the reported reactions. In addition, many of these additives, including monosodium glutamate, aspartame, and most food dyes have been studied extensively, and the results show little scientific evidence exists to suggest they cause any reaction at all.

Avoid Cross Contact: Cross contact of foods with those that may present a food allergy problem is poorly understood and not well communicated. Although food processors are well aware of the dangers of cross contact and manage them appropriately, such caution is not always taken in the home, school cafeteria, or restaurant. Although unintentional, the effects can be devastating. For some food allergic individuals, the most minute particle of the allergen can be fatal. Some examples of mishaps that can induce a food allergic reaction include:

- Plain chocolate brownies are served using the same spatula that was used to serve peanut-containing brownies.
- French fries are prepared in the same oil used to deep fry fish.

Myth: "Tell me about my corn allergy."

Reality: There are those suspected food allergies that are so rare that their existence is questioned. The most common of these are corn and chocolate "allergy," and there are several probable explanations for adverse reactions. Even though many people claim to be allergic to them, allergists can rarely demonstrate allergy to corn or chocolate in double-blind, placebo-controlled food challenges.

Corn "allergy" is often associated with a reaction to another allergenic substance. In some cases soy allergic individuals may react to products containing corn. Occasionally corn is carried, handled, or stored in the same containers used for soy. Although only minute residues of soy may remain, this can be enough to cause an allergic reaction in highly sensitive people.

Chocolate "allergy" is also thought to be extremely rare, and though some are truly chocolate-allergic, most who complain of symptoms have irreproducible reactions. Possibly the reactions are due to another ingredient found in the chocolate product being consumed.

Food allergy is certainly nothing to be taken lightly. Although its prevalence appears to be increasing, overreaction, self-diagnosis, and incorrect assumptions only lead to skepticism of physicians and food service workers—obviously, a less-than-ideal situation for the truly allergic individual. It is vitally important to leave the diagnosis of a food allergy to a board-certified allergist.

Chapter 19

Egg Allergy

Chapter Contents

Section 19.1

What Is Egg Allergy?

"Eggs: One of the nine most common food allergens,"
reprinted with permission from the Canadian Food Inspection Agency,
© 2006.

Allergic Reactions

Anaphylactic reactions are severe allergic reactions that occur when the body's immune system overreacts to a particular allergen. These reactions may be caused by food, insect stings, latex, medications, and other substances. The nine priority food allergens are peanuts, tree nuts, sesame seeds, milk, eggs, seafood (fish, crustaceans, and shellfish), soy, wheat, and sulfites (a food additive).

What are the symptoms of an allergic reaction?

When someone comes in contact with an allergen, the symptoms of a reaction may develop without warning, may be delayed, may happen as two episodes (biphasic), or may develop quickly then rapidly progress from mild to severe. The most dangerous symptoms include breathing difficulties, a drop in blood pressure, or shock, which may result in loss of consciousness and even death. A person experiencing an allergic reaction may have any of the following symptoms:

- trouble breathing, speaking, or swallowing;
- a drop in blood pressure, rapid heartbeat, or loss of consciousness;
- flushed face, hives or a rash, or red and itchy skin;
- swelling of the eyes, face, lips, throat, and tongue;
- anxiousness, distress, faintness, paleness, sense of doom, weakness; and
- cramps, diarrhea, or vomiting.

224

How are food allergies and severe food allergy reactions treated?

Currently there is no cure for food allergies. The only option is complete avoidance of the specific allergen. Appropriate emergency treatment for a severe food allergy reaction includes an injection of epinephrine (adrenalin), which is available in an auto-injector device. Epinephrine must be administered as soon as symptoms of a severe allergic reaction appear. The injection must be followed by further treatment and observation in a hospital emergency room. If your allergist has diagnosed you with a food allergy and prescribed epinephrine, carry it with you all the time and know how to use it. Follow your allergist's advice on how to use an epinephrine auto-injector device.

Frequently Asked Questions about Egg Allergies

I have an egg allergy. How can I avoid an egg-related reaction?

Avoid all food and products that contain egg and egg derivatives, including any product whose ingredient list warns it "may contain" egg.

Can an egg allergy be outgrown?

Studies show that most children outgrow their egg allergy by three years of age. However, a severe egg allergy can last a lifetime. Consult your allergist before reintroducing egg products.

Can a person who is allergic to raw eggs eat cooked eggs?

Usually not. While cooking can alter the protein of a raw egg, it may not be sufficient to prevent a reaction. Consult your allergist before experimenting.

Are flu and MMR shots safe for someone with an egg allergy?

Influenza vaccines are grown on egg embryos and may contain a small amount of egg protein. Consult your allergist before getting a flu shot. Although the MMR (Measles, Mumps, and Rubella) vaccine may contain egg protein, it is considered safe for children.

How can I determine if a product contains egg or egg derivatives?

Always read the ingredient list carefully. Egg and egg derivatives can often be present under different names, e.g., albumin.

What do I do if I am not sure whether a product contains egg or egg derivatives?

If you have an egg allergy, do not eat or use the product. Get ingredient information from the manufacturer.

Watch out for allergen cross contamination!

Cross contamination is the transfer of an ingredient (food allergen) to a product that does not normally have that ingredient in it. Through cross contamination, a food that should not contain the allergen could become dangerous to eat for those who are allergic.

Cross contamination can happen:

- during food manufacturing through shared production and packaging equipment;
- at retail through shared equipment, e.g., cheese and deli meats sliced on the same slicer; and through bulk display of food products, e.g., bins of baked goods, bulk nuts; and
- during food preparation at home or in restaurants through equipment, utensils and hands.

Avoiding Egg and Egg Derivatives

Make sure you read product labels carefully to avoid products that contain egg and egg derivatives. Avoid food and products that do not have an ingredient list and read labels every time you shop. Manufacturers may occasionally change their recipes or use different ingredients for varieties of the same brand. Refer to the following list before shopping:

Other Names for Eggs

- Albumin/Albumen
- Conalbumin
- Egg substitutes, e.g., Egg Beaters®

- Globulin
- Livetin
- Lysozyme
- Meringue
- Ovalbumin
- Ovoglobulin
- Ovolactohydrolyze proteins
- Ovomacroglobulin
- Ovomucin, ovomucoid
- Ovotransferrin
- Ovovitellin
- Silico-albuminate
- Simplesse®
- Vitellin

Possible Sources of Eggs

Note: Avoid all food and products that contain egg in the ingredient list, e.g., powdered egg. The terms "ovo" and "albumin" mean the product contains egg.

- Alcoholic cocktails/drinks
- Baby food
- Baked goods and baking mixes, e.g., breads, cakes, cookies, doughnuts, muffins, pancakes, pastries, pretzels
- Battered/fried foods
- Confectionary, e.g., candy, chocolate
- Cream-filled pies, e.g. banana, chocolate, coconut
- Creamy dressings, salad dressings, spreads, e.g., mayonnaise, Caesar salad dressing, tartar sauce
- Desserts, e.g., custard, dessert mixes, ice cream, meringue, pudding, sorbet
- Egg/fat substitutes
- Fish mixtures, e.g., surimi (used to make imitation crab/lobster meat)
- Foam/milk topping on coffee

- Homemade root beer, malt drink mixes
- Icing, glazes, e.g., egg wash on baked goods, nougat
- Lecithin
- Meat mixtures, e.g., hamburger, hot dogs, meatballs, meatloaf, salami, etc.
- Orange Julep®, Orange Julius® (orange juice beverages)
- Pasta, e.g., egg noodles
- Quiche, soufflé
- Sauces, e.g., béarnaise, hollandaise, Newburgh
- Soups, broths, bouillons

Non-Food Sources of Eggs

- Anesthetic, e.g., Diprivan® (propofol)
- Certain vaccines, e.g., MMR (measles, mumps, and rubella)
- Craft materials
- Hair care products
- Medications

Note: These lists are not complete and may change. Food and food products purchased from other countries, through mail order or the internet, are not always produced using the same manufacturing and labeling standards.

What Can I Do?

Be Informed: See an allergist and educate yourself about food allergies. Contact your local allergy association for further information.

Before Eating: Allergists recommend that if you do not have your epinephrine auto-injector device with you, that you do not eat. If an ingredient list says a product "may contain" or "does contain" egg or egg derivatives, do not eat it. If you do not recognize an ingredient or there is no ingredient list available, avoid the product.

Section 19.2

Tips for Managing an Egg Allergy

Baking

For each egg, substitute one of the following in recipes. These substitutes work well when baking from scratch and substituting 1 to 3 eggs.

- 1 tsp. baking powder, 1 T. liquid, 1 T. vinegar
- 1 tsp. yeast dissolved in ¼ cup warm water
- 1½ T. water, 1½ T. oil, 1 tsp. baking powder
- 1 packet gelatin, 2 T. warm water. Do not mix until ready to use.

Some Hidden Sources of Egg

- Eggs have been used to create the foam or milk topping on specialty coffee drinks and are used in some bar drinks.
- Some commercial brands of egg substitutes contain egg whites.
- Most commercially processed cooked pastas (including those used in prepared foods such as soup) contain egg or are processed on equipment shared with egg-containing pastas. Boxed, dry pastas are usually egg-free, but may be processed on equipment that is also used for egg-containing products. Fresh pasta is sometimes egg-free, too. Read the label or ask about ingredients before eating pasta.

Commonly Asked Questions

Can an MMR Vaccine be given to an individual with an egg allergy?

The recommendations of the American Academy of Pediatrics (AAP) acknowledge that the MMR [measles, mumps, rubella] vaccine can be safely administered to all patients with egg allergy. The AAP recommendations have been based, in part, on overwhelming scientific evidence supporting the routine use of one-dose administration of the MMR vaccine to egg-allergic patients. This includes those patients with a history of severe, generalized anaphylactic reactions to egg.

I've heard the flu vaccine contains egg, is this true?

Yes, influenza vaccines usually contain a small amount of egg protein.

Is a flu shot safe for an individual with an egg allergy?

Influenza vaccines are grown on egg embryos and may contain a small amount of egg protein. If you or your child is allergic to eggs, speak to your doctor before receiving a flu shot.

Can someone who is allergic to eggs have a flu shot?

Scientists suggest individuals with egg allergy be given an allergy test with the vaccine. If the test results are negative, the vaccine may be given in a single dose. If the test results are positive, individual assessment of benefits versus risk should be discussed with a doctor.

Because of a family history of allergy, I have been advised to delay the introduction of egg until my child is 2 years of age. Does this mean my child should not be given the flu shot?

Children under 23 months of age may be at higher risk for complications from influenza and are a group that typically require more hospitalizations from this sometimes fatal disease. You and your child's doctor should discuss the options. The general guideline is to follow the current CDC recommendations regarding the administration of the influenza vaccine to infants 6 to 23 months of age, unless the infant has a known clinical history of egg allergy.

Is an intranasal influenza vaccine an option for someone with an egg allergy?

The intranasal vaccine contains egg protein, and it not recommended for use in individuals with egg allergy. It is approved for use in persons ages 5 to 49 years, but it is not approved for use in patients with asthma.

Chapter 20

Milk Allergy

Almost all infants are fussy at times. But sometimes infants are excessively fussy because they have an allergy to the protein in cow's milk, which is the basis for most commercial baby formulas.

A person of any age can have a milk allergy, but it is more common among infants. Approximately 2% to 3% of infants have a milk allergy, and they typically outgrow it.

If you think that your child has a milk allergy, talk with your child's doctor. There are tests that can diagnose the condition and alternatives to milk-based formulas and dairy products that your doctor can recommend.

What Is a Milk Allergy?

A milk allergy occurs when the child's immune system mistakenly sees the milk protein as dangerous and tries to fight it off. This starts an allergic reaction, which can cause an infant to be fussy and irritable, and cause an upset stomach and other symptoms. Most children who are allergic to cow's milk also react to goat's milk and sheep's milk, and some of them are also allergic to the protein in soy milk.

"Milk Allergy in Infants" was provided by KidsHealth, one of the largest resources online for medically reviewed health information written for parents, kids, and teens. For more articles like this one, visit www.KidsHealth.org, or www.TeensHealth.org. © 2005 The Nemours Foundation. This document was reviewed by Raman Sreedharan, M.D., and Devendra Mehta, M.D., August 2005.

Infants who are breastfed have a lower risk of developing a milk allergy than infants who are formula fed, but researchers don't fully understand why some children develop a milk allergy and others don't. It's believed that in many cases, the allergy is genetic.

Typically, a milk allergy goes away on its own by the time a child is 3 to 5 years old, but some children never outgrow it.

A milk allergy is not the same thing as lactose intolerance, the inability to digest the sugar lactose, which is rare in infants and more common among older kids and adults.

Symptoms of a Milk Allergy

Symptoms of cow's milk protein allergy will generally appear within the first few months of life. An infant can experience symptoms either very quickly after feeding (rapid onset) or not until 7 to 10 days after consuming the cow's milk protein (slower onset).

The slower-onset reaction is more common. Symptoms may include loose stools (possibly containing blood), vomiting, gagging, refusing food, irritability or colic, and skin rashes. This type of reaction is more difficult to diagnose because the same symptoms may occur with other health conditions. Most children will outgrow this form of allergy by 2 years of age.

Rapid-onset reactions come on suddenly with symptoms that can include irritability, vomiting, wheezing, swelling, hives, other itchy bumps on the skin, and bloody diarrhea. In rare cases, a potentially severe allergic reaction called anaphylaxis can occur and affect the baby's skin, stomach, breathing, and blood pressure. Anaphylaxis is more common in other food allergies than in a milk allergy.

Diagnosing a Milk Allergy

If you suspect that your infant is allergic to milk, call your baby's doctor. The doctor will likely ask about any family history of allergies or food intolerance and then do a physical exam. There's no single lab test to accurately diagnose a milk allergy, so your doctor might order several tests to make the diagnosis and rule out any other health problems.

In addition to a stool test and a blood test, the doctor may order an allergy skin test, in which a small amount of the milk protein is inserted just under the surface of the child's skin with a needle. If a red, raised spot called a wheal emerges, the child may have a milk allergy.

The doctor may also request an oral challenge test. After you stop feeding your baby milk for about a week, the doctor will have the infant consume milk, then wait for a few hours to watch for any allergic reaction. Sometimes doctors repeat this test to reconfirm the diagnosis.

Treating a Milk Allergy

If your infant has a milk allergy and you are breastfeeding, it's important to restrict the amount of dairy products that you ingest because the milk protein that's causing the allergic reaction can cross into your breast milk. You may want to talk to a dietitian about finding alternative sources of calcium and other vital nutrients to replace what you were getting from dairy products.

Since January 2006, all food makers must clearly state on package labels whether the foods contain milk or milk-based products, indicating this in or next to the ingredient list on the packaging. Keep in mind, though, that this law applies only to foods packaged after the start of 2006, so some foods packaged before then may not have any information about food allergens.

If you are formula-feeding your infant, your doctor may advise you to switch to a soy protein-based formula. If your infant can't tolerate soy, the doctor may have you switch to a hypoallergenic formula, one in which the proteins are broken down into particles so that the formula is less likely to trigger an allergic reaction.

Two major types of hypoallergenic formulas are available:

- Extensively hydrolyzed formulas have cow's milk proteins that are broken down into small particles so that they are less allergenic than the whole proteins in regular formulas. Most infants who have a milk allergy can tolerate these formulas, but in some cases, they still provoke allergic reactions.

- Amino acid-based infant formulas, which contain protein in its simplest form (amino acids are the building blocks of proteins). This may be recommended if your baby's condition doesn't improve even after a switch to a hydrolyzed formula.

There are also "partially hydrolyzed" formulas on the market, but they are not considered truly hypoallergenic and they can still provoke a significant allergic reaction.

The formulas available in the market today are approved by the U.S. Food and Drug Administration (FDA) and created through a very

233

specialized process that cannot be duplicated at home. Goat's milk, rice milk, or almond milks are not safe and are not recommended for infants.

Once you switch your baby to another formula, the symptoms of the allergy should go away in 2 to 4 weeks. Your child's doctor will probably recommend that you continue with a hypoallergenic formula up until the baby's first birthday, then gradually introduce cow's milk into his or her diet.

If you have any questions or concerns, talk with your child's doctor.

Chapter 21

Tree Nut and Peanut Allergy

Chapter Contents

Section 21.1

Understanding Nut and Peanut Allergy

"Nut and Peanut Allergy" was provided by KidsHealth, one of the largest resources online for medically reviewed health information written for parents, kids, and teens. For more articles like this one, visit www.KidsHealth .org, or www.TeensHealth.org. © 2003 The Nemours Foundation. This document was reviewed by William J. Geimeier, M.D., September 2003.

First grade has been a difficult parenting year for Anne. Her 6-year-old son, Justin, began eating lunch in the cafeteria with hundreds of other students armed with their peanut butter sandwiches, peanut butter crackers, and all those hidden peanuts in their processed foods.

For Justin, who has an extremely severe allergy to peanuts, it means sitting at a separate table with other children who have food allergies. But Justin isn't alone: The U.S. Food and Drug Administration estimates that 6% of children younger than 3 years old have some kind of allergy to food, putting them at risk of an allergic reaction at home, or even more dangerously, away from home.

It seems ironic that one of the most popular, most readily available proteins causes one of the most pervasive and severe allergies among Americans.

What are nut and peanut allergies?

The most common allergy-causing foods are peanuts, tree nuts, milk, eggs, fish, shellfish, wheat, and soy, according to the Food Allergy and Anaphylaxis Network (FAAN). About 1.5 million people in the United States are allergic to peanuts (which are not a true nut, but a legume—in the same family as peas and lentils). Half of those allergic to peanuts are also allergic to tree nuts, such as almonds, walnuts, pecans, cashews, and often sunflower and sesame seeds. The American Academy of Allergy, Asthma, and Immunology estimates that up to 2 million, or 8%, of children in the United States are affected by food allergies, and that six foods account for 90% of those food allergy reactions in kids: milk, eggs, peanuts, wheat, soy, and tree nuts.

Food allergies occur when a person's immune system mistakenly believes that something he or she ate is harmful to the body. In an attempt to protect the body, the immune system produces antibodies called immunoglobulin E (IgE). Those antibodies then cause mast cells (which are allergy cells in the body) to release chemicals into the bloodstream, one of which is histamine. The histamine then acts on a person's eyes, nose, throat, lungs, skin, or gastrointestinal tract and causes the symptoms of the allergic reaction. Future exposure to that same allergen (things like nuts or pollen that you can be allergic to are known as allergens) will trigger this antibody response again. This means that every time that person eats that particular food, he or she will have an allergic reaction.

Unlike allergies to other foods like milk and eggs, children generally don't outgrow allergies to peanuts or nuts. But over time, they should become experienced at avoiding the foods that make them ill.

What are the signs and symptoms?

The first signs of an allergic reaction can be a runny nose, a skin rash all over the body, or a tingly tongue. The symptoms can quickly become more serious—including signs of anaphylaxis (a sudden, potentially severe allergic reaction involving various systems in the body), such as difficulty breathing, swelling of the throat or other parts of the body, a rapid drop in blood pressure, and dizziness or unconsciousness. Other possible symptoms include hives, tightness of the throat, a hoarse voice, nausea, vomiting, abdominal pain, diarrhea, and lightheadedness.

To someone who has no allergies, seeing someone else experiencing anaphylaxis can be just as scary as it is for the allergic person. Anaphylaxis can happen just seconds after being exposed to a triggering substance. It can involve various areas of the body (such as the skin, respiratory tract, gastrointestinal tract, and cardiovascular system), and can be mild to fatal. The annual incidence of anaphylactic reactions is small—about 30 per 100,000 people—although people with asthma, eczema, or hay fever are at greater risk of experiencing them.

How is a nut or peanut allergy diagnosed?

Obviously, babies can't tell their parents when their tummies hurt or their throats itch, so diagnosing food allergies early in a child's life can be difficult. Doctors therefore generally recommend that parents refrain from giving their children peanut butter or other peanut or nut products until after they're 2 years old. If there's a family history of food allergies, parents should wait until the child is 3. And many doctors recommend that their pregnant patients—especially those with food allergies—keep the lid on the peanut butter jar until after the baby's born and they're done nursing.

If your doctor suspects your child might have a peanut or nut allergy, he or she will probably refer you to an allergist or allergy specialist for further testing. The allergy specialist will ask you and your child questions, such as how often does your child have the reaction, how quickly do symptoms start after eating a particular food, and whether any family members have allergies or conditions like eczema and asthma.

Allergies are diagnosed using a skin test or blood test, depending on the age and condition of the patient. Initially, the suspected allergen is placed on the skin and the skin is pricked with a plastic toothpick-like instrument. If the child is allergic, a reaction (a welt that looks like a mosquito bite) will develop in 20 minutes. Skin testing can also be done by injecting the suspected allergen under the skin with a needle.

It's important that your child stop taking antiallergy medications (such as over-the-counter antihistamines) 2 to 3 days before a skin test because they can interfere with the results. Most cold medications, as well as some antidepressants, can also affect skin testing. Check with the allergist's office if you're unsure about what medications need to be stopped and for how long.

Some doctors may also take a blood test that will check for antibodies for specific allergens.

If the results of the skin or blood tests are still unclear, then in select cases, a food challenge may be needed for final diagnosis. During this test, your child might be given gradually increasing amounts of nuts or peanuts to eat, while being watched for symptoms by the doctor. This can only be performed in a clinic or hospital where access to immediate medical care and medications is available. And it should be avoided if your child has experienced a clear-cut anaphylactic reaction to nuts or peanuts in the past.

How is it treated?

There is no real cure for food allergies. The only real way to cope with them on a daily basis is to know the trigger foods and avoid them. So parents must educate their children early and often, not only about the allergy itself but also what reaction they will have if they eat the offending food. The task at hand is to stay vigilant about reading each and every food label and educating others, including relatives, caregivers, neighbors, and teachers.

In case of an emergency, doctors recommend that nut- and peanut-allergic adults and children 12 or 13 and older (depending on the maturity of the child) keep a shot of epinephrine with them in an easy-to-carry container that looks like a pen. Millions of parents across the country carry epinephrine everywhere they go.

With one injection into the thigh, epinephrine, or adrenaline, is administered to ease the allergic reaction. A prescription for epinephrine includes two auto-injections. Your child's doctor can give you instructions on how to use and store the epinephrine injection pen; it's essential that you familiarize yourself with the procedure.

If your child is 12 or older, make sure he or she keeps the pen readily available at all times. If the child is younger than 12, talk to the school nurse, your child's teacher, and your child's child-care provider about keeping one on hand in case of an emergency. Also make sure that epinephrine pens are available at your home, as well as at the homes of friends and family members. Your child's doctor may also encourage your child to wear a medical alert bracelet. It's also a good idea to carry an over-the-counter antihistamine, which can help alleviate allergy symptoms in some people. But antihistamines should not be used as a replacement for the epinephrine.

Kids who have had to take an epinephrine shot should go immediately to a medical facility or hospital emergency department, where additional treatment can be given if needed. Up to one third of anaphylactic reactions can have a second wave of symptoms several hours following the initial attack, so the child might need to be observed in a clinic or hospital for 4 to 8 hours following the reaction.

Caring for Your Child

It's important to be vigilant about your child's food allergies, even during simple, everyday activities. Here are some basic tips:

- Read food labels. Beginning in 2006, food makers are required to clearly state whether a product contains peanuts or tree nuts that could trigger an allergic reaction. The statement should be in or adjacent to the list of ingredients. (Keep in mind though, this rule only applies to foods labeled after the start of 2006. So some of the products that were made before then and are still on the shelves may not say anything about allergens.)

- Avoid cooked foods you didn't make yourself—anything with an unknown list of ingredients. Stay away from baking mixes, chilis, Asian dishes, and buffet restaurants where spoons go in and out of various bowls that may contain nuts or seeds.

- Avoid fried foods (especially in restaurants and fast-food places) that may be made with peanut oil or may contain hidden peanuts or nuts.

- Don't be cavalier about food allergies—tell everyone who handles the food your child eats, from waiters and waitresses to chefs and bakers. If the manager or owner of a restaurant is uncomfortable about your request for peanut- or nut-free food preparation, don't eat there.

- Encourage people not to feed your child. Make your own school lunches, as well as snacks and treats to take to parties, play dates, sleepovers, school functions, and other outings.

- Talk to the daycare supervisor or school principal before your child attends. Then talk to your child's classmates or send home a note explaining that your child has a severe allergy to peanuts or nuts. Ask parents to refrain from sending in snacks that have peanuts.

- Keep epinephrine accessible at all times—not in the glove compartment of your car, but with you, because seconds count during an anaphylaxis episode. It's a good idea to also keep epinephrine in your child's classroom (not just in the nurse's office), or with your child, depending on state laws.

- See a board-certified allergist or your child's doctor regularly.

Here are some other tips that might make life a little easier for you and your nut- or peanut-allergic child:

- Use—and encourage others to use—an antiseptic hand wash after meals.

- Consult with a dietitian to come up with safe but delicious meals and snacks.

- Carry a list of foods to watch out for in your backpack or bag.

- Talk to your child's teachers, relatives, caregivers, and close friends about the allergy. Teach them to recognize the signs of anaphylaxis and show them how to help your child.

Be sure to arm yourself with all of the other need-to-know info that will help keep your nut- or peanut-allergic child safe including a comprehensive list of ingredients and foods to avoid.

Section 21.2

Eating a Nut- and Peanut-Free Diet

"Nut and Peanut Allergy Diet" was provided by KidsHealth, one of the largest resources online for medically reviewed health information written for parents, kids, and teens. For more articles like this one, visit www .KidsHealth.org, or www.TeensHealth.org. © 2003 The Nemours Foundation. This information was reviewed by William J. Geimeier, M.D., in September 2003.

When your child is allergic to nuts or peanuts, any food—even a Valentine's Day chocolate or the hot dog you serve at your Memorial Day picnic—needs to undergo an exhaustive ingredient analysis. And, as any parent who has a child with a nut or peanut allergy knows, Halloween can be an absolute nightmare.

But you don't have to be a chemist to know which foods are OK and which ones could cause a potentially dangerous allergic reaction in your child. Reading labels and just knowing what the hidden ingredients are can go a long way toward keeping your child safe.

What Is a Nut and Peanut Allergy?

About 1.5 million adults and children in the United States have an allergy to peanuts, and 50% of these people also are allergic to nuts or tree nuts. There's no typical age of diagnosis, although research indicates that the median age of first exposure is 14 months. And although many children outgrow allergies to milk, soy, and eggs, those with allergies to peanuts and nuts rarely outgrow their reactions.

Although peanuts aren't true nuts but legumes (in the same family as peas and lentils), the reaction in people allergic to them is similar to the reaction in people who are allergic to tree nuts, such as walnuts, cashews, and pecans.

241

An allergic reaction is when the immune system mistakenly believes that a harmless substance, in this case a nut or peanut, is harmful. It creates specific antibodies to that food to protect your body. The next time you eat that food, your immune system releases huge amounts of chemicals and histamines to protect your body, triggering an allergic reaction.

What Are the Signs and Symptoms?

You may not even recognize an allergic reaction, depending on the severity, the age of the child, and previous exposure to the allergen. The first signs of a reaction could be a runny nose, a skin rash all over the body, or a tingly tongue. Symptoms can quickly become more serious—including difficulty breathing, swelling of the throat or other parts of the body, rapid drop in blood pressure, and dizziness or unconsciousness. Other possible symptoms include hives, vomiting, abdominal cramps, and diarrhea. Symptoms usually appear within a few seconds to 2 hours after ingesting or being exposed to the allergen.

A sudden, potentially severe allergic reaction, called anaphylaxis, can involve various systems in the body (such as the skin, respiratory tract, gastrointestinal tract, and cardiovascular system) and can be fatal. Anaphylaxis can cause a person's blood pressure to drop, airways to narrow, and tongue to swell, resulting in serious breathing difficulty, loss of consciousness, and, in some cases, even death.

Treating a Nut or Peanut Allergy

Unfortunately, there's no cure for food allergies; the only way to help kids who have them is to stay away from the foods that will cause a reaction.

If your child has been diagnosed with a nut or peanut allergy, learn everything you can about what to watch out for and the type of reaction your child will have if you come into contact with a nut or peanut (or nut and peanut ingredients in other foods).

In case of an emergency, doctors recommend that adults and children 12 years and older who have a nut or peanut allergy keep a shot of epinephrine with them in an easy-to-carry container that looks like a pen. If a nut- or peanut-allergic person accidentally eats nuts or peanuts and has an anaphylactic reaction, a shot of epinephrine can be given to help counteract it. Your child's doctor can give you instructions on how to use and store the epinephrine injection pen; it's essential that you familiarize yourself with the procedure.

If your child is 12 years or older, make sure he or she keeps the pen readily available at all times. If the child is younger than 12, talk to the school nurse and your child's teacher about keeping one on hand in case of an emergency. Also make sure that epinephrine pens are available at your home, as well as at the homes of friends and family members. Your child's doctor may also encourage your child to wear a medical alert bracelet. It's also a good idea to carry an over-the-counter antihistamine, which can help alleviate allergy symptoms in some people. But antihistamines should be used in addition to epinephrine and not as a replacement for the shot.

Kids who have had to take an epinephrine shot should go immediately to a medical facility or hospital emergency department, where additional treatment can be given if needed. Up to one third of anaphylactic reactions can have a second wave of symptoms several hours following the initial attack, so the child might need to be observed in a clinic or hospital for 4 to 8 hours following the reaction.

Feeding a Child with a Nut or Peanut Allergy

Doctors advise parents to keep their children away from foods linked to severe allergies—such as eggs, fish, shellfish, peanuts, and nuts—until they're 2. The Food Allergy and Anaphylaxis Network (FAAN) recommends that children not eat eggs before age 2 or any sort of nuts or fish until age 3.

Parents who suspect or know that their child has a nut or peanut allergy must read every food label on every item and educate their children to do the same. Beginning in 2006, food makers are required to clearly state whether a product contains nuts or peanuts. But that only applies to foods labeled after 2006, so there may be some products still on store shelves, which don't have the label.

The problem with peanuts, unlike tree nuts, is that they're used in many, many foods, posing a threat to unwitting consumers. The Food and Drug Administration requires food manufacturers to list every ingredient in a product, with several exceptions—flavors, colors, or spices, and those in insignificant amounts. In addition, ingredient lists still don't cover possible cross contamination when the same equipment that's used to process peanuts for another product is also used to make foods that don't have peanuts as ingredients.

That's why the responsibility falls on parents to make sure their child doesn't eat and isn't exposed to foods with nuts or peanuts.

When reading labels, avoid these ingredients:

* food additive 322 (also often listed as lecithins);

243

- arachis (an alternative term for peanut);
- hydrolyzed vegetable protein (which may be found in some cereals);
- arachis oil (peanut oil);
- emulsified or satay (which could mean that the food was thickened with peanuts); and
- natural and artificial flavoring (which could contain tree nuts and are used in many foods, including barbecue sauce, cereals, crackers, and ice cream).

Foods to avoid include:

- peanut butter;
- mixed nuts;
- crushed nuts in sauces;
- African, Chinese, Indonesian, Japanese, Mexican, and Vietnamese dishes (which often contain peanuts or are contaminated with peanuts during meal preparation);
- pesto (an Italian sauce made with nuts);
- marzipan (a paste made from ground almonds and sugar);
- mandelonas (peanuts soaked in almond flavoring);
- health food bars;
- artificial nuts (which could be peanuts that have been deflavored and reflavored with a nut, such as pecan or walnut);
- all cakes and pastries with unknown ingredients, particularly carrot cake, pumpkin cake or pie, and fruit and nut rolls;
- bouillon and Worcestershire sauce;
- praline and nougat;
- muesli and fruited breakfast cereals;
- vegetarian dishes;
- prepared salads and salad dressings; and
- gravy.

Doctors also advise peanut-allergic patients to avoid chocolate candies, unless they're absolutely certain there's no risk of cross contamination during manufacturing. Many candy companies are very aware of nut and peanut allergy issues. Some even make sure they manufacture candies that contain nuts separately from those that don't, so people with nut allergies can still enjoy their products. To be sure a candy is nut- and peanut-free, log on to the manufacturer's website or call the toll-free number listed on the package. Most companies have customer-service representatives that can answer nut and peanut allergy questions accurately.

Even nonfood items can contain ingredients that could cause a reaction in a nut- or peanut-allergic child:

- Hackysacks, beanbags, and draft dodgers are sometimes filled with crushed nut shells.

- Bird feed, dog food and treats, hamster food and bedding, livestock feed, some cosmetics (especially moisturizers), secondhand toys and furniture, and ant traps and mousetraps could even contain nuts or peanuts.

It's important to be vigilant about your child's food allergies, even during simple, everyday activities. Here are some basic tips allergist Sandra Gawchik, M.D., gives her patients:

- Avoid baked goods you didn't make yourself—anything with an unknown list of ingredients. Stay away from baking mixes, chili mixes, etc.

- Be careful when eating at Asian or buffet restaurants—spoons often go in and out of various bowls that may contain nuts or seeds and could easily cross contaminate foods.

- Don't be cavalier about food allergies—tell everyone who handles the food your child eats, from waiters and waitresses to chefs and bakers. If the manager or owner of a restaurant is uncomfortable about your request for peanut- or nut-free food preparation, don't eat there.

- If you're unsure about whether a food or candy is nut and peanut free, log on to the manufacturer's website or call the toll-free number listed on the package. Most companies have customer service representatives that can answer nut and peanut allergy questions accurately.

- Encourage people not to feed your child. Don't take food from strangers. Make your own snacks and treats to take to parties, play dates, school functions, and other outings.

- Talk to the daycare supervisor or school principal before your child attends. Then talk to your child's classmates or send home a note explaining that your child has a severe allergy to peanuts or nuts. Ask parents to refrain from sending in snacks that contain peanuts. If your child's school doesn't already have one, talk to the school principal, your child's teacher, or cafeteria personnel about setting up a nut- and peanut-free table in the cafeteria.

- Keep epinephrine accessible at all times—not in the glove compartment of your car, but with you because seconds count during an anaphylaxis episode. It's a good idea to also keep epinephrine in your child's classroom (not just in the nurse's office), or in your child's backpack, depending on your state's laws on carrying medicine in classrooms.

- See a board-certified allergist or your child's doctor regularly.

A little bit of knowledge and an ounce of prevention can go a long way in ensuring that your nut- or peanut-allergic child stays free of allergic reactions.

Chapter 22

Seafood Allergy

Chapter Contents

Section 22.1

Understanding Seafood Allergy

"Seafood (Fish, Crustaceans and Shellfish)—One of the nine
most common food allergens," reprinted with permission from the
Canadian Food Inspection Agency, © 2006.

Note: In this text, the term seafood refers to all edible fish, crustaceans, and shellfish from fresh and saltwater.

Allergic Reactions

Anaphylactic reactions are severe allergic reactions that occur when the body's immune system overreacts to a particular allergen. These reactions may be caused by food, insect stings, latex, medications, and other substances. The nine priority food allergens are peanuts, tree nuts, sesame seeds, milk, eggs, seafood (fish, crustaceans, and shellfish), soy, wheat, and sulfites (a food additive).

What are the symptoms of an allergic reaction?

When someone comes in contact with an allergen, the symptoms of a reaction may develop without warning, may be delayed, may happen as two episodes (biphasic), or may develop quickly then rapidly progress from mild to severe. The most dangerous symptoms include breathing difficulties, a drop in blood pressure, or shock, which may result in loss of consciousness and even death. A person experiencing an allergic reaction may have any of the following symptoms:

- trouble breathing, speaking, or swallowing;
- a drop in blood pressure, rapid heartbeat, or loss of consciousness;
- flushed face, hives or a rash, or red and itchy skin;
- swelling of the eyes, face, lips, throat, and tongue;
- anxiousness, distress, faintness, paleness, sense of doom, weakness; and
- cramps, diarrhea, or vomiting.

248

How are food allergies and severe food allergy reactions treated?

Currently there is no cure for food allergies. The only option is complete avoidance of the specific allergen. Appropriate emergency treatment for a severe food allergy reaction includes an injection of epinephrine (adrenalin), which is available in an auto-injector device. Epinephrine must be administered as soon as symptoms of a severe allergic reaction appear. The injection must be followed by further treatment and observation in a hospital emergency room. If your allergist has diagnosed you with a food allergy and prescribed epinephrine, carry it with you all the time and know how to use it. Follow your allergist's advice on how to use an epinephrine auto-injector device.

Frequently Asked Questions about Seafood Allergies

What is the difference between crustaceans and shellfish?

Crustaceans are aquatic animals that have jointed legs, a hard shell, and no backbone, such as crab, crayfish, lobster, prawns, and shrimp. Shellfish (also known as molluscs) have a hinged two-part shell and include clams, mussels, oysters, and scallops, and various types of octopus, snails, and squid. Seafood allergies are one of the most common.

How can I avoid a fish, crustacean, or shellfish-related reaction if I'm allergic to these food?

Avoid all food and products that contain or warn that they "may contain" fish, crustaceans, or shellfish and their derivatives as directed by your allergist.

What is the difference between a fish, crustacean, or shellfish allergy and histamine poisoning?

When someone has a seafood allergy, his or her immune system has an abnormal reaction to either fish, crustacean, or shellfish proteins. Histamine poisoning is caused by eating fish that contain high levels of histamine, a chemical that forms when certain types of fish start to decompose. High levels of histamine develop when fish, such as anchovies, mackerel, mahi-mahi, and tuna, are not properly frozen or refrigerated. Histamine poisoning causes symptoms similar to seafood allergic reactions and can often be mistaken for a fish, crustacean, or shellfish allergic reaction. If you are unsure whether you have a sea-food allergy or histamine poisoning, consult an allergist or seek emergency medical treatment.

If I am allergic to one type of seafood will I be allergic to another?

It is possible for some people who are allergic to one type of sea-food (fish, crustacean, or shellfish) to eat other types of seafood without having a reaction. However, studies show that when a person has a specific seafood allergy, he or she may also be allergic to other species within the same group. For example, if you're allergic to cod, you may also be allergic to pike as both are fish; if you're allergic to shrimp, you may also be allergic to lobster as both are crustaceans; if you're allergic to mussels, you may also be allergic to clams as both are shell-fish. If someone is allergic to one type of seafood—crustaceans or fish or shellfish—he or she will not necessarily be allergic to the other types. Consult your allergist before experimenting.

Can I have a seafood-related reaction even if I do not eat or use seafood and seafood derivatives?

Yes. There have been reported reactions to seafood vapors from cooking, preparing (e.g., sizzling skillets), and handling fish, crusta-ceans, and shellfish and/or products that contain them. Avoid these situations. Seafood and seafood derivatives can often be present under different names, e.g., kamaboko. Always read the ingredient list carefully.

What do I do if I am not sure whether a product contains seafood or seafood derivatives?

If you have a fish, crustacean, or shellfish allergy, do not eat or use the product. Get ingredient information from the manufacturer.

Watch out for Allergen Cross Contamination

Cross contamination is the transfer of an ingredient (food allergen) to a product that does not normally have that ingredient in it. Through cross contamination, a food that should not contain the allergen could become dangerous to eat for those who are allergic.

Cross contamination can happen:

- during food manufacturing through shared production and packaging equipment;

- at retail through shared equipment, e.g., cheese and deli meats sliced on the same slicer; and through bulk display of food products, e.g., bins of baked goods, bulk nuts; and

- during food preparation at home or in restaurants through equipment, utensils, and hands.

Avoiding Fish and Fish Derivatives

Make sure you read product labels carefully to avoid products that contain seafood and seafood derivatives. Avoid food and products that do not have an ingredient list and read labels every time you shop. Manufacturers may occasionally change their recipes or use different ingredients for varieties of the same brand. Refer to the following list before shopping:

Other Names for Fish, Crustaceans, and Shellfish

- **Fish:** Anchovy, bass, bluefish, bream, carp, catfish (channel cat, mudcat), char, chub, cisco, cod, eel, flounder, grouper, haddock, hake, halibut, herring, mackerel, mahi-mahi, marlin, monkfish (angler fish, lotte), orange roughy, perch, pickerel (dore, walleye), pike, plaice, pollock, pompano, porgy, rockfish, salmon, sardine, shark, smelt, snapper, sole, sturgeon, swordfish, tilapia (St. Peter's fish), trout, tuna (albacore, bonito), turbot, white fish, whiting.

- **Crustaceans:** Crab, crayfish (crawfish, écrevisse), lobster (langouste, langoustine, coral, tomalley), prawns, shrimp (crevette).

- **Shellfish:** Abalone, clam, cockle, conch, limpets, mussels, octopus, oysters, periwinkle, quahaugs, scallops, snails (escargot), squid (calamari), whelks.

Possible Sources of Fish, Crustaceans, and Shellfish

- Coffee

- Deli meats, e.g., bologna, ham

- Dips, spreads, kamaboko (imitation crab/lobster meat)

- Ethnic foods, e.g., fried rice, paella, spring rolls

251

- Fish mixtures, e.g., surimi (used to make imitation crab/lobster meat)
- Garnishes, e.g., antipasto, caponata (Sicilian relish), caviar, roe (unfertilized fish eggs)
- Gelatin, marshmallows
- Hot dogs
- Pizza toppings
- Salad dressings
- Sauces, e.g., fish, marinara, steak, Worcestershire
- Soups
- Spreads, e.g., taramasalata (contains salted carp roe)
- Sushi
- Tarama (salted carp roe)
- Wine
- Non-food sources of fish, crustaceans and shellfish
- Fish food
- Lip balm/lip gloss
- Pet food

Note: These lists are not complete and may change. Food and food products purchased from other countries, through mail order or the internet, are not always produced using the same manufacturing and labeling standards.

What Can I Do?

Be Informed: See an allergist and educate yourself about food allergies. Contact your local allergy association for further information.

Before Eating: Allergists recommend that if you do not have your epinephrine auto-injector device with you, that you do not eat. If an ingredient list says a product "may contain" or "does contain" seafood or seafood derivatives, do not eat it. If you do not recognize an ingredient or there is no ingredient list available, avoid the product.

Section 22.2

Tips for Managing a Fish or Shellfish Allergy

© 2006. Used with permission from The Food Allergy & Anaphylaxis Network.

Allergic reactions to fish and shellfish are commonly reported in both adults and children. It is generally recommended that individuals who have had an allergic reaction to one species of fish, or positive skin tests to fish, avoid all fish. The same rule applies to shellfish. If you have a fish allergy but would like to have fish in your diet, speak with your allergist about the possibility of being tested with various types of fish.

Some Hidden Sources of Fish

- Caponata, a traditional sweet-and-sour Sicilian relish, can contain anchovies.
- Caesar salad dressings and steak or Worcestershire sauce often contain anchovies.
- Surimi (imitation crab meat) contains fish.

Commonly Asked Questions

Should carrageenan be avoided by a fish- or shellfish-allergic individual?

Carrageenan is not fish. Carrageenan, or "Irish moss," is a red marine algae. This food product is used in a wide variety of foods, particularly dairy foods, as an emulsifier, stabilizer, and thickener. It appears safe for most individuals with food allergies. Carrageenan is not related to fish or shellfish and does not need to be avoided by those with food allergies.

Should iodine be avoided by a fish- or shellfish-allergic individual?

Allergy to iodine, allergy to radiocontrast material (used in some lab procedures), and allergy to fish or shellfish are not related. If you have an allergy to fish or shellfish, you do not need to worry about cross reactions with radiocontrast material or iodine.

Keep in Mind

- Fish-allergic individuals should avoid fish and seafood restaurants because of the risk of contamination in the food-preparation area of their "non-fish" meal from a counter, spatula, cooking oil, fryer, or grill exposed to fish.

- Fish protein can become airborne during cooking and cause an allergic reaction.

- Some individuals have had reactions from walking through a fish market.

- Allergic reactions to fish and shellfish can be severe and are often a cause of anaphylaxis.

Chapter 23

Wheat Allergy

Chapter Contents

Section 23.1

What Is Wheat Allergy?

"Wheat—One of the nine most common food allergens,"
reprinted with permission from the Canadian Food Inspection Agency,
© 2006.

Allergic Reactions

Anaphylactic reactions are severe allergic reactions that occur when the body's immune system overreacts to a particular allergen. These reactions may be caused by food, insect stings, latex, medications, and other substances. The nine priority food allergens are peanuts, tree nuts, sesame seeds, milk, eggs, seafood (fish, crustaceans and shellfish), soy, wheat, and sulfites (a food additive).

What are the symptoms of an allergic reaction?

When someone comes in contact with an allergen, the symptoms of a reaction may develop without warning, may be delayed, may happen as two episodes (biphasic), or may develop quickly then rapidly progress from mild to severe. The most dangerous symptoms include breathing difficulties, a drop in blood pressure, or shock, which may result in loss of consciousness and even death. A person experiencing an allergic reaction may have any of the following symptoms:

- trouble breathing, speaking, or swallowing;

- a drop in blood pressure, rapid heartbeat, or loss of consciousness;

- flushed face, hives or a rash, or red and itchy skin;

- swelling of the eyes, face, lips, throat, and tongue;

- anxiousness, distress, faintness, paleness, sense of doom, weakness; and

- cramps, diarrhea, or vomiting.

How are food allergies and severe food allergy reactions treated?

Currently there is no cure for food allergies. The only option is complete avoidance of the specific allergen. Appropriate emergency treatment for a severe food allergy reaction includes an injection of epinephrine (adrenalin), which is available in an auto-injector device. Epinephrine must be administered as soon as symptoms of a severe allergic reaction appear. The injection must be followed by further treatment and observation in a hospital emergency room. If your allergist has diagnosed you with a food allergy and prescribed epinephrine, carry it with you all the time and know how to use it. Follow your allergist's advice on how to use an epinephrine auto-injector device.

Frequently Asked Questions about Wheat Allergies

I have a wheat allergy. How can I avoid a wheat-related reaction?

Avoid all food and products that contain wheat and wheat derivatives, including any product whose ingredient list warns it "may contain" wheat.

What is the difference between a wheat allergy and celiac disease?

Wheat allergy and celiac disease are two different conditions. When someone has a wheat allergy, his or her immune system has an abnormal reaction to proteins from wheat, with symptoms similar to that of other allergic food reactions. When a person with celiac disease eats food containing the protein gluten (found in wheat and some other grains) it damages the lining of the small intestine, which stops the body from absorbing nutrients. This can lead to diarrhea, weight loss, and eventually malnutrition. If you are unsure whether you have a wheat allergy or celiac disease, consult an allergist or a physician.

How can I determine if a product contains wheat or wheat derivatives?

Always read the ingredient list carefully. Wheat and wheat derivatives can often be present under different names, e.g., semolina.

What do I do if I am not sure whether a product contains wheat or wheat derivatives?

If you have a wheat allergy, do not eat or use the product. Get ingredient information from the manufacturer.

Watch out for Allergen Cross Contamination

Cross contamination is the transfer of an ingredient (food allergen) to a product that does not normally have that ingredient in it. Through cross contamination, a food that should not contain the allergen could become dangerous to eat for those who are allergic.

Cross contamination can happen:

- during food manufacturing through shared production and packaging equipment;
- at retail through shared equipment, e.g., cheese and deli meats sliced on the same slicer; and through bulk display of food products, e.g., bins of baked goods, bulk nuts; and
- during food preparation at home or in restaurants through equipment, utensils, and hands.

Avoiding Wheat and Wheat Derivatives

Make sure you read product labels carefully to avoid products that contain wheat and wheat derivatives. Avoid food and products that do not have an ingredient list and read labels every time you shop. Manufacturers may occasionally change their recipes or use different ingredients for varieties of the same brand. Refer to the following list before shopping:

Other Names for Wheat

- Atta
- Bulgur
- Couscous
- Durum
- Einkorn
- Emmer
- Enriched/white/whole wheat flour

- Farina
- Gluten
- Graham flour, high gluten/protein flour
- Kamut
- Seitan
- Semolina
- Spelt (dinkel, farro)
- Triticale (a cross between wheat and rye)
- Triticum aestivum
- Wheat bran/flour/germ/starch

Possible Sources of Wheat

Note: Avoid all food and products that are made from wheat and/or contain wheat in the ingredient list including baked goods, baking mixes, breads, cakes, cookies, doughnuts, muffins, battered/fried foods, bread crumbs, cereals, crackers, croutons, creamed (thickened) soups, gravy mixes, and pasta.

- Baking powder, flour
- Beer
- Coffee substitutes made from cereal
- Falafel
- Gelatinized starch, modified starch, modified food starch
- Host (communion/altar bread/wafers)
- Hydrolyzed plant protein
- Ice cream
- Imitation bacon
- Meat, fish, and poultry binders and fillers, e.g., deli meats, hot dogs, surimi (used to make imitation crab/lobster meat)
- Pie fillings
- Prepared ketchup, mustard
- Salad dressings
- Sauces, e.g., chutney, soy sauce, tamari sauce
- Seasonings
- Snack foods, e.g., candy, chocolate bars

- Non-food sources of wheat
- Cosmetics, hair care products
- Medications, vitamins
- Modeling compound, e.g., PLAY-DOH©
- Pet food
- Wreath decorations

Note: These lists are not complete and may change. Food and food products purchased from other countries, through mail order or the internet, are not always produced using the same manufacturing and labeling standards. For example, some gluten-free products from Europe may contain wheat starch.

What Can I Do?

Be Informed: See an allergist and educate yourself about food allergies. Contact your local allergy association for further information.

Before Eating: Allergists recommend that if you do not have your epinephrine auto-injector device with you, that you do not eat. If an ingredient list says a product "may contain" or "does contain" wheat or wheat derivatives, do not eat it. If you do not recognize an ingredient or there is no ingredient list available, avoid the product.

Section 23.2

Tips for Managing a Wheat Allergy

© 2006. Used with permission from
The Food Allergy & Anaphylaxis Network.

Baking

When baking with wheat-free flours, a combination of flours usually works best. Experiment with different blends to find one that will give you the texture you are trying to achieve. Try substituting 1 cup wheat flour with one of the following:

- 7/8 cup rice flour
- 5/8 cup potato starch flour
- 1 cup soy flour plus 1/4 cup potato starch flour
- 1 cup corn flour

Commonly Asked Questions

What is the difference between celiac disease and wheat allergy?

Celiac disease and wheat allergy are two distinct conditions. Celiac disease, or "celiac sprue," is a permanent adverse reaction to gluten. Those with celiac disease will not lose their sensitivity to this substance. This disease requires a lifelong restriction of gluten.

The major grains that contain gluten are wheat, rye, oats, and barley. These grains and their by-products must be strictly avoided by people with celiac disease.

Wheat-allergic people have an IgE-mediated response to wheat protein. These individuals must only avoid wheat. Most wheat-allergic children outgrow the allergy.

Are kamut and spelt safe alternatives to wheat?

No. Kamut is a cereal grain, which is related to wheat. Spelt is an

261

ancient wheat that has recently been marketed as safe for wheat-allergic individuals. This claim is untrue, however. Wheat-allergic patients can react as readily to spelt as they do to common wheat.

Keep in Mind

- Read labels carefully. At least one brand of hot dogs and one brand of ice cream contains wheat. It is listed on the label.
- Many country-style wreaths are decorated with wheat products.
- Some types of imitation crab meat contain wheat.
- Wheat flour is sometimes flavored and shaped to look like beef, pork, and shrimp, especially in Asian dishes.

Chapter 24

Other Types of Food Allergy

Chapter Contents

Section 24.1

Soy Allergy

What Does a Soy Allergy Mean?

Soybeans belong to the legume family and have an almost identical protein structure to peanut. However, a person will not necessarily be allergic to peanut if they have an allergic reaction to soy and vice versa.

Symptoms of a soy allergy include asthma, rhinitis (stuffy nose), hives (urticaria), eczema, tissue swelling, and digestive disturbances. In infants a soy allergy can cause diarrhea, vomiting, abdominal pain, crying, and a tendency to gain very little weight. Symptoms of soy allergy often present as similar symptoms to a milk allergy.

Soy is used in many processed foods. Products that say high protein often contain soy flour or other soy derivatives. Soy oil and soy lecithin are the two most commonly used soy products in processed food and thankfully they do not usually cause allergic reactions in children (the soy protein that causes the allergic reaction has been removed.)

Read Labels Carefully

Common names of soy products/always contains it:

- Edamame
- Miso
- Natto
- Shoyu
- Tamari
- Tempeh
- Texturized vegetable protein (TVP)

- Tofu
- Soy milk
- Soy sauce
- Soy nuts
- Soy grits
- Soy protein
- Soy protein isolate
- Soybean paste/curd
- Sobee
- Kyodofu (freeze-dried tofu)
- Soy sprouts
- Soy flour

These ingredients may contain soy if the source has not been specified:

- Bulking agent
- Emulsifier
- Guar gum
- Gum Arabic
- Hydrolyzed vegetable protein (HVP)
- Hydrolyzed plant protein (HPP)
- Lecithin
- Protein filler/extender
- Mono- and diglycerides
- MSG (monosodium glutamate)
- Seasoned salt
- Shortenings
- Stabilizer
- Thickener
- Vegetable gum/starch/oil/protein

Common sources/foods containing soy:

- Baby food

- Canned fish
- Chocolates (creamed centers)
- Cooking oils
- High protein bars/foods
- Ice cream/frozen desserts
- Dessert mixes
- Margarine
- Mayonnaise
- Meat products
- Powdered meal replacers
- Sauces (Asian, gravy, soy, Worcestershire)
- Shortenings
- Soy/tofu cheese
- Soy yogurt
- Baked goods
- Breakfast cereals (mixed grain/multigrain)
- Infant cereals
- High protein flour and bread
- Stuffings
- Mixed sprouts
- Salad sprouts
- Salad dressings
- Canned soup/dried soup mixes
- Vegetarian meat replacers
- Frozen dinners
- Mixed bean preparation
- Prepared sauces, e.g., barbecue, oriental
- Chocolate

As always, use extra precaution when eating out at restaurants or eating foods prepared by others.

Section 24.2

Sesame Seed Allergy

"Sesame seeds—One of the nine most common food allergens" is reprinted with permission from the Canadian Food Inspection Agency, © 2006.

Allergic Reactions

Anaphylactic reactions are severe allergic reactions that occur when the body's immune system overreacts to a particular allergen. These reactions may be caused by food, insect stings, latex, medications, and other substances. The nine priority food allergens are peanuts, tree nuts, sesame seeds, milk, eggs, seafood (fish, crustaceans, and shellfish), soy, wheat, and sulfites (a food additive).

What are the symptoms of an allergic reaction?

When someone comes in contact with an allergen, the symptoms of a reaction may develop without warning, may be delayed, may happen as two episodes (biphasic), or may develop quickly then rapidly progress from mild to severe. The most dangerous symptoms include breathing difficulties, a drop in blood pressure, or shock, which may result in loss of consciousness and even death. A person experiencing an allergic reaction may have any of the following symptoms:

- trouble breathing, speaking, or swallowing;

- a drop in blood pressure, rapid heartbeat, or loss of consciousness;

- flushed face, hives or a rash, or red and itchy skin;

- swelling of the eyes, face, lips, throat, and tongue;

- anxiousness, distress, faintness, paleness, sense of doom, weakness; and

- cramps, diarrhea, vomiting.

How are food allergies and severe food allergy reactions treated?

Currently there is no cure for food allergies. The only option is complete avoidance of the specific allergen. Appropriate emergency treatment for a severe food allergy reaction includes an injection of epinephrine (adrenalin), which is available in an auto-injector device. Epinephrine must be administered as soon as symptoms of a severe allergic reaction appear. The injection must be followed by further treatment and observation in a hospital emergency room. If your allergist has diagnosed you with a food allergy and prescribed epinephrine, carry it with you all the time and know how to use it. Follow your allergist's advice on how to use an epinephrine auto-injector device.

Frequently Asked Questions about Sesame Seed Allergies

I have a sesame seed allergy. How can I avoid a sesame seed-related reaction?

Avoid all food and products that contain sesame seeds and sesame derivatives, including any product whose ingredient list warns it "may contain" sesame.

How can I determine if a product contains sesame seeds or sesame derivatives?

Always read the ingredient list carefully. Sesame seeds and sesame derivatives can often be present under different names, e.g., tahini.

What do I do if I am not sure whether a product contains sesame seeds or sesame derivatives?

If you have a sesame seed allergy, do not eat or use the product. Get ingredient information from the manufacturer.

Watch out for Allergen Cross Contamination

Cross contamination is the transfer of an ingredient (food allergen) to a product that does not normally have that ingredient in it. Through cross contamination, a food that should not contain the allergen could become dangerous to eat for those who are allergic.

Cross contamination can happen:

- during food manufacturing through shared production and packaging equipment;
- at retail through shared equipment, e.g., cheese and deli meats sliced on the same slicer; and through bulk display of food products, e.g., bins of baked goods, bulk nuts; and
- during food preparation at home or in restaurants through equipment, utensils, and hands.

Avoiding Sesame Seeds and Sesame Derivatives

Make sure you read product labels carefully to avoid products that contain sesame seeds and sesame derivatives. Avoid food and products that do not have an ingredient list and read labels every time you shop. Manufacturers may occasionally change their recipes or use different ingredients for varieties of the same brand. Refer to the following list before shopping.

Other Names for Sesame Seeds

- Benne/benne seed/benniseed
- Gingelly/gingelly oil
- Seeds
- Sesamol/sesamolina
- Sesamum indicum
- Sim sim
- Tahina
- Tahini
- Til
- Vegetable oil

Possible Sources of Sesame Seeds

- Aqua Libra® (herbal drink)
- Baked goods, e.g., breads, cookies, pastries, bagels, buns
- Bread crumbs, bread sticks, cereals, crackers, melba toast, muesli
- Dips, pâtés, spreads, e.g., hummus, chutney
- Dressings, gravies, marinades, salads, sauces, soups

- Ethnic foods, e.g., flavored rice, noodles, shish kebabs, stews, stir fry
- Flavor(ing)
- Herbs, seasoning, spice
- Margarine
- Processed meats, sausages
- Risotto (rice dish)
- Sesame oil, sesame salt (gomasio)
- Snack foods, e.g., bagel/pita chips, candy, granola bars, halvah, pretzels, rice cakes, sesame snap bars
- Tahini
- Tempeh
- Vegetarian burgers

Non-Food Sources of Sesame Seeds

- Adhesive bandages
- Cosmetics, hair care products, perfumes, soaps, sunscreens
- Drugs
- Fungicides, insecticides
- Lubricants, ointments, topical oils
- Pet food
- Sesame meal, e.g., poultry and livestock feed

Note: These lists are not complete and may change. Food and food products purchased from other countries, through mail order or the internet, are not always produced using the same manufacturing and labeling standards.

What Can I Do?

Be informed: See an allergist and educate yourself about food allergies. Contact your local allergy association for further information.

Before Eating: Allergists recommend that if you do not have your epinephrine auto-injector device with you, that you do not eat. If an ingredient list says a product "may contain" or "does contain" sesame or sesame derivatives, do not eat it. If you do not recognize an ingredient or there is no ingredient list available, avoid the product.

Chapter 25

Food Additives and Chemicals That May Cause Allergic Reactions

Chapter Contents

Section 25.1

Facts about Food Additives

Many people believe that food additives cause most food reactions. In fact, natural foods cause most reactions. Studies have found, though, that a few additives do cause problems in a few people.

What is a food additive?

Thousands of man-made and natural substances are added to the food and drink we consume. Some of these additives are vitamins and minerals to improve our health and preservatives to slow decay. Others enhance flavor or color, add texture, and make foods less acidic.

Who has adverse reactions to food additives?

It is unclear how many people have adverse reactions to food additives. Many people claim to have them, but study results have confirmed that food additives cause reactions in only a few people. And of the thousands of additives used, only a handful have been identified as possible causes of adverse reactions.

A report that sparked public interest in adverse reactions to additives was published in 1959. It reported that three patients developed hives after taking tablets that contained tartrazine. Tartrazine, also known as FD&C yellow No. 5, is used to add yellow color to food. Today, scientists question the process used by those researchers to connect taking tartrazine with developing hives. At that time, though, the report convinced more people they should look into additives as the possible source of various reactions.

In 1973, Benjamin Feingold, M.D., claimed that some food additives cause children to be hyperactive. Symptoms of hyperactivity, or attention deficit disorder, include nervousness, short attention span, and aggressiveness. Feingold developed a diet low in salicylic acid (a salt), artificial colors, and artificial flavors such as aspartame. He claimed that close adherence to the diet reduced hyperactivity in children.

Other researchers have been unable to show that the diet works for more than a few children. In 1982, a National Institutes of Health (NIH) team of experts concluded that scientific findings do not support the claim that food additives cause hyperactivity. Studies since then support those findings.

The Feingold diet does not cause physical harm. Children who are needlessly on the diet, though, may be emotionally and socially harmed, pediatricians warn.

What are the symptoms of food additive reactions?

Symptoms vary in type and degree. They depend on the additive causing the reaction, how sensitive the patient is to the product, and the amount consumed. Most reactions are chemical, not allergic reactions. People who react to one chemical are not likely to react to others.

The most serious reaction to a food additive is anaphylactic shock. This is a life-threatening condition that includes breathing problems and loss of consciousness, among other physical reactions. It usually occurs within minutes after consuming the additive. When this happens, blood vessels widen so much that blood pressure plummets. Symptoms include sweating, paleness, panting, nausea, rapid pulse, faintness, confusion, and even passing out. Without speedy treatment, this intense allergic reaction can cause death.

What additives cause reactions?

There are eight additives that may cause reactions:

- Sulfites can cause mild to life-threatening symptoms in approximately 5 percent of people with asthma. Symptoms include chest tightness, hives, stomach cramps, diarrhea, breathing problems, and other symptoms of anaphylactic shock. Experts suspect that the reactions are caused by a hyper-reaction to inhaled sulfur dioxide. Some products sulfites can be found in include wine, dried fruits, white grape juice, frozen potatoes, maraschino cherries, fresh shrimp, and certain jams and jellies. Sulfites at one time were used on fresh fruits and vegetables to retain color and freshness. The Food and Drug Administration, which governs the use of food additives, has banned them from such use.

- Aspartame (NutraSweet®) is a calorie-free sweetener. Most reported reactions include hives; swelling of the eyelids, lips, or hands; and headaches. But these reactions have not been verified.

273

People who have a problem breaking down the amino acid phenylalanine should not consume aspartame. Some claim the product also causes hyperactivity in children, but study results do not support these claims.

- Parabens are used to preserve foods and medications. Some examples of parabens are ethyl, methyl, propyl, butylparabens, and sodium benzoate. In sunscreens and shampoos, they can cause severe contact dermatitis. This is a skin condition that causes redness, swelling, itching, and pain. But adverse reactions to foods containing parabens have not been clearly shown in studies.

- Tartrazine is a dye used in beverages, candy, ice cream, desserts, cheese, canned vegetables, hot dogs, salad dressings, seasoning salts, catsup, and some other foods. It may be associated with hives or swelling; although suspected of causing asthma attacks, recent studies suggest that this is unlikely. A 1983 scientific review of studies led experts to conclude that no more than 2 percent of children react to dye additives. These reactions are very rare in recent studies.

- MSG (monosodium glutamate, or glutamic acid) forms 20 percent of dietary protein. MSG is used in Oriental foods and in manufactured meat, poultry, and other products by manufacturers and restaurants to enhance flavors. It is believed to cause "Chinese Restaurant Syndrome." A patient may have a headache, a burning sensation on the back of the neck, chest tightness, nausea, diarrhea, and sweating. There have been rare reports that people with asthma who have consumed MSG have more severe asthma attacks. This is still being researched.

- Nitrates and nitrites are used to preserve foods, prevent deadly botulism infection, enhance flavors, and color foods. They may rarely cause headaches and hives in some people. Nitrates and nitrites are used in hot dogs, bologna, salami, and other processed meats and fish.

- BHT (butylated hydroxytoluene) and BHA (butylated hydroxyanisole) are added to breakfast cereals and other grain products to prevent them from taking in oxygen and changing color, odor, and flavor. They have been linked to chronic hives and other skin reactions on rare occasions.

- Benzoates are preservatives for some foods including cakes, cereals, salad dressings, candy, margarine, oils, and dry yeast. Benzoate reactions are very rare.

How are reactions to food additives diagnosed?

Today, scientists would demand stricter control of the process reported in 1959 to diagnose tartrazine as the cause of the hives. They question if other claims of adverse reactions to food additives are based on properly controlled studies showing a relationship.

You may have reason to believe that you have adverse reactions to certain food additives. If you do, remove the additives from your diet for a few days. Your symptoms should promptly go away if the additive is the cause. There is no evidence that any food additive causes a reaction that lasts more than one day.

To confirm that an additive is causing a reaction, a controlled study can be done. The food additive should be added and removed from the diet. Neither the patient nor the physician should know if the additive is in the diet. The patient should then be watched to see if there is a change in symptoms. Symptoms should improve when the food is removed from the diet.

How can I prevent a reaction?

The only way to prevent a reaction is to avoid the cause. To make sure you do not unknowingly consume the product, carefully read ingredient lists on food labels, and question restaurant staff about cooking methods.

To avoid sulfiting agents, look for sulfur dioxide, sodium or potassium sulfite, bisulfite, or metabisulfite in ingredient lists.

Tips for Follow-Up

If you have had a serious adverse reaction to a food additive, wear a Medic-Alert bracelet or necklace to alert health care providers of your allergy in case of an emergency. If anaphylaxis is a concern, always carry adrenaline in a syringe, such as EpiPen or Ana-Kit, for injecting in an emergency.

Report adverse reactions to the Food and Drug Administration's Adverse Reaction Monitoring System. The agency will look into the possibility that the additive is a public health hazard.

If you use the internet to read about reactions to food additives, look closely at the source of the information to judge the validity of the information.

Section 25.2

Histamine Intolerance

Histamine is a natural substance produced by the body and is also present in many foods. It is released by the body during times of stress and allergy.

What Is Histamine?

In an allergic response, an allergen stimulates the release of antibodies, which attach themselves to mast cells. When histamine is released from the mast cells it may cause one or more of the following symptoms:

- Eyes to itch, burn, or become watery
- Nose to itch, sneeze, and produce more mucus
- Skin to itch or develop rashes or hives
- Sinuses to become congested and cause headaches
- Lungs to wheeze or have spasms
- Stomach to experience cramps and diarrhea

This chemical (vasoactive amine) is able to create such havoc with the many body functions because it is contained in almost all body tissues.

The main body tissues include the lungs, skin, intestinal mucosa, mast cells, and basophils.

The release of histamine can be induced by almost any allergen. Examples include inhalant allergens, drugs, chemicals, insect venoms, and even some foods.

Histamine in Foods

There are many foods that contain histamine or cause the body to release histamine when ingested. Histamine in food may be

276

responsible for some cases of food intolerance. Histamine-rich foods include:

- Anchovies
- Avocados
- Beer
- Canned foods
- Cheeses
- Ciders
- Eggplant
- Fermented beverages
- Fermented foods
- Fish
- Herring
- Jams and preserves
- Mackerel
- Meats
- Processed meats
- Salami
- Sardines
- Sauerkraut
- Sausage
- Some oriental foods
- Sour cream
- Spinach
- Tomatoes
- Tuna
- Vegetables
- Vermouth
- Vinegars
- Wines
- Yeast extract
- Yogurt

Foods that release histamine into the body include the following:

- Alcohol
- Bananas
- Certain nuts
- Chocolate
- Eggs
- Fish
- Milk
- Papayas
- Pineapple
- Shellfish
- Strawberries
- Tomatoes

Histamine Poisoning

At times the ingestion of high concentrations of histamine may lead to histamine poisoning. It is also known as scombroid poisoning. High levels of histamine occur in spoilage of foods such as fish products.

Section 25.3

Sulfite Sensitivity

"Sulfites: Safe for Most, Dangerous for Some," by Ruth Papazian, from the *FDA Consumer* magazine (www.fda.gov/fdac), published by the U.S. Food and Drug Administration (FDA), December 1996. Revised by David A. Cooke, M.D., October 26, 2006.

It wasn't a special occasion—or even a fancy restaurant—but Karen, 37, will never forget that meal.

"My boyfriend and I were at a hamburger joint, and I had a burger and fries. About 10 minutes after we finished eating, my throat began to itch. I grabbed my [asthma] inhaler but I could feel my throat constricting. I couldn't breathe and started to panic. When I passed out, my boyfriend flagged down a passing police car. The officer radioed for an ambulance, and I was rushed to the hospital. I was revived with a massive dose of epinephrine to counteract the reaction caused by the sulfite solution the potatoes had been soaked in before frying."

"I know enough to stay away from wine, shrimp, and other foods that contain sulfites, and take note whenever I don't feel right after eating something. But I never expected french fries to be sulfited. I've had allergic reactions to sulfites before, but this time I came close to dying."

"I was angry that this happened to me. I felt powerless—I was careful and knowledgeable, and yet I couldn't protect myself. Who ever heard of a lethal french fry? Afterward, I refused to eat out in restaurants for almost two years, and I still can't visit people or go on vacation without knowing there is a hospital nearby."

The Food and Drug Administration estimates that one out of a hundred people is sulfite-sensitive, and that 5 percent of those who have asthma, like Karen (who asked that her last name not be used), are also at risk of suffering an adverse reaction to the substance. "By law, adverse reactions to drugs must be reported to FDA by doctors or pharmaceutical companies. But with sulfites and other food ingredients, reporting is voluntary so it's difficult to say just how many people may be at risk," cautions FDA consumer safety officer JoAnn Ziyad, Ph.D.

Complicating matters, scientists have not pinpointed the smallest concentration of sulfites needed to provoke a reaction in a sensitive or allergic person. Recent research indicates that sulfur dioxide is the actual cause of sulfite sensitivity, but identifying it can be challenging because it can be generated by chemical reactions of other substances in foods. FDA requires food manufacturers and processors to disclose the presence of sulfiting agents in concentrations of at least 10 parts per million, but the threshold may be even lower. The assay used to detect the level of sulfites in food is not sensitive enough to detect amounts less than 10 ppm in all foods (that's 1 part sulfite to 100,000 parts of food—the equivalent of a drop of water in a bathtub) so that's what the regulation has to be based on, explains Ziyad.

"The most rapid reactions occur when sulfites are sprayed onto foods or are present in a beverage, but the most severe reactions occur when sulfites are constituents of the food itself," says Ron Simon, M.D., head of Allergy, Asthma and Immunology at Scripps Clinic and Research Foundation in La Jolla, California.

A person can develop sulfite sensitivity at any point in life, and no one knows what triggers onset or the mechanism by which reactions occur. "Doctors believe that asthmatics develop difficulty breathing by inhaling sulfite fumes from treated foods," notes Dan Atkins, M.D., a pediatrician at the National Jewish Medical and Research Center in Denver, Colorado. He says that in a severe reaction an overwhelming degree of bronchial constriction occurs, causing breathing to stop. This can lead to lack of oxygen reaching the brain, heart, and other organs and tissues and, possibly, a fatal heart rhythm irregularity.

"We now know that asthmatics who have more severe symptoms and are dependent on corticosteroids, such as prednisone or methylprednisolone, are especially prone to sulfite sensitivity and are most at risk of having a severe reaction," notes Atkins. But it's a chicken-and-egg situation, notes Simon: "We don't know which comes first, the asthma or the sulfite sensitivity, because some people's first experience with asthma is a sulfite reaction, and as their asthma becomes more severe they eventually become steroid-dependent."

Sulfite sensitivity can be tricky to diagnose. Karen went to an internist and two pulmonary specialists without getting to the bottom of her problem.

"People who do experience adverse reactions to sulfites know that it's something they ate, but might not know what that something is," says Atkins. "I'll ask a patient complaining of an adverse reaction what he or she ate and drank when it occurred. If beer or wine doesn't seem to be the problem, I tend to dismiss sulfite sensitivity. But if I think sulfites may be the culprit, I'll do a challenge [a type of allergy test in which a small amount of the suspect substance is administered in a capsule or in a drink and the patient is monitored to see whether there is a reaction]."

If a person develops hives after ingesting sulfites, the doctor will do a prick test (a small concentration of sulfite is placed on the skin, which is then pricked; the test is positive if a welt develops on the spot). "People who have positive skin tests to sulfites are likely to be allergic to the additive, rather than have a sensitivity. These people, who are usually not asthmatic, are most at risk of anaphylactic shock [a life-threatening reaction]," says Simon.

Regulatory Status in Flux

Sulfur-based preservatives, or sulfites, have been used around the world for centuries to:

- inhibit oxidation (browning) of light-colored fruits and veg-etables, such as dried apples and dehydrated potatoes;
- prevent melanosis (black spot) on shrimp and lobster;
- discourage bacterial growth as wine ferments;
- condition dough;
- bleach food starches; and
- maintain the stability and potency of some medications.

When the Federal Food, Drug, and Cosmetic Act was amended in 1958 to regulate preservatives and other food additives, FDA considered sulfites to be generally recognized as safe (GRAS). But when FDA reevaluated their safety and proposed to affirm the GRAS status of sulfiting agents in 1982, the agency received numerous reports from consumers and the medical community regarding adverse health reactions. In response, FDA contracted with the Federation of American Societies for Experimental Biology (FASEB) to examine the link between sulfites and reported health problems that ranged from chest tightness or difficulty breathing to hives to fatal anaphylactic shock.

In 1985, FASEB concluded that sulfites are safe for most people, but pose a hazard of unpredictable severity to asthmatics and others who are sensitive to these preservatives. Based on this report, FDA took the following regulatory actions in 1986:

- Prohibited the use of sulfites to maintain color and crispness on fruits and vegetables meant to be eaten raw (for instance, restaurant salad bars or fresh produce in the supermarket).

- Required companies to list on product labels sulfiting agents that occur at concentrations of 10 ppm or higher, and any sulfiting agents that had a technical or functional effect in the food (for instance, as a preservative) regardless of the amount present. (This labeling requirement was extended to standardized foods, such as pickles and bottled lemon juice, in 1993.)

FDA requires that the presence of sulfites be disclosed on labels of packaged food (although manufacturers need not specify the particular agent used). This information will be included in the ingredient portion of the label, along with the function of the sulfiting agent in the food (for instance, a preservative).

When food is sold unpackaged in bulk form (as with a barrel of dried fruit or loose, raw shrimp at the fresh fish counter), store managers must post a sign or some other type of labeling that lists the food's ingredients on the container or at the counter so that consumers can determine whether the product was treated with a sulfiting agent.

In 1987, FDA proposed to revoke the GRAS status of sulfiting agents on "fresh" (not canned, dehydrated or frozen) potatoes intended to be cooked and served unpackaged and unlabeled to consumers (french fries, for example), and issued a final ruling to this effect in 1990. However, the rule was held null and void in 1990 after a protracted court battle in which the "fresh" potato industry prevailed on procedural grounds.

This legal setback notwithstanding, "the agency continues to have concerns about the safety of sulfiting agents, and plans further action to protect the consumer," notes Ziyad. Steps the agency is considering include establishing maximum residual levels for specific foods and additional labeling rules.

"The ultimate goal of sulfite regulation is to make sure that there is no higher level of sulfite residues in food than is absolutely necessary and to encourage the use of substitutes for sulfites in food processing," says Ziyad.

Sniffing out Sulfites

Since 1985, FDA's Adverse Reaction Monitoring System has been tracking reactions to sulfites. Over a 10-year period, 1,097 such cases have been reported. However, thanks to regulatory action taken by FDA over the years, coupled with increased consumer savvy, the number of reported sulfite-related health incidents has been dropping steadily. In 1995, just six cases were reported.

Twenty years ago, FDA banned the use of sulfites on fruits and vegetables that are to be eaten raw (as with a salad bar)—and the vast majority of those in the food service industry honor the prohibition—but consumers who are sulfite-sensitive "shouldn't take anything for granted," says Ziyad.

Current FDA regulations do not require managers of food service establishments to disclose whether sulfites were used in food preparation. "Consumers continually request FDA to extend the regulation to include food service establishments because either waiters and other staff members didn't know whether the food was treated with sulfites, or gave erroneous information," notes Ziyad. "FDA's position on the issue has been that consumers who see sulfites listed on the label of a packaged food should be able to deduce that the same food sold in a food service establishment would also contain sulfites," she explains.

In addition, sulfites are still found in a variety of cooked and processed foods (including baked goods, condiments, dried and glacéed fruit, jam, gravy, dehydrated or pre-cut or peeled "fresh" potatoes, molasses, shrimp, and soup mixes) and beverages (such as beer, wine, hard cider, fruit and vegetable juices, and tea).

Since sulfites are added to so many foods, someone who is sensitive to the additive must not assume that a food is safe to eat, says Atkins. He recommends these measures to avoid sulfites when buying unlabeled foods at the deli or supermarket and ordering at a restaurant:

- If the food is packaged, read the label. If it is being sold loose or by the portion, ask the store manager or waiter to check the ingredient list on the product's original bulk-size packaging.

- Avoid processed foods that contain sulfites, such as dried fruits, canned vegetables, maraschino cherries, and guacamole. If you want to eat a potato, order a baked potato rather than hash browns, fries, or any dish that involves peeling the potato first.

- If you have asthma, have your inhaler with you when you go out to eat. Similarly, if you've experienced a severe reaction to sulfites in the past (such as breaking out in hives), carry an antihistamine and make sure you have handy a self-administering injectable epinephrine, such as EpiPen, so that if you have a reaction you can stabilize your condition until you get to an emergency room.

"It takes some doing, but you can take steps to minimize your contact with sulfites if you are diagnosed with asthma or sulfite sensitivity," says Ziyad. "But you may not even know you have a problem with sulfites until a reaction occurs. Undiagnosed people are at risk because even if they know that sulfites can cause adverse reactions, they often don't associate sulfites with their own health problems," says Ziyad.

"Regulations can go a long way towards protecting people, but there's no substitute for knowledge."

Chapter 26

Oral Allergy Syndrome

Oral allergy syndrome is an allergy to certain raw fruits, vegetables, seeds, spices, and nuts causing allergic reactions in the mouth and throat. These allergic reactions happen mostly in people with hay fever, especially spring hay fever due to birch pollen, and late summer hay fever due to ragweed pollen.

An allergic reaction happens while eating the raw food and causes itchy, tingly mouth, lips, throat, and palate. There may be swelling of the lips, tongue, and throat, and watery itchy eyes, runny nose, and sneezing. Handling the raw fruit or vegetable—e.g., peeling it or touching the juice to the lips—may cause rash, itching, or swelling where the juice touches the skin or sneezing, runny nose, and water eyes. Sometimes, more severe symptoms can happen such as vomiting, cramps, and diarrhea, and, on rare occasions, life-threatening reactions with swelling of the throat, wheezing, trouble breathing, and anaphylaxis may occur.

Fruit, Vegetable, and Nut Allergies Associated with Oral Allergy Syndrome

Fruits

- Apple family (apple, pear)

- Plum family (plum, peach, prune, nectarine, apricot, cherry)
- Kiwifruit

Vegetables

- Parsley family (carrot, celery, dill, anise, cumin, coriander, caraway)
- Potato family (potato, tomato, green pepper)

Nuts

- Hazelnut
- Walnut
- Almond

Legumes

- Peas
- Beans
- Peanut

Seeds

- Sunflower seeds

Ragweed allergy (which causes hay fever in August and September) can be associated with allergies to raw bananas and the members of the gourd family (melon, watermelon, honeydew, cantaloupe, zucchini, and cucumber).

Grass allergy can be associated with allergies to orange, melon, watermelon, tomato, kiwi, and peanut.

These allergic reactions usually occur only when the food is raw. People who are allergic to the raw food can eat it cooked, canned, microwaved, processed, or baked. For example, someone allergic to raw apples can eat applesauce, apple jelly, apple juice, apple pie, and dried apples. However, nuts may cause allergic reactions whether raw or cooked. This problem is usually life-long. Allergy tests to these foods may sometimes be negative unless a fresh fruit is used for the test (instead of a commercial allergy extract). The allergic reaction to these foods can occur any time of the year when eating the foods but can be worse during the pollen season and especially if hay fever is very troublesome that year.

The allergic reaction is not due to pesticides, chemicals, or wax on the fruit. However, because the more allergic part of the fruit may be in the skin, some people allergic to fruits, e.g., peaches, can eat the flesh without reaction if the skin is peeled away. For apples, some brands of apples cause more allergic reactions than others. Freshly picked apple, e.g., straight from the tree or an unripe apple, may cause fewer allergic reactions than ones that are very ripe or ones that have been stored for weeks after picking.

Severe allergic reactions to foods causing oral allergy syndrome are most likely to occur with celery, kiwifruit, peaches, apricots, apples, and nuts, especially hazelnuts.

Management of Oral Allergy Syndrome

- These allergies are caused by the raw fruit or vegetable and therefore, once they are cooked or processed, they can usually be eaten.

- You do not need to avoid all the foods listed above. Avoid only those particular ones which have caused allergic reactions.

- Be aware, however, that if you do have oral allergy syndrome to some of the foods, you can develop allergies to other foods listed.

- If an allergic reaction occurs to one of these foods, stop eating it immediately. Severe reactions may happen if you keep eating that food. Allergic reactions may be treated with antihistamines.

- If you have had severe symptoms including trouble breathing when eating the foods, you may need to carry injectable medication with you to treat these reactions (e.g., EpiPen®).

- For mild oral allergy syndrome, try peeling the fruit, eating unripe or partially ripe fruits, or picking them directly from the tree so that they are quite fresh. If you react, do not keep eating the food.

- Microwaving briefly to a temperature of 80 to 90 degrees Fahrenheit (26 to 32 degrees Celsius) may allow you to eat the food.

- Nuts which cause oral allergy syndrome should be totally avoided, whether fresh or cooked, because of the higher risk of severe reactions.

- Allergy shots for hay fever may sometimes help associated food allergies.

Substitute Raw Fruits

[Instead of eating fruits that cause oral allergy syndrome, try] berries* (strawberry, blueberry, raspberries, etc.), citrus* (orange, mandarins, etc.), grapes, currants, gooseberries, guava, mango, figs, pineapple, papaya, avocado, persimmon, pomegranates, or watermelon.*

Substitute Raw Vegetables

[Instead of eating vegetables that cause oral allergy syndrome, try foods from the] mustard family (cabbage, cauliflower, broccoli, watercress, radish; goose foot family (spinach, swiss chard); or composite family (green onions).

Substitute Nuts

[Instead of eating nuts that cause oral allergy syndrome, try varieties such as the] peanut*, cashew, pistachio, brazil, macadamia, or pine nut.

Note: May occasionally cause oral allergy syndrome.

Chapter 27

Eosinophilic Esophagitis and Its Relationship to Food Allergies

Chapter Contents

Section 27.1

What Is Eosinophilic Esophagitis?

"About EE," reprinted with permission from the
American Partnership for Eosinophilic Disorders website, © 2006.

What is an eosinophil?

Eosinophils, a type of white blood cell, are an important part of the immune system, helping us fight off certain types of infections, such as parasites. Many different problems can cause high numbers of eosinophils in the blood including allergies (food and environmental), certain infections (caused by parasites), eosinophil-associated gastrointestinal disorders, leukemia, and other problems. When eosinophils occur in higher than normal numbers in the body, without a known cause, an eosinophilic disorder may be present.

Eosinophilic disorders are further defined by the area affected. For instance, eosinophilic esophagitis means abnormal numbers of eosinophils in the esophagus.

What is EE?

Eosinophilic esophagitis is characterized by the infiltration of a large number of eosinophils, a type of white blood cell, in the esophagus (the tube connecting the mouth to the stomach). Eosinophils are an important part of the immune system, helping us fight off certain types of infections, such as parasites. A variety of stimuli may trigger this abnormal production and accumulation of eosinophils, including certain foods. Eosinophilic esophagitis means eosinophils infiltrating the esophagus; –itis means inflammation.

People with EE commonly have other allergic diseases such as asthma or eczema. EE affects people of all ages, gender, and ethnic backgrounds. In certain families, there may be an inherited (genetic) tendency. EE is thought to be the most common type of eosinophil-associated gastrointestinal disorder.

Eosinophils are not normally present in the esophagus, although they may be found in small numbers in other areas of the gastrointestinal tract. Diseases other than EE can cause eosinophils in the esophagus including gastroesophageal reflux diseases (GERD), food allergy, and inflammatory bowel disease.

What are the symptoms of EE?

Symptoms vary from one individual to the next and may differ depending on age. Vomiting may occur more commonly in young children and difficulty swallowing may occur in older individuals.

Common symptoms include:

- reflux that does not respond to usual therapy (which includes proton pump inhibitors, a medicine which stops acid production in the stomach);
- dysphagia (difficulty swallowing);
- food impactions (food gets stuck in the throat);
- nausea and vomiting;
- failure to thrive (poor growth or weight loss);
- abdominal or chest pain;
- poor appetite;
- malnutrition; and
- difficulty sleeping.

How is EE diagnosed?

In individuals with symptoms consistent with EE, an upper endoscopy with biopsies is needed for the diagnosis. The endoscopy is often performed after treatment with reflux medications have failed to relieve the symptoms. Medications for reflux include proton pump inhibitors or histamine-2 receptor blockers.

During an upper endoscopy, the gastroenterologist looks at the esophagus, stomach and duodenum (first part of the small bowel) through an endoscope (small tube inserted through the mouth) and takes multiple small tissue samples (biopsies) which the pathologist reviews under the microscope. Even if the esophagus appears normal, the biopsies may show EE. A high number of eosinophils (counted per high power field) suggest the diagnosis of EE. GERD also causes eosinophils in the esophagus, but typically far fewer. The pathologist will also look for tissue injury, swelling, and thickening of the esophageal layers. With EE, the eosinophils are limited to the esophagus and not

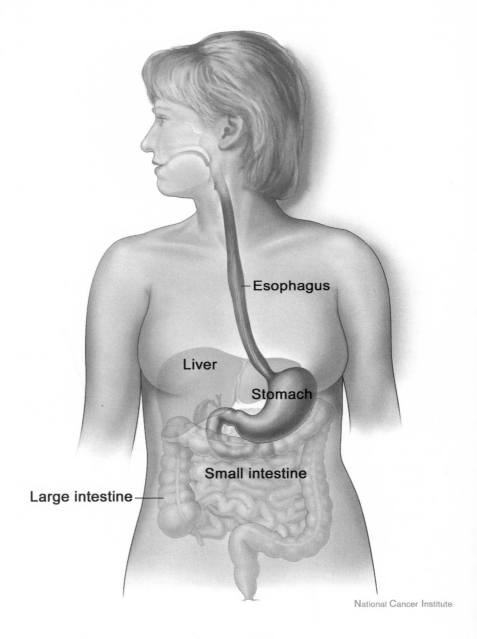

National Cancer Institute

Figure 27.1. *The upper gastrointestinal tract.*

found in other areas. Once the diagnosis of EE is confirmed, food allergy testing is typically recommended to guide treatment. Skin prick testing to different foods is the most common type of allergy testing.

Allergy testing (skin prick, patch testing and RAST): Once the diagnosis of EE is confirmed, allergy testing is typically requested. In many situations, avoiding allergens that trigger the eosinophils will be effective treatment. The reactions to foods are not always immediate hypersensitivity (IgE-mediated). This means that a food can be consumed with no obvious reaction to it, but over a period of days to weeks the eosinophils triggered by the food will cause inflammation and injury to the esophagus. For this reason, food logs (keeping track of foods and symptoms) may not identify the offending food. The skin testing will include skin prick testing and may also include patch testing (to look for delayed reactions).

Skin prick testing is for IgE-mediated reactions (immediate hypersensitivity). Skin prick testing involves scratching small amounts of pure food or environmental allergens into the skin. A wheal (bump) greater than the negative control indicates a positive test. Both a positive control (one that should cause a wheal) and negative control (should not cause a wheal) are used.

Skin patch testing can be used when testing for delayed food reactions. Skin patch testing is most commonly used to test for dermatologic (skin) reactions. When used for food reactions, small amounts of a pure food are placed in tiny cups, which are then taped to the back. The foods will be chosen based on the patient's diet, previous reactions, and prior skin prick test results. The patches are removed after 48 hours and read at 72 hours.

RAST (radioallergosorbent test) is not as helpful for identifying foods that cause EE. Instead, RAST may be used to confirm an immediate reaction to a food (for instance, hives following a peanut butter sandwich). RAST testing identifies IgE antibodies for a specific food.

Why is it so difficult to obtain a diagnosis?

EE is a relatively uncommon disorder that doctors may not encounter often. The diagnosis of EE is often delayed, sometimes for years, because of lack of awareness of these disorders.

Although doctors may have minor disagreements concerning specific criteria, the diagnosis can be confirmed with biopsies in the majority of cases. In rare situations, it may be difficult to distinguish eosinophilic esophagitis from gastroesophageal reflux disease (GERD). Working closely with your health care team is the best way to ensure a proper and timely diagnosis.

What is the treatment?

- Dietary
- Medications

Most children and adults with EE respond favorably to dietary treatments. The dietary restrictions are guided by food allergy testing and fine-tuned with food trials once the symptoms have resolved.

Elimination diets, in which all "positive" foods on allergy testing are removed from the diet, are one type of dietary treatment. An elimination diet may be the only treatment needed for some individuals with eosinophilic esophagitis.

Elemental diets, in which all sources of protein are removed from the diet, are another dietary therapy. The elemental diet includes only an amino acid formula (building blocks of protein), no whole or partial proteins. Simple sugars, salt, and oils are permitted on an elemental diet.

Children and adults who rely in part, or completely, on an elemental amino acid-based formula may have a difficult time drinking enough of the formula. To maintain proper nutrition, some may require tube feedings directly into the stomach (enteral feeds).

Food trials involve adding back one ingredient at a time to determine specific foods causing a reaction. Food trials begin after symptoms resolve and eosinophils have cleared.

Medications for EE most commonly include steroids to control inflammation and suppress the eosinophils. Steroids are used if dietary measures do not resolve the symptoms. Steroids can be taken orally or topically (swallowed from an asthma inhaler).

Patients with EE may require additional endoscopies and biopsies to assess how the esophagus is responding to specific treatment. The initial diagnosis of EE can be overwhelming and often affects the entire family. A positive attitude and a focus on non-food activities go a long way in learning to live with EE. With proper treatment, individuals with EE can lead a normal life.

Section 27.2

Scientists Discover Genetic Profile of Eosinophilic Esophagitis

"Scientists Discover Genetic Profile of an Often-Misdiagnosed Chronic Allergic Disease of Children," National Institute of Allergy and Infectious Diseases (NIAID, www.niaid.nih.gov), part of the National Institutes of Health, February 1, 2006.

Though many parents may never have heard of it, a severe and chronic condition called eosinophilic esophagitis (EE) is recognized by doctors as an emerging health problem for children. A disease that was often misdiagnosed in the past, EE has been increasingly recognized in the United States, Europe, Canada, and Japan in the last few years. Cases of the disease can be devastating since children who suffer from it may have a host of lifelong problems.

Now, an interdisciplinary team of scientists funded in part by the National Institute of Allergy and Infectious Diseases (NIAID) and the National Institute of Diabetes and Digestive and Kidney Diseases (NIDDK), both components of the National Institutes of Health (NIH), has published a major advance in understanding EE. In the February 2006 issue of the *Journal of Clinical Investigation,* the team reveals that a highly specific subset of human genes plays a role in this complicated disease.

"Understanding the genetic profile of a disease such as EE is an important first step towards developing new ways to diagnose and treat it," says NIAID Director Anthony S. Fauci, M.D.

In EE, the esophagus (the muscular tube that connects the end of the throat with the opening of the stomach) becomes inflamed—often, but not always, due to allergic reactions to food. This inflammation causes nausea, heartburn, vomiting, and difficulty swallowing. In advanced cases, children may suffer from malnutrition, often require special liquid diets, and may need to have a feeding tube inserted in order to receive nourishment. EE, first identified in 1977, has been increasingly recognized since the advent of diagnostic endoscopy, a procedure in which a flexible fiberoptic tube is inserted down the throat to directly image and biopsy the esophagus.

Historically, part of the reason why the disease has been misdiagnosed is that its symptoms are very similar to those of acid reflux disease. However similar the two diseases are in terms of symptoms, their underlying physiology is vastly different. Drugs on the market for treating acid reflux do not abate the symptoms of EE, which is not caused by production of stomach acid, but likely by inflammation in the esophagus resulting from the abnormal accumulation of immune cells know as eosinophils—hence its name eosinophilic esophagitis. Eosinophils are white blood cells that contain inflammatory chemicals, highly reactive proteins, destructive enzymes, toxins, muscle contractors, and signaling molecules that can guide immune defenses to the site of infection.

At the Cincinnati Children's Hospital Medical Center, Professor of Pediatrics Marc E. Rothenberg, M.D., Ph.D., has seen patients with EE for a number of years and pursued clinical and laboratory research on the disease as well. To better understand the disease, Dr. Rothenberg and his colleagues examined the gene expression in tissue samples taken directly from the esophagus of individuals with EE as well as from people without the disease. These individuals were selected to represent a diverse sample with respect to age, sex, and disease state. Dr. Rothenberg and his colleagues found that a particular set of 574 genes was expressed differently in people with EE than in those without the illness.

This transcript signature, as they call it, yielded some surprising findings; it was largely the same for every person with EE, regardless of age and whether or not these people had food allergies. This transcript signature was quite distinct from the signature observed in patients with acid reflux disease, thus allowing the two diseases to be easily discriminated. Although EE is more common in males than in females, the genes expressed in the esophagus did not vary dramatically between males and females with EE. Of the 574 genes, the investigators found that the expression of one gene in particular, termed eotaxin-3, was elevated in people with EE compared to people without the disease—at up to more than 100-fold greater amounts in EE than in controls. Eotaxin-3, a factor released from certain cells and tissues, acts to attract circulating eosinophils, yet no one had previously observed that the local levels of eotaxin-3 correlated directly with the number of eosinophils in the esophagus.

In their paper, Dr. Rothenberg and his colleagues also demonstrated that, in a mouse model of EE, mice lacking receptors for eotaxin were protected against developing EE. These results, when taken with those of the human studies, suggest that a drug to block eotaxin-3 might have therapeutic value. Finally, by sequencing the eotaxin-3 genes of all the people in their study, the investigators identified certain genetic variations known as single nucleotide polymorphisms (SNPs)—particular spots within the DNA sequence of the gene where a single base of DNA may vary from person to person. One particular SNP in the gene appears to occur more frequently in patients with EE than in controls, and, if this is confirmed, SNPs may provide a way to determine if people are at risk for EE.

Reference: Blanchard et al. Eotaxin-3 and a uniquely conserved gene expression profile in eosinophilic esophagitis. *Journal of Clinical Investigation* DOI: 10.1172/JCI26679 (2006).

Chapter 28

Avoiding Food Allergy Triggers

Chapter Contents

Section 28.1

Decoding Food Labels:
Tools for People with Food Allergies

Background

True food allergies are immune-mediated systemic allergic reactions to certain foods. According to the U.S. Food and Drug Administration (FDA), true food allergies affect less than 2% of the adult population and 2% to 8% of children. However, the impact of true allergies can be quite severe. Most childhood food allergies are found in young infants and children under 3 years old. Food allergies have a genetic component and may be more common among those with asthma.

Reactions to a food allergen can range from uncomfortable skin irritations to gastrointestinal distress to respiratory involvement to life-threatening anaphylaxis—a systemic allergic reaction that generally involves several of these areas as well as the cardiovascular system. The number of people with food allergies appears to be increasing, especially among children. To keep pace with this trend, there is an increasing need for preemptive food selection strategies.

Currently, an individual with a food allergy must learn to read labels carefully and critically. This is because a food allergen may take on an unfamiliar name when used for processing purposes. For example, if eggs, one of the most allergenic foods, are used as a binder to retain water in a food product, the term binder rather than egg will appear on the food label. Similarly, soy protein may be used for flavoring and listed on the label as natural flavoring.

New legislation, The Food Allergen Labeling and Consumer Protection Act (FALCPA), would require food manufacturers to use common names to identify major allergens. If approved by the House of Representatives, the FALCPA should provide consistent ingredient information, understandable at-a-glance to the average consumer, by January 2006. Until that time, understanding current labeling information is vital to allergic individuals.

The goal of this text is to provide information to help consumers understand ingredient statements on food packages, so they can avoid foods and food products that might contain specific allergens. It also differentiates between allergies and intolerances and discusses the potential for cross contamination of foods both in and away from the home.

Food Allergy versus Food Intolerance versus Histamine Sensitivity

Most people experience an adverse reaction to some food at some point in their life. This does not necessarily mean that the individual is allergic to that food. Food intolerances, including sensitivity to elevated levels of histamine in foods, can produce a response similar to an allergic reaction. Adverse reactions and suspected allergens can be identified through a detailed history and specific allergy testing by a physician or qualified specialist to exclude other causes.

The difference between food allergies and food intolerance is how the body handles the offending food. In the case of an allergy, the immune system recognizes a chemical in the food (usually a protein) as an allergen and produces antibodies against it.

A response to an allergen may manifest as:

- swelling of the lips;

- stomach cramps, vomiting, diarrhea;

- hives, rashes, eczema;

- wheezing or breathing problems; or

- severely reduced blood pressure.

Most common allergens are found in the following food groups:

1. Cow's milk (especially among children)

2. Wheat (especially among children)

3. Soy (especially among children)

4. Eggs

5. Peanuts

301

6. Tree nuts

7. Fish/shellfish

8. Food additives (not true allergens, but capable of causing re-
    action or illness specific to a given person)

In most cases, children will outgrow their allergies to milk, wheat, soy, and eggs, but not to peanuts. Adults do not usually grow out of or lose their allergies.

Food intolerance is more common than a true allergy and does not involve the immune system. Intolerance is a metabolic problem in which the body cannot adequately digest the offending food. This is usually because of a chemical deficiency (i.e., an enzyme deficiency).

An individual with food intolerance can generally consume a small amount of the offending food without becoming symptomatic. However, that specific amount may be different for each individual. Intolerances, unlike allergies, seem to intensify with age.

Histamine sensitivity may be considered a type of food intolerance. Because histamine is a primary mediator of an allergic response in the body, consumption of histamine can elicit a similar response. Histamine toxicity is most frequently associated with the consumption of spoiled fish, but has also been associated with aged cheeses and red wines. Elevated levels of histamine occur naturally in these foods.

Decoding Allergens in Foods

Eggs

If you are allergic to egg protein, you should avoid any product with the word egg on the label. You should also avoid products with the following terms on their label:

*   Albumin

*   Lysozyme

*   Binder

*   Ovalbumin

*   Coagulant

*   Ovomucin

*   Emulsifier

*   Ovomucoid

*   Globulin/ovoglobulin

- Ovovitellin
- Lecithin
- Vitellin
- Livetin
- Simplesse (Simplesse™ is a fat substitute made from egg white and milk protein.)

Types of foods that likely contain egg protein include:

- Baked goods and packaged mixes
- Marshmallows
- Creamy fillings and sauces
- Processed meat products
- Breakfast cereals
- Pastas/egg noodles
- Malted drinks and mixes
- Salad dressing/mayonnaise
- Pancakes and waffles
- Soups
- Marzipan (Marzipan might be made with egg whites)
- Meringue
- Custard
- Pudding

Milk

Milk and milk proteins are also found in a variety of processed foods. Individuals with milk protein allergies should avoid all types of milk, ice cream, and yogurt and cheese, including vegetarian cheese. Allergic individuals should avoid foods with the terms butter, cream, casein, caseinate, whey, or emulsifier on the label. Additional labeling terms indicating the presence of milk proteins in a food product include:

- Caramel color or flavoring
- Lactose
- High protein flavor
- Natural flavoring

303

- Lactalbumin/lactalbumin phosphate
- Solids
- Lactoglobulin
- Simplesse (Simplesse™ is a fat substitute made from egg white and milk protein.)

Types of foods that likely contain milk protein include:

- Battered foods
- Custard, puddings, and sherbet
- Baked goods and mixes
- Imitation sour cream
- Breakfast cereals
- Instant mashed potatoes
- Chocolate
- Margarine
- Cream sauces, soups, and mixes
- Sausages
- Gravies and mixes
- Sweets/candies
- Ghee (Ghee is clarified butter frequently used in Indian cuisine.)

Wheat

Individuals who are allergic to wheat proteins should avoid any product that contains the term wheat, bulgur, couscous, bran, gluten, bread crumbs, or hydrolyzed wheat proteins on the label. Wheat has binding properties that are very useful in the food processing industry and has been extended for use in the pharmaceutical industry. Individuals with wheat allergies should discuss the composition of prescription or over-the-counter medications with a pharmacist prior to use. The presence of wheat protein in a food product may be indicated by the following label terms:

- Flour—bleached, unbleached, white, whole wheat, all-purpose, enriched, graham, durum, high gluten, high protein
- MSG (monosodium glutamate)
- Cornstarch

- Vegetable starch/gum
- Farina
- Gelatinized starch
- Semolina
- Hydrolyzed vegetable protein
- Modified food starch
- Miso (Fermented soy product with up to 50% wheat)
- Spelt
- Kamut
- Triticale

Spelt and kamut are both relatives of wheat; triticale is a wheat/rye hybrid. These grains are gaining popularity as wheat substitutes. Spelt, kamut, and triticale-containing products are marketed primarily through health/natural food stores.

Types of foods that likely contain wheat proteins include:

- Ale/beer/wine/bourbon/whiskey
- Gravy
- Baked goods and mixes—including barley products
- Ice cream and cones
- Battered or breaded foods
- Malts and flavorings
- Breakfast cereals
- Pasta/egg noodles
- Candy/chocolate
- Soup and soup mixes
- Processed meats
- Soy sauce
- Coffee substitutes
- Pretzels, chips, and crackers

Soy

Soy can be consumed as a whole bean, a nut, or a cow's-milk alternative. Soy can be processed into foods such as tofu, soy curd, yuba (soy film), and soy flour. Soy can be fermented into products such as tempeh, natto, miso, and soy sauce. Soy has a variety of supportive uses in the food industry as well. It can be a thickener, stabilizer, emulsifier, and a protein extender. Allergic individuals should avoid products with these terms on the label in addition to products containing the terms soy and soybean.

Soybean oil should be protein free, but this is not always the case and some allergic individuals must avoid soybean oil and products made with soybean oil (margarine and products made with margarine, salad dressings, and baby foods). The presence of the following terms on the product label may also indicate the presence of soy protein:

- Guar gum
- Miso (Miso is a paste made from fermented soybeans; used as a flavoring agent in Japanese cuisine.)
- Bulking agent
- Monosodium glutamate (MSG)
- Carob
- Protein
- Gum Arabic
- Starch
- Hydrolyzed vegetable protein (HVP)/hydrolyzed soy protein
- Textured vegetable protein (TVP)
- Lecithin
- Vegetable broth/gum/starch

Types of foods that likely contain soy protein include:

- Baked goods
- Oriental foods
- Some breakfast cereals
- Processed meats
- Hamburger patties
- Ice cream
- Butter substitutes/shortening
- Liquid/powdered meal replacers
- Chocolates/candy

- Seasoning sauces
- Canned meat/fish in sauces
- Seasoned salt
- Canned/packaged soups
- Snack bars
- Canned tuna
- Bouillon cubes
- Crackers
- TV dinners
- Gravies/mixes
- Tamari (Tamari is a dark sauce, similar to but thicker than soy sauce)

Peanuts and Tree Nuts

Peanuts are one of the most severely allergenic foods available in the market place. Peanuts are frequently used as a flavoring/seasoning agent in a variety of products. Peanuts and peanut oil are commonly used in Oriental cooking. As with soy oil, peanut oil (occasionally referred to as arachic oil) may very well contain an amount of peanut protein sufficient to elicit an allergic reaction. The terms peanut, peanut butter, ground-nut, flavoring, extract, and oriental sauce on a product label generally indicates the presence of peanut protein.

Types of foods that may contain peanut protein include:

- Baked goods/mixes
- Chili
- Battered foods
- Soups
- Some breakfast cereals
- Marzipan (Marzipan is a paste made of almond and sugar, used on pastry or molded into candy. Marzipan might be made with egg white as well)
- Cereal-based products
- Satay sauce (Satay sauce is made with peanuts or peanut butter and soy sauce. It might also be made with other allergenic ingredients such as shrimp paste or fish sauce.)

- Candy/candy bars/sweets (read label)
- Milk formula
- Ice cream
- Chinese dishes/egg roll
- Margarine/vegetable oil/vegetable fat
- Asian dishes (e.g., Thai/Indonesian)
- Some grain breads
- African dishes
- Snack foods
- Energy bars
- Barbecue/Worcestershire sauce
- Meat substitutes
- Sunflower seeds (Sunflower seeds may be processed on equipment shared with peanuts.)

Individuals with a peanut allergy may or may not be allergic to tree nuts (e.g., almonds, cashews, pecans, walnuts) as well. Individuals with tree-nut allergies should be cautious of the foods listed above as well as the following: mixed nuts, artificial nuts, nut oils, nut pastes, nut butters, nut extracts, salad dressings, and amaretto products.

Fish and Seafood

Seafood refers to fish and shellfish. Fish is a potent allergen among children. Shellfish tends to be a more potent allergen among adults. Although seafood might be incorporated into a variety of foods during processing, the products' label generally states this clearly. Certain species of fish contain high levels of histidine (an amino acid), which can be converted into histamine by bacteria. Reactions to histamine can mimic allergic reactions, but are not indicative of a true allergy.

Types of foods that might contain fish/seafood proteins include:

- Worcestershire/steak sauce
- Surimi (Surimi is a fish protein [most commonly made from pollack], marketed as imitation seafood. Surimi may contain artificial flavor, sweeteners, egg white, starch, and small amounts of real shellfish.)

308

- Caesar salad dressing
- Caponata (Caponata is an eggplant relish that can contain anchovies.)
- Hot dogs/bologna/ham
- Marinara sauce
- Pizza toppings
- Vitamin supplements (read label)
- Fish sauce
- Curry paste
- Fish stock

Food Additives

Food additives are frequently incorporated into food products during processing. They may be used as a product preservative, a flavor enhancer or sweetener, a coloring agent, a conditioner, or a stabilizer. Over the years, adverse reactions to certain food additives, casually referred to as allergies, have been reported. Most notably, these include:

- sulfite induced asthma;
- monosodium glutamate–induced asthma or MSG Symptom Complex;
- aspartame-induced hives and/or migraines; and
- FD&C Yellow No. 5 (Tartrazine)–induced hives and/or asthma.

Reactions to these additives are not immunologically mediated. Rather, reactions to these food additives are considered idiosyncratic (affecting different people in different ways) in that the mechanism of these reactions remains unknown.

Sulfites: Sulfites are used as preservatives to prevent browning reactions. Although sulfite-induced asthma is well documented, its mechanisms are not well understood by experts. So sulfite sensitive individuals should avoid foods with the following terms listed on their label: sulfur dioxide, potassium metabisulfite, sodium metabisulfite, potassium bisulfite, sodium bisulfite, and sodium sulfite.

Monosodium Glutamate (MSG): Glutamate, an amino acid, occurs naturally in many foods, with particularly high levels in dairy

309

products, meat, fish, and some vegetables. Glutamate has a distinct flavor. Monosodium glutamate (MSG) is added to food as a flavor enhancer. MSG Symptom Complex includes headaches, nausea, rapid heartbeat, vomiting, a tingling/numbness/burning sensation along the back, neck, arms, face, and chest pains. These MSG-induced symptoms tend to occur in sensitive individuals within 1 hour of consuming large amounts (more than 3 grams) of MSG or consuming MSG in a liquid (e.g., soup). Individuals with asthma may be predisposed to this syndrome as well as MSG-induced asthma attacks. Food products containing MSG will list it on the label. However, MSG may be used in restaurants, especially in Oriental cooking.

Aspartame: Aspartame is an artificial sweetener made from two amino acids: phenylalanine and aspartic acid. Aspartame is marketed as a low-calorie sweetener (NutraSweet and Equal are among its popular names). Associations have been reported between aspartame and a list of adverse symptoms including: headaches or migraines; dizziness; rashes; swelling of the lips or eyelids; difficulty breathing; rapid heartbeat; and depression. Individuals with mood disorders may be particularly vulnerable to these reactions. Aspartame is listed on the label of food products, beverages, and in medications, where it may also be used as a sweetening agent.

FD&C Yellow No. 5 (Tartrazine): FD&C Yellow No. 5, or tartrazine, is a dye used as a coloring agent in food processing. Among sensitive individuals, tartrazine appears to be a trigger for asthma, runny nose, and hives. The presence of this dye in a food or drug should be clearly indicated by the terms FD&C Yellow No. 5, tartrazine, or possibly E102 on the food product label or drug package insert. Individuals who are sensitive to aspirin may be sensitive to tartrazine as well.

Cross Contamination of Foods in and away from Home

If you are or live with an allergic individual, then cross contamination becomes a daily issue. Cross contamination refers to the situation through which a "safe" food comes in contact with an allergen—even a small amount. At home, this could occur by cutting a peanut butter sandwich on a cutting board. The board is effectively contaminated with enough peanut allergen to elicit a reaction from the next allergic user. In a bakery, this could occur when an employee removes a sugar cookie for an allergic customer with the same tongs that were used to remove a peanut-butter cookie. In a restaurant, this could occur if the steak you ordered is grilled alongside the fish you are allergic to.

To avoid cross contamination at home:

- Separate allergenic foods from other foods by storing them in a plastic box or container in the refrigerator or on the pantry shelf.

- Clean all pots, pans, and utensils thoroughly with soap and hot water, immediately after use with an allergen.

- Wash plates and utensils used with allergenic foods, separately and with a separate set of washing and drying cloths.

- Do not use wooden bowls or utensils because they absorb contaminants.

- Wash hands after contact with an allergen or wear nonlatex food gloves during food preparation.

To avoid cross contamination in restaurants:

- Avoid buffet-style dining.

- Avoid stores or cafes where food products are stored in bulk bins.

- Avoid sliced deli meats because slicers are used with a variety of products.

- Avoid seafood restaurants if you are allergic to any type of seafood.

- Avoid Asian restaurants (such as Thai or Indonesian) if you have a peanut or soy allergy.

- Tell your server about your allergy.

- Ask about possible hidden ingredients, especially in salad dressings and sauces.

- Ask about other foods being prepared in the kitchen simultaneously.

- Order simple dishes with sauces on the side.

- Carry a Chef Card—a personalized card with simple instructions to the chef and others, describing your allergy, related ingredients, and cross-contamination issues.

- Don't be afraid to leave a restaurant if you don't feel safe.

Not all foods and potential allergens have been included in this text. Check with your physician/specialist to make sure you have a complete, individualized list. If you are in doubt regarding food label information or product ingredients, contact the food manufacturer.

By Elizabeth A. Gollub, Ph.D., M.P.H., R.D., OPS professional, Amy Simonne, Ph.D., assistant professor and extension specialist, Department of Family, Youth and Community Sciences, University of Florida, Gainesville, FL 32611.

References

1. Food Allergen Labeling and Consumer Protection Act of 2003 (HR 3684 IH).

2. IFT—Scientific Status Summary: Seafood Allergy and Allergens—A review. October 1995.

3. Sicherer SH, Sampson HA. Prevalence of peanut and tree nut allergy in the United States determined by means of a random digit dial telephone survey: a five-year follow-up study. *Journal of Allergy and Clinical Immunology.* 2003;112(6):1203–1207.

4. Steinman HA. Hidden allergens in foods. *Journal of Allergy and Clinical Immunology.* 1996;98(2):241–250.

5. Taylor SL, Hefle SL. Food allergies and other food sensitivities. *Food Technology.* 2001;55(9):68–83.

6. Taylor SL, Stratton JE, Nordlee JA. Histamine poisoning (scombroid fish poisoning): an allergy-like intoxication. *J Toxicol Clin Toxicol.* 1989;27(4-5):225–240.

7. U.S. Food and Drug Administration. *FDA Medical Bulletin.* Monosodium Glutamate. 1996; vol. 26(1). http://www.fda.gov/medbull/january96/msg.html

8. U.S. Food and Drug Administration. Food allergies rare but risky. *FDA Consumer* May 1994. http://vm.cfsan.fda.gov/~dms/wh-alrg1.html

9. U.S. Food and Drug Administration. When food becomes the enemy. *FDA Consumer* July-August 2001 revised April 2004. www.fda.gov/fdac/features/2001/401_food.html

10. Walton RG, Hudak R, Green-Waite RJ. Adverse reactions to aspartame: double-blind challenge in patients from a vulnerable population. *Biol Psychiatry.* 1993 Jul 1-15; (34(1-2): 13–17.

11. William, J., Jr. Food Allergens: Effectively managing processing risks. *Food Protection Trends.* 2004. Vol. 24(1):20–22.

Section 28.2

Consumers with Allergies Will Benefit from Improved Food Labels

Excerpted from "FDA to Require Food Manufacturers to List Food Allergens: Consumers with Allergies Will Benefit From Improved Food Labels," by the Food and Drug Administration (www.fda.gov), December 20, 2005.

Effective January 1, 2006, the Food and Drug Administration (FDA) is requiring food labels to clearly state if food products contain any ingredients that contain protein derived from the eight major allergenic foods. As a result of the Food Allergen Labeling and Consumer Protection Act of 2004 (FALCPA), manufacturers are required to identify in plain English the presence of ingredients that contain protein derived from milk, eggs, fish, crustacean shellfish, tree nuts, peanuts, wheat, or soybeans in the list of ingredients or to say "contains" followed by name of the source of the food allergen after or adjacent to the list of ingredients.

This labeling will be especially helpful to children who must learn to recognize the presence of substances they must avoid. For example, if a product contains the milk-derived protein, casein, the product's label will have to use the term "milk" in addition to the term "casein" so that those with milk allergies can clearly understand the presence of the allergen they need to avoid.

It is estimated that 2 percent of adults and about 5 percent of infants and young children in the United States suffer from food allergies. Approximately 30,000 consumers require emergency room treatment and 150 Americans die each year because of allergic reactions to food.

"The eight major food allergens account for 90 percent of all documented food allergic reactions, and some reactions may be severe or life-threatening," said Robert E. Brackett, PhD, Director of FDA's Center for Food Safety and Applied Nutrition. "Consumers will benefit from improved food labels for products that contain food allergens."

FALCPA does not require food manufacturers or retailers to relabel or remove from grocery or supermarket shelves products that do not reflect the additional allergen labeling as long as the products were labeled before the effective date. As a result, FDA cautions consumers that there will be a transition period of undetermined length during which it is likely that consumers will see packaged food on store shelves and in consumers' homes without the revised allergen labeling.

Chapter 29

Reducing Allergy Risk and Caring for Your Child with Food Allergies

Chapter Contents

315

Section 29.1

The Timing of Solids Introduction to Infants and the Relationship to Food Allergies

"Introducing Cereal to Infants: Delaying Past 6 Months May Increase the Risk of Allergy" was provided by KidsHealth, one of the largest resources online for medically reviewed health information written for parents, kids, and teens. For more articles like this one, visit www.KidsHealth.org, or www.TeensHealth.org. © 2006 The Nemours Foundation. This document was reviewed by Steven Dowshen, M.D., June 2006.

Introducing solid foods to infants too soon—before 3 to 4 months—is associated with a higher risk of developing food allergies, which affect about 6% of children under 3. But delaying the introduction of cereal past 6 months of age may also increase a child's risk of allergy to wheat, say researchers from the National Jewish Medical and Research Center and the University of Colorado in Denver, Colorado.

In this small study, the parents of 1,612 infants reported when they introduced certain grains, such as wheat, barley, rye, and oats, into their child's diet. From birth to 4 years of age, the parents also noted whether a physician had diagnosed their child with allergies to foods such as:

- wheat;
- cow's milk;
- dairy products;
- infant formula;
- peanuts/peanut butter/nuts;
- eggs; and
- shellfish.

Parents also noted whether other family members had asthma, eczema, hives, or other conditions associated with allergy. In addition, children underwent periodic physical exams and blood testing to check for signs of allergy to wheat.

Overall, about 1% of children developed an allergy to wheat (children with celiac disease, a digestive disorder that's caused by a sensitivity to foods containing gluten, weren't included in this study). Researchers discovered that children who had their first taste of cereal after 6 months of age had more than four times the risk of developing wheat allergy compared with kids who were introduced to cereal prior to 6 months of age. Having a relative with an allergic condition also increased a child's risk of developing wheat allergy.

What This Means to You

According to the results of this small study, waiting until after 6 months of age to introduce cereal doesn't protect kids—in fact, it could increase their risk of developing an allergy to wheat. Symptoms of wheat allergy include skin swelling, hives, or itching; cramps, nausea, or vomiting; or wheezing and runny nose after eating or inhaling products made with wheat. Generally, doctors recommend that parents introduce cereals around 6 months of age. If you have any questions about when to introduce solid foods or if you think your child is showing signs of a food allergy, talk to your doctor.

Source: Jill A. Poole, M.D.; Kathy Barriga, MSPH; Donal Y. M. Leung, M.D., Ph.D.; Michelle Hoffman, RN; George S. Eisenbarth, M.D., Ph.D.; Marian Rewers, M.D., Ph.D.; Jill M. Norris, MPH, Ph.D.; *Pediatrics,* June 2006.

Section 29.2

Babies at High Risk for Allergies May Benefit from Formulas Free of Cow's Milk and Soy Proteins

"Hydrolyzed Casein or Whey Formula May Benefit Babies at Risk for Allergies" was provided by KidsHealth, one of the largest resources online for medically reviewed health information written for parents, kids, and teens. For more articles like this one, visit www.KidsHealth.org, or www.TeensHealth.org. © 2005 The Nemours Foundation. This document was reviewed by Steven Dowshen, M.D., October 2005.

Hydrolyzed formulas, originally developed as an alternative to infant formulas containing cow's milk or soy proteins, have been used to treat food allergies in infants with moms who can't breastfeed. But do they help to reduce the risk of allergies in infants with a family history of allergies?

Researchers from the Johns Hopkins University School of Medicine examined 22 previously published studies that evaluated the effectiveness of hydrolyzed formulas in infants. The studies compared the allergy-preventing effectiveness of hydrolyzed formulas, compared to breastfeeding, cow's milk formulas, soy formulas, and combinations of these other formulas.

In general, children who consumed only hydrolyzed formula had a lower rate of allergies for up to 5 years after birth, compared to infants fed traditional cow's milk formulas. Researchers concluded that using hydrolyzed formulas reduced the risk of allergies among infants whose parents had allergies (having a family history of allergies puts an infant at high risk for developing them, too).

What This Means to You

According to the results of this study, babies at high risk may have a reduced risk of developing allergies if they are fed hydrolyzed formulas. Hydrolyzed formulas marketed in the United States include the brand names Nutramigen, Alimentum, Pregestimil, and Nestle Good Start Supreme. If your child has an increased risk of allergies because of a family history of the disease, you can reduce your child's risk by breastfeeding as long as possible. If breastfeeding isn't possible, discuss with your child's doctor the potential benefits of using a hydrolyzed formula.

Source: Tiffani Hays, MS, RD, LN; Robert A. Wood, M.D.; *Archives of Pediatrics and Adolescent Medicine,* September 2005.

Section 29.3

Feeding Your Food-Allergic Child

"Food Allergies" was provided by KidsHealth, one of the largest resources online for medically reviewed health information written for parents, kids, and teens. For more articles like this one, visit www.KidsHealth.org, or www.TeensHealth.org. © 2005 The Nemours Foundation. This document was reviewed by William J. Geimeier, M.D., July 2005.

When Marcy prepared a peanut butter and jelly sandwich for her son Ben's lunch that morning, she did it because they were running late for day care and it was the quickest thing she could put together. But shortly after Ben began eating his lunch, his child-care provider noticed he seemed to be trying to scratch an itch in his mouth. After he vomited and began wheezing, the care provider sought medical treatment for Ben, who was later diagnosed with a food allergy, in this case to peanuts.

Along with milk, eggs, wheat, soy, and shellfish, peanuts are among the most common foods that cause allergies. For some kids, food allergies can cause only minor discomfort, like a little tingling in the mouth. But for others they can be severe, causing difficulty breathing, for example.

Learning how to recognize an allergic reaction will help you get your child the medical care needed if a reaction occurs. If your child has already been diagnosed with a food allergy, it's important to know:

- how to accommodate your child's dietary needs and
- what emergency preparations to make in case your child has an allergic reaction

What Is a Food Allergy?

With a food allergy, the body reacts as though that particular food product is harmful. As a result, the body's immune system (which fights infection and disease) creates antibodies to fight the food allergen, the substance in the food that triggers the allergy. The next time a person comes in contact with that food by touching or eating it or inhaling its particles, the body releases chemicals, including one called histamine, to "protect" itself. These chemicals trigger allergic symptoms that can affect the respiratory system, gastrointestinal tract, skin, or cardiovascular system. These symptoms might include a runny nose, an itchy skin rash, a tingling in the tongue, lips, or throat, swelling, abdominal pain, or wheezing.

People often confuse food allergies with food intolerance because of similar symptoms. Food intolerance:

- doesn't involve the immune system;

- can be caused by a person's inability to digest certain substances, such as lactose; and

- can be unpleasant but is rarely dangerous.

The symptoms of food intolerance can include burping, indigestion, flatulence, loose stools, headaches, flushing, or nervousness. A person with food intolerance can usually eat small amounts of the particular food without having any symptoms.

According to the U.S. Food and Drug Administration (FDA), up to 6% of children in the United States under age 3 have food allergies. They are less common in adults but, overall, food allergies affect nearly 4 million people.

Doctors can't predict which kids will have food allergies and which kids won't, but some factors may place a child at higher risk for developing food allergies. The tendency to become allergic in general is inherited. Many kids with food allergies come from families whose members have a history of other allergies.

Certain other health conditions are associated with severe allergic reactions to foods. For example, people with asthma are at greater risk for developing severe reactions from food allergies.

There's nothing you can do to completely eliminate the possibility that your child will develop food allergies. However, breastfeeding (especially exclusive breastfeeding that is not supplemented with infant formula) can help infants who are especially prone to milk or soy allergies avoid allergic reactions. When an infant consumes only breast milk, he or she has a decreased exposure to foods that can cause allergies. Some doctors also recommend that allergy-prone babies not be fed solid foods until 6 months of age or later to avoid exposure to allergenic foods.

Some Common Food Allergens

A child could be allergic to any food, but there are eight common allergens that account for 90% of all reactions in children:

1. milk
2. eggs
3. peanuts
4. tree nuts (such as walnuts and cashews)
5. fish
6. shellfish (such as shrimp)
7. soy
8. wheat

In general, most common food allergies are outgrown in childhood. Of kids who are allergic to milk, eggs, wheat, and soy, 55% of them outgrow those allergies by the time they are 3 years old. When it comes to nuts and seafood, 25% of kids with those allergies outgrow them by the time they are 3 years old.

Because allergens affect multiple parts of the body, an allergic child may experience a wide variety of symptoms within a few minutes or up to 2 hours after coming into contact with the food. Typically the first symptom is itching; other symptoms involve a rash, gastrointestinal symptoms, nausea, diarrhea, respiratory symptoms, and swelling.

A common skin symptom of a food allergy is hives, or raised red itchy bumps on the skin. Swelling of the face, throat, lips, and tongue also may occur, often within minutes of contact with the food. Respiratory symptoms such as wheezing and trouble breathing or gastrointestinal symptoms such as sudden abdominal pain and vomiting also are common reactions.

When a child has a serious allergic reaction with widespread effects on the body, this condition is known as anaphylaxis. A child with anaphylaxis, which can involve the heart, lungs, blood vessels, and other body systems, may:

- feel dizzy or lightheaded;
- lose consciousness;
- have a rapid heart rate;
- have difficulty breathing because of a swelling in the throat and airways; or
- have a life-threatening drop in blood pressure (also known as anaphylactic shock).

Without rapid emergency medical treatment, children with anaphylaxis can die if they are unable to breathe or if they collapse due to shock.

Medications that increase the heart rate and blood pressure, such as epinephrine, are often needed to control any kind of severe allergic reaction.

Diagnosing a Food Allergy

If your child has ever experienced any allergy symptoms or you suspect your child may have a food allergy, it's a good idea to contact your child's doctor or an allergy specialist. The doctor will take your child's medical history and ask questions about specific symptoms and your child's diet. To help identify specific allergens, the doctor may ask you to keep a food diary for your child with details on what foods are eaten and when symptoms occur.

Before diagnosing your child with a food allergy, the doctor will look for any other conditions that could be causing symptoms. For example, if your child seems to have diarrhea after drinking milk, the doctor may check to see if lactose intolerance could be causing this instead of a food allergy. In rare cases, a child is sensitive to dyes or food additives such as yellow #5 or monosodium glutamate (or MSG, a flavor enhancer commonly used in Asian and other foods), which can cause symptoms similar to those of a food allergy.

Another condition that may mimic food allergy symptoms is celiac disease, in which the child is not able to tolerate gluten, a protein found in wheat and certain other grains. Occasionally, a reaction can be caused by eating cheese, wine, or fish with high levels of histamine, a chemical occurring naturally in the body that in larger amounts may cause symptoms such as hives and rashes.

After other possible causes of the child's symptoms are ruled out, the doctor may recommend an elimination diet to help diagnose and identify a food allergy. During an elimination diet, a child avoids eating any food that is suspected of causing an allergy and the doctor follows the results to see if allergy symptoms disappear. If they do, the food will then be reintroduced to see if the child's symptoms reappear.

Skin testing also may be done to diagnose a food allergy. This procedure is usually performed in the doctor's office. The doctor will prick or scratch the child's skin with a plastic or metal prong with a small amount of allergen on it, placing the suspected allergic substance on the skin. If the child develops an itchy bump surrounded by redness (also called a wheal) within 15 minutes of the skin prick, the child is considered allergic to that substance.

For children who have extremely severe allergic reactions or other skin conditions such as eczema, the skin test may cause irritation or other more serious reactions. Your child's doctor may also do blood tests that check for antibodies for specific allergens.

Treating a Food Allergy

After diagnosing your child with a food allergy, the doctor will help you create a treatment plan. No medication can cure food allergies, so treatment usually means avoiding the allergen and all the foods that contain it.

Often, allergists will instruct parents to completely restrict the allergen from the child's diet. But it can be difficult to eliminate the offending food and maintain an otherwise nutritious, balanced diet, so it may be helpful to consult a registered dietitian about your child's diet.

Your child also may be advised to avoid foods containing similar allergens because they could cause a reaction as well. For example, a child who experiences hives and wheezing after eating shrimp probably will be told to avoid other shellfish such as lobster and crab. Your child's doctor should provide you with information about foods to avoid, ingredients to be careful of, and support groups for parents of children with food allergies.

Although there's no cure for food allergies, medications can treat both minor and severe symptoms. Antihistamines may be used to treat symptoms such as hives, runny nose, and abdominal pain associated with an allergic reaction. If your child wheezes or has asthma flares (also called attacks) as the result of a food allergy, the doctor will likely recommend that a bronchodilator such as albuterol (which can be inhaled from a handheld pump device) be taken right away to reduce breathing difficulties. But remember: If your child experiences an allergy-triggered breathing problem, it's important to seek emergency medical treatment immediately, even if your child has been given breathing medications at home or school to treat the reaction.

Epinephrine is often used to treat severe allergic reactions. If your child has severe food allergies, it's a good idea to have epinephrine within easy reach for quick use at all times. This may mean keeping epinephrine in your home, car, briefcase or purse, and also at relatives' homes, and your child's day care or school.

Signs and symptoms of a severe allergic reaction include:

- feeling of warmth, flushing, or tickling in the mouth;
- red, itchy rash;
- hives;
- feeling of lightheadedness;
- shortness of breath;
- wheezing;
- severe sneezing;
- anxiety;
- cramps in the stomach or uterus; and
- vomiting or diarrhea.

If your child has a food allergy reaction severe enough to cause wheezing, you should seek emergency care immediately instead of using an inhaler to treat the wheezing. As soon as you recognize that your child is having a severe reaction, call 911 and explain your child's condition. Quick treatment can mean the difference between life and death for children with the most severe food allergies.

Feeding Your Child with Food Allergies

Feeding a child with food allergies can be challenging. You'll need to familiarize yourself with food labels and ingredients lists so you can avoid your child's particular allergen. Below are a few suggestions of what to watch out for.

If your child is allergic to:

- **Milk:** Avoid cheeses, butter, creams, and yogurt. Also avoid lactose-free milk as well as foods with ingredients such as casein and whey.

- **Eggs:** Avoid cakes, cookies, pastries, mayonnaise, and egg substitutes. Also avoid foods that contain ovalbumin, often abbreviated as Ov. Some fresh pastas and soups may also be prepared with eggs. In addition, the doctor may advise against a flu shot for a child with an egg allergy because the flu vaccine contains small amounts of egg protein.

- **Soy:** Avoid soybeans, soy nut butter, soy sauce, soy protein, soy oil, and tofu. Also avoid any food with lecithin in the ingredients list.

- **Peanuts:** Avoid any food that contains nuts, as well as peanut flour or peanut oil. You will also want to prevent your child from eating Asian foods (which are often cooked in peanut oil), egg rolls, chocolate, candy bars, and any pastries that may contain nuts. If a food's ingredients include hydrolyzed plant or vegetable protein, avoid it because it may contain peanuts. Although peanuts and tree nuts are two different foods and are not actually related, children who have peanut allergies are advised to avoid tree nuts (and vice versa) because about 30% react to both allergens.

- **Tree nuts:** Avoid almonds, Brazil nuts, walnuts, pecans, cashews, and macadamia nuts. You'll also want to keep your child away from nut butters or any product that mentions nuts in the ingredients list, including ice cream or crackers, unless you know them to be nut-free.

- **Shellfish:** Avoid crab, lobster, shrimp, snails, clams, and oysters, as well as other types of shellfish. Children who are allergic to shellfish may be able to tolerate fish that swim, such as flounder or cod, but testing may be needed to determine any sensitivity to those foods. Alternatively, children who are allergic to fish that swim may tolerate shellfish. Marinara sauce, Worcestershire sauce, salad dressings, and hot dogs and deli meats may also contain fish or shellfish ingredients.

In general, if your child has severe food allergies, it's a good idea to be cautious about allowing your child to eat processed foods. If you cook with whole-food ingredients and bake from scratch, you'll greatly decrease your child's risk of exposure to an allergen.

And just because your child has a food allergy doesn't mean that favorite kid foods have to be out of reach. Many of your favorite family recipes can be easily modified to fit your child's special needs. For example, in recipes calling for milk, substitute equal amounts of juice or water to preserve consistency. If your child has an egg allergy, you can substitute a mixture of 1 teaspoon (5 milliliters) of baking powder,

1 tablespoon (15 milliliters) of water or milk, and 1 tablespoon (15 milliliters) of vinegar for each egg. For more information about food substitutions and allergen-free recipes, look to food allergy organizations such as the Food Allergy & Anaphylaxis Network, which publishes cookbooks and recipes for parents of children with food allergies.

Beginning in 2006, packaged foods that contain some of the most common allergens must be clearly labeled. Food makers are required to clearly state, in or adjacent to the list of ingredients, whether the product contains milk, eggs, fish, shellfish, tree nuts, peanuts, wheat, or soybeans. This new law only applies to foods labeled after the start of 2006, so there may still be products on the grocery store shelves that were packaged before then, which don't have information about allergens.

Even so, eating packaged foods or dining in schools or restaurants could bring your child into contact with hidden sources of the allergen. Even if a food does not initially contain the allergenic food as an ingredient, your child could be exposed to it due to cross-contamination. In cross-contamination, a pan, utensil, dish, or surface used to prepare an allergenic food could contaminate a food that wouldn't normally cause a reaction. For example, cheeses and deli meats might be cut with the same slicer, which could be dangerous for a child with a milk allergy who orders a cheese-free sandwich.

Planning is key to helping your child enjoy meals and snacks and avoid allergic reactions. In general, it's safer to pack your child's food yourself than to rely on restaurants. If you do visit a restaurant with your child, it's important to ask detailed questions about the preparation techniques and ingredients used to make the food. And consider choosing simply prepared menu items such as cuts of meat, steamed vegetables, or baked potatoes instead of complicated dishes that contain many ingredients.

Traveling with a child who has food allergies can be challenging, but many hotels and airlines offer options to make it a little easier. When making reservations with an airline, it's a good idea to tell the representative that your child has food allergies. With prior notice, some airlines will avoid serving peanut snacks during the flight and most will serve your child allergen-free meals. To ensure your child's safety, confirm your child's special meal before boarding the plane and ask the flight attendants how the food is prepared so you're sure there's no chance of cross-contamination. At your destination, consider staying in a hotel or motel offering small refrigerators or hot plates that will allow you to prepare meals in your room.

Although packing your child's lunch will avoid cross-contamination and ensure that your child eats only allergen-free foods, you also may be able to work with your child's school cafeteria to manage your child's allergy. Talk to the school's nutritionist for detailed information about the ingredients in breakfast or lunch menus, and discuss food preparation practices to determine if cross-contamination could take place. Some schools even provide peanut-free tables or rooms for children with severe peanut allergies. It's important to be open with teachers and school administrators about your child's allergy so they can help keep your child safe.

Other Tips for Avoiding Reactions

The key to successful management of your child's food allergy is being prepared. Depending on the severity of the allergy, your child's doctor may recommend that your child carry prescription medication, such as epinephrine, in case of a severe allergic reaction. You may also be instructed to keep antihistamines close at hand to treat your child in case of an emergency.

Unfortunately, mistakes can happen even when you and your child are being careful. Because of the potential severity of allergic reactions to food, your child should wear a medical alert bracelet or necklace with the allergic condition inscribed on it. In an emergency, medical personnel or doctors will know that your child has a food allergy.

Try to work with your child's school or child-care center to find ways your child can be supervised to prevent contact with allergenic foods. Find out who would give your child treatment and discuss your child's allergies with that person, making sure that they have any necessary medications.

Although breastfeeding is one way to delay a child's exposure to allergens, certain allergens from foods in a mother's diet can be passed through breast milk and cause a reaction in an infant. If your family has a history of food allergies and you are breastfeeding your child, discuss your situation with an allergy specialist or your child's doctor. The doctor may recommend that you eliminate major allergenic foods such as dairy products, eggs, peanuts and tree nuts, fish and shellfish, and soy from your own diet.

If you must eliminate a major component of your diet—such as dairy products—consider consulting a registered dietitian to ensure that your diet is balanced and provides enough calories for good health while you're nursing.

A final crucial step in protecting your child is stressing the importance of healthy habits. Teach your child to never share or trade food at school or at a friend's house. If the allergy isn't outgrown, you'll need to teach your child how to read food labels and ingredients lists and to ask how food is prepared when eating away from home.

Part Four

Airborne, Chemical, and Other Environmental Allergy Triggers

Chapter 30

Airborne Allergens: Something in the Air

Introduction

Sneezing is not always the symptom of a cold. Sometimes, it is an allergic reaction to something in the air. Health experts estimate that 35 million Americans suffer from upper respiratory tract symptoms that are allergic reactions to airborne allergens. Pollen allergy, commonly called hay fever, is one of the most common chronic diseases in the United States. Worldwide, airborne allergens cause the most problems for people with allergies. The respiratory symptoms of asthma, which affect approximately 11 million Americans, are often provoked by airborne allergens.

Overall, allergic diseases are among the major causes of illness and disability in the United States, affecting as many as 40 to 50 million Americans.

The National Institute of Allergy and Infectious Diseases (NIAID) of the National Institutes of Health (an agency of the U.S. Department of Health and Human Services) supports and conducts research on allergic diseases. The goals of this research are to provide a better understanding of the causes of allergy, to improve methods for diagnosing and treating allergic reactions, and eventually to prevent allergies.

From a booklet by the National Institute of Allergy and Infectious Diseases (NIAID, www.niaid.nih.gov), part of the National Institutes of Health, April 2003. Table 30.1 is also a publication of the NIAID titled "Is It a Cold or an Allergy?" dated September 2005.

This text summarizes what health experts know about the causes and symptoms of allergic reactions to airborne allergens, how health care providers diagnose and treat these reactions, and what medical researchers are doing to help people who suffer from these allergies.

What is an allergy?

An allergy is a specific reaction of the body's immune system to a normally harmless substance, one that does not bother most people. People who have allergies often are sensitive to more than one substance. Types of allergens that cause allergic reactions include:

- pollens;
- house dust mites;
- mold spores;
- food;
- latex rubber;
- insect venom; and
- medicines.

Why are some people allergic?

Scientists think that some people inherit a tendency to be allergic from one or both parents. This means they are more likely to have allergies. They probably, however, do not inherit a tendency to be allergic to any specific allergen. Children are more likely to develop allergies if one or both parents have allergies. In addition, exposure to allergens at times when the body's defenses are lowered or weakened, such as after a viral infection or during pregnancy, seems to contribute to developing allergies.

What is an allergic reaction?

Normally, the immune system functions as the body's defense against invading germs such as bacteria and viruses. In most allergic reactions, however, the immune system is responding to a false alarm. When an allergic person first comes into contact with an allergen, the immune system treats the allergen as an invader and gets ready to attack.

The immune system does this by generating large amounts of a type of antibody called immunoglobulin E, or IgE. Each IgE antibody is specific for one particular substance. In the case of pollen allergy, each antibody is specific for one type of pollen. For example, the immune system may produce one type of antibody to react against oak pollen and another against ragweed pollen.

The IgE molecules are special because IgE is the only type of antibody that attaches tightly to the body's mast cells, which are tissue cells, and to basophils, which are blood cells. When the allergen next encounters its specific IgE, it attaches to the antibody like a key fitting into a lock. This action signals the cell to which the IgE is attached to release (and, in some cases, to produce) powerful chemicals like histamine, which cause inflammation. These chemicals act on tissues in various parts of the body, such as the respiratory system, and cause the symptoms of allergy.

Table 30.1. Is It a Cold or an Allergy?

Symptoms	Cold	Airborne Allergy
Cough	Common	Sometimes
General Aches, Pains	Slight	Never
Fatigue, Weakness	Sometimes	Sometimes
Itchy Eyes	Rare or Never	Common
Sneezing	Usual	Usual
Sore Throat	Common	Sometimes
Runny Nose	Common	Common
Stuffy Nose	Common	Common
Fever	Rare	Never
Duration	3 to 14 days	Weeks (for example, 6 weeks for ragweed or grass pollen seasons)
Treatment	Antihistamines, decongestants, nonsteroidal anti-inflammatory medicines	Antihistamines, nasal steroids, decongestants
Prevention	Wash your hands often; avoid close contact with anyone with a cold	Avoid those things you are allergic to such as pollen, house dust mites, mold, pet dander, cockroaches
Complications	Sinus infection, middle ear infection, asthma	Sinus infection, asthma

Source: U.S. Department of Health and Human Services, National Institutes of Health, National Institute of Allergy and Infectious Diseases, September 2005.

Symptoms

The signs and symptoms of airborne allergies are familiar to many:

- sneezing, often with a runny or clogged nose;
- coughing and postnasal drip;
- itching eyes, nose, and throat;
- watering eyes;
- conjunctivitis;
- "allergic shiners" (dark circles under the eyes caused by increased blood flow near the sinuses); and/or
- "allergic salute" (in a child, persistent upward rubbing of the nose that causes a crease mark on the nose).

In people who are not allergic, the mucus in the nasal passages simply moves foreign particles to the throat, where they are swallowed or coughed out. But something different happens in a person who is sensitive to airborne allergens.

In sensitive people, as soon as the allergen lands on the lining inside the nose, a chain reaction occurs that leads the mast cells in these tissues to release histamine and other chemicals. The powerful chemicals contract certain cells that line some small blood vessels in the nose. This allows fluids to escape, which causes the nasal passages to swell—resulting in nasal congestion. Histamine also can cause sneezing, itching, irritation, and excess mucous production, which can result in allergic rhinitis.

Other chemicals released by mast cells, including cytokines and leukotrienes, also contribute to allergic symptoms.

Some people with allergy develop asthma, which can be a very serious condition. The symptoms of asthma include:

- coughing;
- wheezing; and
- shortness of breath.

The shortness of breath is due to a narrowing of the airways in the lungs and to excess mucous production and inflammation. Asthma can be disabling and sometimes fatal. If wheezing and shortness of breath accompany allergy symptoms, it is a signal that the airways also have become involved.

Is it an allergy or a cold?

There is no good way to tell the difference between allergy symptoms of runny nose, coughing, and sneezing and cold symptoms. Allergy symptoms, however, may last longer than cold symptoms. Anyone who has any respiratory illness that lasts longer than a week or two should consult a health care provider.

Pollen Allergy

Each spring, summer, and fall, tiny pollen grains are released from trees, weeds, and grasses. These grains hitch rides on currents of air. Although the mission of pollen is to fertilize parts of other plants, many never reach their targets. Instead, pollen enters human noses and throats, triggering a type of seasonal allergic rhinitis called pollen allergy. Many people know this as hay fever.

Of all the things that can cause an allergy, pollen is one of the most common. Many of the foods, medicines, or animals that cause allergies can be avoided to a great extent. Even insects and household dust are escapable. But short of staying indoors, with the windows closed, when the pollen count is high—and even that may not help—there is no easy way to avoid airborne pollen.

What is pollen?

Plants produce tiny—too tiny to see with the naked eye—round or oval pollen grains to reproduce. In some species, the plant uses the pollen from its own flowers to fertilize itself. Other types must be cross-pollinated. Cross-pollination means that for fertilization to take place and seeds to form, pollen must be transferred from the flower of one plant to that of another of the same species. Insects do this job for certain flowering plants, while other plants rely on wind for transport.

The types of pollen that most commonly cause allergic reactions are produced by the plain-looking plants (trees, grasses, and weeds) that do not have showy flowers. These plants make small, light, dry pollen grains that are custom-made for wind transport.

Amazingly, scientists have collected samples of ragweed pollen 400 miles out at sea and 2 miles high in the air. Because airborne pollen can drift for many miles, it does little good to rid an area of an offending plant. In addition, most allergenic pollen comes from plants that produce it in huge quantities. For example, a single ragweed plant can generate a million grains of pollen a day.

The type of allergens in the pollen is the main factor that determines whether the pollen is likely to cause hay fever. For example, pine tree pollen is produced in large amounts by a common tree, which would make it a good candidate for causing allergy. It is, however, a relatively rare cause of allergy because the type of allergens in pine pollen appear to make it less allergenic.

Among North American plants, weeds are the most prolific producers of allergenic pollen. Ragweed is the major culprit, but other important sources are sagebrush, redroot, pigweed, lamb's quarters, Russian thistle (tumbleweed), and English plantain.

Grasses and trees, too, are important sources of allergenic pollens. Although more than 1,000 species of grass grow in North America, only a few produce highly allergenic pollen.

It is common to hear people say they are allergic to colorful or scented flowers like roses. In fact, only florists, gardeners, and others who have prolonged, close contact with flowers are likely to be sensitive to pollen from these plants. Most people have little contact with the large, heavy, waxy pollen grains of such flowering plants because this type of pollen is not carried by wind but by insects such as butterflies and bees.

Some grasses that produce pollen:

- Timothy grass
- Kentucky bluegrass
- Johnson grass
- Bermuda grass
- Redtop grass
- Orchard grass
- Sweet vernal grass

Some trees that produce pollen:

- Oak
- Ash
- Elm
- Hickory
- Pecan
- Box elder
- Mountain cedar

When do plants make pollen?

One of the most obvious features of pollen allergy is its seasonal nature—people have symptoms only when the pollen grains to which they are allergic are in the air. Each plant has a pollinating period that is more or less the same from year to year. Exactly when a plant starts to pollinate seems to depend on the relative length of night and day—and therefore on geographical location—rather than on the weather. On the other hand, weather conditions during pollination can affect the amount of pollen produced and distributed in a specific year. Thus, in the Northern Hemisphere, the farther north you go, the later the start of the pollinating period and the later the start of the allergy season.

A pollen count, familiar to many people from local weather reports, is a measure of how much pollen is in the air. This count represents the concentration of all the pollen (or of one particular type, like ragweed) in the air in a certain area at a specific time. It is shown in grains of pollen per square meter of air collected over 24 hours. Pollen counts tend to be the highest early in the morning on warm, dry, breezy days and lowest during chilly, wet periods. Although the pollen count is an approximate measure that changes, it is useful as a general guide for when it may be wise to stay indoors and avoid contact with the pollen.

Mold Allergy

What is mold?

There are thousands of types of molds and yeasts in the fungus family. Yeasts are single cells that divide to form clusters. Molds are made of many cells that grow as branching threads called hyphae. Although both can probably cause allergic reactions, only a small number of molds are widely recognized offenders.

The seeds or reproductive pieces of fungi are called spores. Spores differ in size, shape, and color among types of mold. Each spore that germinates can give rise to new mold growth, which in turn can produce millions of spores.

What is mold allergy?

When inhaled, tiny fungal spores, or sometimes pieces of fungi, may cause allergic rhinitis. Because they are so small, mold spores also can reach the lungs.

In a small number of people, symptoms of mold allergy may be brought on or worsened by eating certain foods such as cheeses processed with fungi. Occasionally, mushrooms, dried fruits, and foods containing yeast, soy sauce, or vinegar will produce allergy symptoms.

Where do molds grow?

Molds can be found wherever there is moisture, oxygen, and a source of the few other chemicals they need. In the fall, they grow on rotting logs and fallen leaves, especially in moist, shady areas. In gardens they can be found in compost piles and on certain grasses and weeds. Some molds attach to grains such as wheat, oats, barley, and corn, which makes farms, grain bins, and silos likely places to find mold.

Hot spots of mold growth in the home include damp basements and closets, bathrooms (especially shower stalls), places where fresh food is stored, refrigerator drip trays, house plants, air conditioners, humidifiers, garbage pails, mattresses, upholstered furniture, and old foam rubber pillows.

Molds also like bakeries, breweries, barns, dairies, and greenhouses. Loggers, mill workers, carpenters, furniture repairers, and upholsterers often work in moldy environments.

What molds are allergenic?

Like pollens, mold spores are important airborne allergens only if they are abundant, easily carried by air currents, and allergenic in their chemical makeup. Found almost everywhere, mold spores in some areas are so numerous they often outnumber the pollens in the air. Fortunately, however, only a few dozen different types are significant allergens.

In general, *Alternaria* and *Cladosporium* (Hormodendrum) are the molds most commonly found both indoors and outdoors in the United States. *Aspergillus*, *Penicillium*, *Helminthosporium*, *Epicoccum*, *Fusarium*, *Mucor*, *Rhizopus*, and *Aurebasidium* (*Pullularia*) are common as well.

There is no relationship, however, between a respiratory allergy to the mold *Penicillium* and an allergy to the drug penicillin, which is made from mold.

Are mold counts helpful?

Similar to pollen counts, mold counts may suggest the types and number of fungi present at a certain time and place. For several reasons, however, these counts probably cannot be used as a constant guide for daily activities.

One reason is that the number and types of spores actually present in the mold count may have changed considerably in 24 hours because weather and spore distribution are directly related. Many common allergenic molds are of the dry spore type—they release their spores during dry, windy weather. Other fungi need high humidity, fog, or dew to release their spores. Although rain washes many larger spores out of the air, it also causes some smaller spores to be propelled into the air.

In addition to the effect of weather changes during 24-hour periods on mold counts, spore populations may also differ between day and night. Dry spore types are usually released during daytime, and wet spore types are usually released at night.

Are there other mold-related disorders?

Fungi or organisms related to them may cause other health problems similar to allergic diseases. Some kinds of *Aspergillus* may cause several different illnesses, including both infections and allergies. These fungi may lodge in the airways or a distant part of the lung and grow until they form a compact sphere known as a "fungus ball." In people with lung damage or serious underlying illnesses, *Aspergillus* may grasp the opportunity to invade the lungs or the whole body.

In some people, exposure to these fungi also can lead to asthma or to a lung disease resembling severe inflammatory asthma called allergic bronchopulmonary aspergillosis. This latter condition, which occurs only in a small number of people with asthma, causes wheezing, low-grade fever, and coughing up of brown-flecked masses or mucous plugs. Skin testing, blood tests, x-rays, and examination of the sputum for fungi can help establish the diagnosis. Corticosteroid drugs usually treat this reaction effectively. Immunotherapy (allergy shots) is not helpful.

Dust Mite Allergy

Dust mite allergy is an allergy to a microscopic organism that lives in the dust found in all dwellings and workplaces. House dust, as well as some house furnishings, contains microscopic mites. Dust mites are perhaps the most common cause of perennial allergic rhinitis. House dust mite allergy usually produces symptoms similar to pollen allergy and also can produce symptoms of asthma.

House dust mites, which live in bedding, upholstered furniture, and carpets, thrive in summer and die in winter. In a warm, humid house, however, they continue to thrive even in the coldest months. The particles seen floating in a shaft of sunlight include dead dust mites and their waste products. These waste products, which are proteins, actually provoke the allergic reaction.

What is house dust?

Rather than a single substance, so-called house dust is a varied mixture of potentially allergenic materials. It may contain fibers from different types of fabrics and materials such as:

- cotton lint, feathers, and other stuffing materials;
- dander from cats, dogs, and other animals;
- bacteria;
- mold and fungus spores (especially in damp areas);
- food particles;
- bits of plants and insects; or
- other allergens peculiar to an individual house or building.

Cockroaches are commonly found in crowded cities and in the southern United States. Certain proteins in cockroach feces and saliva also can be found in house dust. These proteins can cause allergic reactions or trigger asthma symptoms in some people, especially children. Cockroach allergens likely play a significant role in causing asthma in many inner-city populations.

Animal Allergy

Household pets are the most common source of allergic reactions to animals.

Many people think that pet allergy is provoked by the fur of cats and dogs. Researchers have found, however, that the major allergens are proteins in the saliva. These proteins stick to the fur when the animal licks itself.

Urine is also a source of allergy-causing proteins, as is the skin. When the substance carrying the proteins dries, the proteins can then float into the air. Cats may be more likely than dogs to cause allergic reactions because they lick themselves more, may be held more, and spend more time in the house, close to humans.

Some rodents, such as guinea pigs and gerbils, have become increasingly popular as household pets. They, too, can cause allergic reactions in some people, as can mice and rats. Urine is the major source of allergens from these animals.

Allergies to animals can take 2 years or more to develop and may not decrease until 6 months or more after ending contact with the animal. Carpet and furniture are a reservoir for pet allergens, and the allergens can remain in them for 4 to 6 weeks. In addition, these allergens can stay in household air for months after the animal has been removed. Therefore, it is wise for people with an animal allergy to check with the landlord or previous owner to find out if furry pets lived on the premises.

Chemical Sensitivity

Some people report that they react to chemicals in their environments and that these allergy-like reactions seem to result from exposure to a wide variety of synthetic and natural substances. Such substances can include those found in:

- paints;
- carpeting;
- plastics;
- perfumes;
- cigarette smoke; and
- plants.

Although the symptoms may resemble those of allergies, sensitivity to chemicals does not represent a true allergic reaction involving IgE and the release of histamine or other chemicals. Rather than a reaction to an allergen, it is a reaction to a chemical irritant, which may affect people with allergies more than others.

Diagnosis

People with allergy symptoms—such as the runny nose of allergic rhinitis—may at first suspect they have a cold, but the "cold" lingers on. Testing for allergies is the best way to find out if a person is allergic.

Skin Tests

Allergists (doctors who specialize in allergic diseases) use skin tests to determine whether a person has IgE antibodies in the skin that react to a specific allergen. The allergist will use weakened extracts from allergens such as dust mites, pollens, or molds commonly found in the local area. The extract of each kind of allergen is injected under a person's skin or is applied to a tiny scratch or puncture made on the arm or back.

Skin tests are one way of measuring the level of IgE antibody in a person. With a positive reaction, a small, raised, reddened area, called a wheal (hive), with a surrounding flush, called a flare, will appear at the test site. The size of the wheal can give the doctor an important diagnostic clue, but a positive reaction does not prove that a particular allergen is the cause of symptoms. Although such a reaction indicates that IgE antibody to a specific allergen is present, respiratory symptoms do not necessarily result.

Blood Tests

Skin testing is the most sensitive and least costly way to identify allergies. People with widespread skin conditions like eczema, however, should not be tested using this method.

There are other diagnostic tests that use a blood sample to detect levels of IgE antibody to a particular allergen. One such blood test is called the radioallergosorbent test (RAST), which can be performed when eczema is present or if a person has taken medicines that interfere with skin testing.

Some ways to handle airborne allergies:

- avoid the allergen;
- take medicine; or
- get allergy shots.

Prevention

Avoidance

Pollen and Molds: Complete avoidance of allergenic pollen or mold means moving to a place where the offending substance does not grow and where it is not present in the air. Even this extreme solution may offer only temporary relief because a person sensitive to a specific pollen or mold may develop allergies to new allergens after repeated exposure to them. For example, people allergic to ragweed may leave their ragweed-ridden communities and relocate to areas where ragweed does not grow, only to develop allergies to other weeds or even to grasses or trees in their new surroundings. Because relocating is not a reliable solution, allergy specialists do not encourage this approach.

There are other ways to reduce exposure to offending pollens.

- Remain indoors with the windows closed in the morning, for example, when the outdoor pollen levels are highest. Sunny, windy days can be especially troublesome.

- Wear a face mask designed to filter pollen out of the air and keep it from reaching nasal passages, if you must work outdoors.

- Take your vacation at the height of the expected pollinating period and choose a location where such exposure would be minimal.

Vacationing at the seashore or on a cruise, for example, may be effective retreats for avoiding pollen allergies.

House Dust: If you have dust mite allergy, pay careful attention to dust-proofing your bedroom. The worst things to have in the bedroom are:

- wall-to-wall carpet;
- blinds;
- down-filled blankets;
- feather pillows;
- stuffed animals;
- heating vents with forced hot air;
- dogs and cats; and
- closets full of clothing.

Carpets trap dust and make dust control impossible.

- Shag carpets are the worst type of carpet for people who are sensitive to dust mites.

- Vacuuming doesn't get rid of dust mite proteins in furniture and carpeting, but redistributes them back into the room, unless the vacuum has a special HEPA (high-efficiency particulate air) filter.

- Rugs on concrete floors encourage dust mite growth.

If possible, replace wall-to-wall carpets with washable throw rugs over hardwood, tile, or linoleum floors, and wash the rugs frequently.

Reducing the amount of dust mites in your home may mean new cleaning techniques as well as some changes in furnishings to eliminate dust collectors. Water is often the secret to effective dust removal.

- Clean washable items, including throw rugs, often, using water hotter than 130 degrees Fahrenheit. Lower temperatures will not kill dust mites.

- Clean washable items at a commercial establishment that uses high water temperature, if you cannot or do not want to set water temperature in your home at 130 degrees. (There is a danger of getting scalded if the water is more than 120 degrees.)

- Dust frequently with a damp cloth or oiled mop.

If cockroaches are a problem in your home, the U.S. Environmental Protection Agency suggests some ways to get rid of them.

- Do not leave food or garbage out.

- Store food in airtight containers.

- Clean all food crumbs or spilled liquids right away.

- Try using poison baits, boric acid (for cockroaches), or traps first, before using pesticide sprays.

If you use sprays:

- Do not spray in food preparation or storage areas.

- Do not spray in areas where children play or sleep.

- Limit the spray to the infested area.

- Follow instructions on the label carefully.

- Make sure there is plenty of fresh air when you spray.

- Keep the person with allergies or asthma out of the room while spraying.

Pets: If you or your child is allergic to furry pets, especially cats, the best way to avoid allergic reactions is to find them another home. If you are like most people who are attached to their pets, that is usually not a desirable option. There are ways, however, to help lower the levels of animal allergens in the air, which may reduce allergic reactions.

- Bathe your cat weekly and brush it more frequently (ideally, a non-allergic person should do this).

- Keep cats out of your bedroom.

- Remove carpets and soft furnishings, which collect animal allergens.

- Use a vacuum cleaner and room air cleaners with HEPA filters.

- Wear a face mask while house and cat cleaning.

Chemicals: Irritants such as chemicals can worsen airborne allergy symptoms, and you should avoid them as much as possible. For example, if you have pollen allergy, avoid unnecessary exposure to irritants such as insect sprays, tobacco smoke, air pollution, and fresh tar or paint during periods of high pollen levels.

Air Conditioners and Filters: When possible, use air conditioners inside your home or car to help prevent pollen and mold allergens from entering. Various types of air-filtering devices made with fiberglass or electrically charged plates may help reduce allergens produced in the home. You can add these to your present heating and cooling system. In addition, portable devices that can be used in individual rooms are especially helpful in reducing animal allergens.

An allergist can suggest which kind of filter is best for your home. Before buying a filtering device, rent one and use it in a closed room (the bedroom, for instance) for a month or two to see whether your allergy symptoms diminish. The airflow should be sufficient to exchange the air in the room five or six times per hour. Therefore, the size and efficiency of the filtering device should be determined in part by the size of the room.

You should be wary of exaggerated claims for appliances that cannot really clean the air. Very small air cleaners cannot remove dust and pollen. No air purifier can prevent viral or bacterial diseases such as the flu, pneumonia, or tuberculosis.

Before buying an electrostatic precipitator, you should compare the machine's ozone output with Federal standards. Ozone can irritate the noses and airways of people with allergies, especially those with asthma, and can increase their allergy symptoms. Other kinds of air filters, such as HEPA filters, do not release ozone into the air. HEPA filters, however, require adequate air flow to force air through them.

Treatment

Medicines

If you cannot adequately avoid airborne allergens, your symptoms often can be controlled by medicines. You can buy medicines without a prescription that can relieve allergy symptoms. If, however, they don't give you relief or they cause unwanted side effects such as sleepiness, your health care provider can prescribe antihistamines and topical nasal steroids. You can use either medicine alone or together.

Antihistamines

As the name indicates, an antihistamine counters the effects of histamine, which is released by the mast cells in your body's tissues and contributes to your allergy symptoms. For many years, antihistamines have proven useful in relieving itching in the nose and eyes; sneezing; and in reducing nasal swelling and drainage.

Many people who take antihistamines have some distressing side effects such as drowsiness and loss of alertness and coordination. Adults may interpret such reactions in children as behavior problems.

Antihistamines that cause fewer of these side effects are available over-the-counter or by prescription. These non-sedating antihistamines are as effective as other antihistamines in preventing histamine-induced symptoms, but most do so without causing sleepiness.

Topical Nasal Steroids

You should not confuse topical nasal steroids with anabolic steroids, which athletes sometimes use to enlarge muscle mass and which can have serious side effects. The chemicals in nasal steroids are different from those in anabolic steroids.

Topical nasal steroids are anti-inflammatory medicines that stop the allergic reaction. In addition to other helpful actions, they decrease the number of mast cells in the nose and reduce mucous secretion and nasal swelling. The combination of antihistamines and nasal steroids is a very effective way to treat allergic rhinitis, especially if you have moderate or severe allergic rhinitis. Although topical nasal steroids can have side effects, they are safe when used at recommended doses.

Cromolyn Sodium

Cromolyn sodium is a nasal spray that in some people helps prevent allergic rhinitis from starting. When used as a nasal spray, it can safely stop the release of chemicals like histamine from mast cells. It has few side effects when used as directed and significantly helps some people manage their allergies.

Decongestants

Sometimes helping the nasal passages to drain away mucus will help relieve symptoms such as congestion, swelling, excess secretions, and discomfort in the sinus areas that can be caused by nasal allergies. Your doctor may recommend using oral or nasal decongestants to reduce congestion along with an antihistamine to control allergic symptoms.

You should not, however, use over-the-counter or prescription decongestant nose drops and sprays for more than a few days. When used for longer periods, these medicines can lead to even more congestion and swelling of the nasal passages. Because of recent concern about the bad effects of decongestant sprays and drops, some have been removed from store shelves.

Immunotherapy

Immunotherapy, or a series of allergy shots, is the only available treatment that has a chance of reducing your allergy symptoms over a longer period of time. You would receive subcutaneous (under the skin) injections of increasing concentrations of the allergen(s) to which you are sensitive. These injections reduce the level of IgE antibodies in the blood and cause the body to make a protective antibody called IgG.

About 85 percent of people with allergic rhinitis will see their hay fever symptoms and need for medicines drop significantly within 12 months of starting immunotherapy. Those who benefit from allergy shots may continue it for 3 years and then consider stopping. While many are able to stop the injections with good results lasting for several years, others do get worse after the shots are stopped.

One research study shows that children treated for allergic rhinitis with immunotherapy were less likely to develop asthma. Researchers need to study this further, however.

As researchers produce better allergens for immunotherapy, this technique will be become an even more effective treatment.

Allergy Research

Research on allergies is focused on understanding what happens to the human body during the allergic process—the sequence of events leading to the allergic response and the factors responsible for allergic diseases.

Scientists supported by NIAID found that, during the first years of their lives, children raised in a house with two or more dogs or cats may be less likely to develop allergic diseases as compared with children raised without pets. The striking finding here is that high pet exposure early in life appears to protect some children from not only pet allergy but also other types of common allergies, such as allergy to house dust mites, ragweed, and grass. This new finding is changing the way scientists think about pet exposure. Scientists must now figure out how pet exposure causes a general shift of the immune system away from an allergic response.

The results of this and a number of other studies suggest that bacteria carried by pets may be responsible for holding back the immune system's allergic response. These bacteria release molecules called endotoxin. Some researchers think endotoxin is the molecule responsible for shifting the developing immune system away from responding to allergens through a class of lymphocytes called Th-2 cells. (These cells are associated with allergic reactions.) Instead, endotoxin may stimulate the immune system to block allergic reactions.

If scientists can find out exactly what it is about pets or the bacteria they carry that prevents the allergic response, they might be able to develop a new allergy treatment.

Some studies are seeking better ways to diagnose as well as treat people with allergic diseases and to better understand the factors that regulate IgE production to reduce the allergic response. Several research institutions are focusing on ways to influence the cells that participate in the allergic response.

NIAID supports a network of Asthma, Allergic and Immunologic Diseases Cooperative Research Centers throughout the United States. The centers encourage close coordination among scientists studying basic and clinical immunology, genetics, biochemistry, pharmacology, and environmental science. This interdisciplinary approach helps move research knowledge as quickly as possible from the lab into the hands of doctors and their allergy patients.

Educating patients and health care providers is an important tool in controlling allergic diseases. All of these research centers conduct and evaluate education programs focused on methods to control allergic diseases.

Since 1991, researchers participating in NIAID's Inner-City Asthma Study have been examining ways to treat asthma in minority children living in inner-city environments. Asthma, a major cause of illness and hospitalizations among these children, is provoked by a number of possible factors, including allergies to airborne substances.

The success of NIAID's model asthma program led the U.S. Centers for Disease Control and Prevention to award grants to help community-based health organizations throughout the United States implement the program.

Based on the success of the first National Cooperative Inner-City Asthma Study, NIAID and the National Institute of Environmental Health Sciences, also part of NIH, started a second cooperative multicenter study in 1996. This study recruited children with asthma, aged 4 to 11, to test the effectiveness of two interventions. One intervention uses a novel communication and doctor education system. Information about the children's asthma severity is provided to their primary care physicians, with the intent that this information will help the doctors give the children the best care possible.

The other intervention involves educating families about reducing exposure to passive cigarette smoke and to indoor allergens, including cockroach, house dust mite, and mold. Researchers are assessing the effectiveness of both interventions by evaluating their capacity to reduce the severity of asthma in these children.

Early data show that by reducing allergen levels in children's beds by one third, investigators reduced by nearly one quarter (22 percent) both the number of days the children wheezed and the number of days the children missed school.

Although several factors provoke allergic responses, scientists know that heredity plays a major role in determining who will develop an allergy. Therefore, scientists are trying to identify and describe the genes that make a person susceptible to allergic diseases.

Because researchers are becoming increasingly aware of the role of environmental factors in allergies, they are evaluating ways to control environmental exposures to allergens and pollutants to prevent allergic disease.

These studies offer the promise of improving the treatment and control of allergic diseases and the hope that one day allergic diseases will be preventable.

Chapter 31

Pollen and Ragweed

Chapter Contents

Section 31.1

What Is Ragweed Allergy?

Come late summer, some 10 to 20 percent of Americans begin to suffer from ragweed allergy, or hay fever. Sneezing; stuffy or runny nose; itchy eyes, nose, and throat; and trouble sleeping make life miserable for these people. Some of them also must deal with asthma attacks.

All this misery can begin when ragweed releases pollen into the air and continues almost until frost kills the plant.

What is ragweed?

Ragweeds are weeds that grow throughout the United States. They are most common in the Eastern states and the Midwest. A plant lives only one season, but that plant produces up to 1 billion pollen grains. Pollen-producing and seed-producing flowers grow on the same plant but are separate organs. After midsummer, as nights grow longer, ragweed flowers mature and release pollen. Warmth, humidity, and breezes after sunrise help the release. The pollen must then travel by air to another plant to fertilize the seed for growth the coming year.

Ragweed plants usually grow in rural areas. Near the plants, the pollen counts are highest shortly after dawn. The amount of pollen peaks in many urban areas between 10 a.m. and 3 p.m., depending on the weather. Rain and low morning temperatures (below 50 degrees Fahrenheit) slow pollen release. Ragweed pollen can travel far. It has been measured in the air 400 miles out to sea and 2 miles up in the atmosphere, but most falls out close to its source.

These annual plants are easily overgrown by turf grasses and other perennial plants that come up from established stems every year. But where the soil is disturbed by streams of water, cultivation, or chemical effects such as winter salting of roads, ragweed will grow. It is often found along roadsides and river banks, in vacant lots and fields. Seeds in the soil even after many decades will grow when conditions are right.

What is ragweed allergy?

The job of immune system cells is to find foreign substances such as viruses and bacteria and get rid of them. Normally, this response protects us from dangerous diseases. People with allergies have specially sensitive immune systems that react when they contact certain harmless substances called allergens. When people who are allergic to ragweed pollen inhale its allergens from air, the common hay fever symptoms develop.

Seventeen species or types of ragweed grow in North America. Ragweed also belongs to a larger family called *Compositae*. Other members of the family that spread pollen by wind can cause symptoms. They include sage, burweed marsh elder and rabbit brush, mugworts, groundsel bush and eupatorium. Some family members spread their pollen by insects rather than wind, and cause few allergic reactions. But sniffing these plants can cause symptoms.

Who gets ragweed allergy?

Of Americans who are allergic to pollen-producing plants, 75 percent are allergic to ragweed. People with allergies to one type of pollen tend to develop allergies to other pollens as well.

People with ragweed allergy may also get symptoms when they eat cantaloupe and banana. Chamomile tea, sunflower seeds and honey containing pollen from *Compositae* family members occasionally cause severe reactions, including shock.

What are its symptoms?

The allergic reaction to all plants that produce pollen is commonly known as hay fever. Symptoms include eye irritation, runny nose, stuffy nose, puffy eyes, sneezing, and inflamed, itchy nose and throat. For those with severe allergies, asthma attacks, chronic sinusitis, headaches, and impaired sleep are symptoms.

How is it diagnosed?

To identify an allergy to ragweed or one of its relatives requires a careful medical history, a physical exam, and testing. The main approach to confirm a suspected allergy is the skin sensitivity test.

For this, the skin is scratched or pricked with extract of ragweed pollen. In sensitive people, the site will turn red, swollen, and itchy. Sometimes blood tests are used to see if an antibody to ragweed is present. This is sometimes necessary, but it takes longer for processing by a laboratory and it is more expensive.

What can I do about it?

There is no cure for ragweed allergy. The best control is to avoid contact with the pollen. This is difficult given the amount of ragweed pollen in the air during pollination time. There is help, though.

- Track the pollen count for your area. The news media often reports the count, especially when pollen is high. You also can call the National Allergy Bureau at 800-9-POLLEN or reach it through the American Academy of Allergy, Asthma and Immunology on the internet (www.aaaai.org). It will give you the pollen count for your region.

- Stay indoors in central air conditioning with a HEPA (high efficiency particulate air) filter attachment when the pollen count is high. This will remove pollen from the indoor air.

- Get away from the pollen where possible. People in the Eastern and Midwestern states may get some relief by going west to the Rocky Mountains and beyond. Going to sea or abroad in late summer can greatly reduce exposure. But check the area abroad you plan to visit. It may have a ragweed season as well.

- You might even consider moving to get away from ragweed. Although this often helps people feel better for a short time, it is common for them to develop allergies to plants in the new location within a few years. A well thought-out treatment plan is a better way to live with your allergies.

- Take antihistamine medications. These work well to control hay fever symptoms, whatever the cause. The drowsiness caused by older products is less of a problem with antihistamines now on the market. Anti-inflammatory nose sprays or drops also help and have few side effects. Similar agents can reduce eye symptoms, but other remedies are needed for the less common, pollen-induced asthma.

- If medication does not give enough relief, consider immunotherapy (allergy shots). This approach reduces the allergic response to specific allergens. For it to work, the allergens must be carefully identified. The allergens are injected over several months or years. If diagnosis and treatment are well directed, you may see major improvements in symptoms.

Section 31.2

Experimental Ragweed Therapy Offers Relief with Fewer Shots

From "Experimental Ragweed Therapy Offers Allergy Sufferers Longer Relief with Fewer Shots," National Institutes of Health and the National Institute of Allergy and Infectious Diseases (NIAID), October 4, 2006.

Americans accustomed to the seasonal misery of sneezing, runny noses, and itchy, watery eyes caused by ragweed pollen might one day benefit from an experimental allergy treatment that not only requires fewer injections than standard immunotherapy, but leads to a marked reduction in symptoms that persists for at least a year after therapy has stopped, according to a new study in the October 5 issue of the *New England Journal of Medicine* (NEJM). The research was sponsored by the Immune Tolerance Network, which is funded by the National Institute of Allergy and Infectious Diseases (NIAID) and the National Institute of Diabetes and Digestive and Kidney Diseases (NIDDK), both components of the National Institutes of Health (NIH), and the Juvenile Diabetes Research Foundation International.

"As many as 40 million Americans suffer from seasonal allergies caused by airborne pollens produced by grasses, trees and weeds," says NIH Director Elias A. Zerhouni, M.D. "Finding new therapies for allergy sufferers is certainly an important research goal."

"This innovative research holds great promise for helping people with allergies," says NIAID Director Anthony S. Fauci, M.D. "A short course of immunotherapy that reduces allergic symptoms over an extended period of time will significantly improve the quality of life for many people."

Ragweed is one of the most common pollens in the United States and is prevalent in the Northeast, Midwest, and the South. In Baltimore, where the *NEJM* study was conducted, the ragweed pollen season lasts from mid-August to October.

Physicians treat people suffering from mild and moderate ragweed allergies with antihistamines or nasal corticosteroids. However, when people with allergies do not respond to these treatments or experience severe symptoms, the next therapeutic option is a course of subcutaneous injections of the allergen, which is called allergen immunotherapy. Although this standard immunotherapy is often effective, it has two major drawbacks. First, it can cause systemic allergic reactions, such as anaphylaxis, a hypersensitivity reaction that can lead to severe and sometimes life-threatening physical symptoms. Second, to provide long-lasting relief, standard immunotherapy may require frequent injections over a 3- to 5-year period. The large number of injections over such an extended period of time often results in many people not completing the treatment.

In the study detailed in *NEJM*, lead investigator Peter Creticos, M.D., medical director of the Johns Hopkins Asthma and Allergy Center in Baltimore, and his research team found that an investigational therapy based on the major ragweed allergen, Amb a 1 (*Ambrosia artemisiifolia* 1), coupled to a unique short, synthetic sequence of DNA that stimulates the immune system, reduced allergy symptoms in adults for at least one year when given just once a week over a 6-week period. The therapeutic agent was provided by Dynavax Technologies Corp., based in Berkeley, California.

"For almost 100 years, we've been using the tedious process of giving allergy sufferers one to two shots a week for up to 4 to 5 years to ensure its success," Dr. Creticos says. "This study is an important immunotherapy advance in that we've shown you can induce long-lasting relief from allergic rhinitis with just a few weeks of injections."

The study initially involved 25 adult volunteers, ages 23 to 60, with a history of seasonal allergic rhinitis, positive skin test reactions to ragweed pollen, and an immediate reaction when nasally challenged with ragweed. Prior to the start of the 2001 fall ragweed season, the study participants received six injections, each a week apart, of either the investigational therapy in increasingly higher doses or a placebo. They received no other injections throughout the course of the study. Fourteen volunteers received the study drug; 11 were given the placebo. The therapy was well-tolerated and caused only limited local reactions, which required neither medication nor change in treatment dose. No clinically significant, therapy-related adverse events occurred.

Throughout the 2001 and 2002 ragweed seasons, the volunteers were monitored for allergy-related symptoms, including the number of sneezes and the degree of postnasal drip, allergy medication use, and quality-of-life scores. Compared with the placebo recipients, the group that received the therapy experienced dramatically better outcomes that continued throughout the 2002 ragweed season even though therapy ended one year earlier.

Clearly, the regimen of only six injections showed therapeutic promise when compared with the current therapy, the study authors note. However, because the results are based on a small number of volunteers and the long-term safety of the therapy is unknown, they say additional clinical trials with longer-term follow-up to adequately assess the therapy's safety and effectiveness are necessary.

How the experimental therapy relieves ragweed allergy symptoms is not fully understood at this time. When exposed to ragweed pollen, people who are allergic to ragweed experience an increase in IgE (immunoglobulin) antibodies; immunotherapy blocks this increase in IgE. Researchers believe the experimental therapy tempers the release of immune regulatory proteins called cytokines, which blocks increases in the level of IgE antibodies.

"Using ragweed as a model allergen system with a predictable seasonal pattern of symptoms and pollen counts, it is possible to correlate pollen levels with symptoms and measure treatment effects on symptoms. This enables us to better understand immune response to allergens and serves as an approach to similar therapies to manage other allergic reactions for which there are currently no treatments, such as food allergies," says Marshall Plaut, M.D., chief of the Allergic Mechanisms Section of NIAID's Division of Allergy, Immunology and Transplantation.

NIAID is a component of the National Institutes of Health. NIAID supports basic and applied research to prevent, diagnose and treat infectious diseases such as HIV/AIDS and other sexually transmitted infections, influenza, tuberculosis, malaria and illness from potential agents of bioterrorism. NIAID also supports research on basic immunology, transplantation and immune-related disorders, including autoimmune diseases, asthma and allergies. For more information about NIAID and its programs, visit http://www.niaid.nih.gov

Reference

PS Creticos et al. Immunotherapy with a ragweed-TLR9 agonist vaccine for allergic rhinitis. The *New England Journal of Medicine* DOI: 10.1056/NEJMoa052196 (2006).

Chapter 32

Common Indoor Triggers: Mold, Dust Mites, and Cockroach Allergens

Chapter Contents

Section 32.1

Mold

Facts about Allergies

The tendency to develop allergies may be inherited. If you have allergic tendencies and are exposed to certain things in your environment (allergens), you may develop allergies to some of those things. Examples of allergy symptoms include itchy eyes, runny nose, asthma symptoms, eczema, and rash. The timing of the allergic response may be immediate or delayed. Allergy testing may be recommended to help identify your allergies.

What Are Allergies to Mold?

Many types of molds live in our environment. Mold grows in indoor and outdoor areas that are warm, dark, and/or moist. Molds reproduce and grow by sending tiny spores into the air. Inhaled spores cause allergy and asthma symptoms.

What about Environmental Control?

Once an allergy has been identified, the next step is to decrease or eliminate exposure to the allergen. This is called environmental control. Evidence shows that allergy and asthma symptoms may improve over time if the recommended environmental control changes are made. Many of the changes are for the entire home. The bedroom is the most important, because the bedroom is where people usually spend one third to one half of their time.

Steps to Control Mold Allergens

- In the bathroom—use an exhaust fan or open a window to remove moisture after showering. Wipe down the damp surfaces after showering. Wash bathrooms with a mold-preventing or mold-killing solution at least once a month.

- In the kitchen—use an exhaust fan to remove water vapor when cooking. Discard spoiled foods immediately. Empty the garbage daily. Empty water pans below self-defrosting refrigerators frequently.

- Remove moldy stored items.

- Vent the clothes dryer outside.

- Remove leaves, clippings and compost from around your house.

- The person with a mold allergy should avoid cutting grass and raking leaves or wear a face mask for these activities.

Other Helpful Suggestions

- Keep the indoor moisture low. The ideal humidity level is 30% to 40%. Use an air conditioner or dehumidifier in warm climates to decrease the humidity.

- Clean the dehumidifier regularly.

- Humidifiers and vaporizers are not recommended because they will increase humidity in the room and create a favorable environment for mold growth. If you must use a humidifier, clean it daily to prevent mold growth.

Your health care provider may recommend additional medications, therapies, or other environmental controls. Exposure to mold can make allergy and/or asthma symptoms worse in some people. To avoid these problems follow the above steps to decrease or eliminate exposure.

Section 32.2

Dust Mites

Facts about Allergies

The tendency to develop allergies may be inherited. If you have allergic tendencies and are exposed to certain things in your environment (allergens), you may develop allergies to some of those things. Examples of allergy symptoms include itchy eyes, runny nose, asthma symptoms, eczema and rash. The timing of the allergic response may be immediate or delayed. Allergy testing may be recommended to help identify your allergies.

What Are Allergies to Dust Mites?

Dust mites are microscopic animals, too small to be seen with the naked eye. The droppings and decaying bodies of dust mites are common allergens. These dust mites live in bedding, carpets, stuffed furniture, old clothing, and stuffed toys. They feed on human skin scales. Dust mites are most common in humid climates. They don't survive when the humidity is below 50%. If droppings of dust mites are inhaled or come in contact with the skin, they may cause allergy, asthma, and/or eczema symptoms.

What about Environmental Control?

Once an allergy has been identified, the next step is to decrease or eliminate exposure to the allergen. This is called environmental control. Evidence shows that allergy and asthma symptoms may improve over time, if the recommended environmental control changes are made. Many of the changes are for the entire home. The bedroom is the most important, because the bedroom is where people usually spend one third to one half of their time.

Steps to Control Dust Mite Allergens

- Enclose the mattress and box springs in a zippered dust-proof encasing. Dust-proof encasings have a layer of material that keeps the dust mites inside the encasing. Encasings are usually made of plastic or plastic-like materials. If there is more than one mattress in the bedroom all mattresses should be encased. It is recommended that cloth tape be placed over the encasing zipper.

- Wash all bedding in hot (130 degrees Fahrenheit) water weekly.

- Put the pillows in zippered dust proof encasings and/or wash the pillows weekly with the bedding.

- Avoid lying on upholstered furniture or carpet.

Other Helpful Suggestions

- Remove carpeting from the bedroom. Instead, use area rugs that can be washed.

- Use wood, leather or vinyl furniture instead of upholstered furniture in the bedroom.

- The person with a dust mite allergy should not vacuum or be in a room while it is being vacuumed.

- Keep the indoor moisture low. The ideal humidity level is 30% to 40%. Use an air conditioner or dehumidifier in warm climates to decrease the humidity.

- Clean the dehumidifier regularly.

- Humidifiers/vaporizers are not recommended because they will increase humidity in the room and create a favorable environment for dust mites. If you must use a humidifier, clean it daily to prevent mold growth.

- Chemical solutions may be helpful. Acaricides (a chemical that kills dust mites) must be applied regularly to carpeting or upholstered furniture. This solution will not remove any preexisting mite droppings. A tannic acid solution, applied as directed, can help neutralize the allergen in mite droppings.

Your health care provider may recommend additional medications, therapies, or other environmental controls. Exposure to dust mites can make allergy, asthma, and/or eczema symptoms worse in some people.

To avoid these problems follow the above steps to decrease or eliminate exposure.

Section 32.3

Facts about Cockroach Allergy

What is cockroach allergy?

When most people think of allergy triggers, they often focus on plant pollens, dust, animals, and stinging insects. In fact, cockroaches also can trigger allergies and asthma.

Cockroach allergy was first reported in 1943, when skin rashes appeared immediately after the insects crawled over patients' skin. Skin tests first confirmed patients had cockroach allergy in 1959.

In the 1970s, studies made it clear that patients with cockroach allergies develop acute asthma attacks. The attacks occur after inhaling cockroach allergens and last for hours. Asthma has steadily increased over the past 30 years. It is the most common chronic disease of childhood. Now we know that the frequent hospital admissions of inner-city children with asthma often is directly related to their contact with cockroach allergens—the substances that cause allergies. From 23 percent to 60 percent of urban residents with asthma are sensitive to the cockroach allergen.

The increase in asthma is not fully understood. Experts think one reason for the increase among children is that they play indoors more than in past years and thus have increased contact with the allergen. This is especially true in the inner cities where they stay inside because of safety concerns.

What causes the allergic reaction?

The job of immune system cells is to find foreign substances such as viruses and bacteria and get rid of them. Normally, this response

protects us from dangerous diseases. People with allergies have su-
persensitive immune systems that react when they inhale, swallow,
or touch certain harmless substances such as pollen or cockroaches.
These substances are the allergens.

Cockroach allergen is believed to derive from feces, saliva, and the
bodies of these insects. Cockroaches live all over the world, from tropical areas to the coldest spots on earth. Studies show that 78 percent
to 98 percent of urban homes have cockroaches. Each home has from
900 to 330,000 of the insects.

Private homes also harbor them, especially if the homes are well
insulated. When one roach is seen in the basement or kitchen, it is
safe to assume that at least 800 roaches are hidden under the kitchen
sink, in closets, and the like. They are carried in with groceries, furniture, and luggage used on trips. Once they are in the home, they
are hard to get rid of.

The amount of roach allergen in house dust or air can be measured.
In dwellings where the amount is high, exposure is high and the rate
of hospitalization for asthma goes up. Allergen particles are large and
settle rapidly on surfaces. They become airborne when the air is
stirred by people moving around or by children at play.

Who develops cockroach allergy?

People with chronic severe bronchial asthma are most likely to
have cockroach allergy. Also likely to have it are people with a chronic
stuffy nose, skin rash, constant sinus infection, repeat ear infection.
and asthma.

Cockroach allergy is a problem among people who live in inner cities or in the South and are of low socioeconomic status. In one study
of inner-city children, 37 percent were allergic to cockroaches, 35 percent to dust mites, and 23 percent to cats. Those who were allergic to
cockroaches and were exposed to the insects were hospitalized for
asthma 3.3 times more often than other children. This was true even
when compared with those who were allergic to dust mites or cats.

Cockroach allergy is more common among poor African Americans.
Experts believe that this is not because of racial differences; rather,
it is because of the disproportionate number of African Americans living in the inner cities.

What are its symptoms?

Symptoms vary. They may be a mildly itchy skin, scratchy throat,
or itchy eyes and nose. Or the allergy symptoms can become stronger,

including severe, persistent asthma in some people. Asthma symptoms often are a problem all year, not just in some seasons. This can make it hard to determine that a cockroach allergy is the cause of the asthma.

How is cockroach allergy diagnosed?

The National Heart, Lung, and Blood Institute recommends that all patients with persistent asthma be tested for allergic response to cockroach as well as to the other chief allergens, dust mites, cats, dogs, and mold.

Diagnosis can be made only by skin tests. The doctor scratches or pricks the skin with cockroach extract. Redness, an itchy rash, or swelling at the site suggests you are allergic to the insect.

Cockroaches should be suspected, though, when allergy symptoms—stuffy nose, inflamed eyes or ears, skin rash, or bronchial asthma—persist year-round.

How can I manage cockroach allergy?

If you have cockroach allergy, avoid contact with roaches and their droppings.

- The first step is to rid your home of the roaches. Because they resist many control measures, it is best to call in pest control experts.

- For ongoing control, use poison baits, boric acid, and traps.

- Don't use chemical agents. They can irritate allergies and asthma.

- Do not leave food and garbage uncovered.

- To manage nasal and sinus symptoms, use antihistamines, decongestants, and anti-inflammatory medications. Your doctor will also prescribe anti-inflammatory medications and bronchodilators if you have asthma.

- If you keep having serious allergic symptoms, see an allergist about allergy injections with the cockroach extract. They can reduce symptoms over time.

Section 32.4

Cockroach Allergens Have the Greatest Impact on Childhood Asthma in Many U.S. Cities

From the National Institute of Environmental Health Sciences
(NIEHS, www.niehs.nih.gov), March 8, 2005.

New results from a nationwide study on factors that affect asthma in inner-city children show that cockroach allergen appears to worsen asthma symptoms more than either dust mite or pet allergens. This research, funded by the National Institute of Environmental Health Sciences (NIEHS) and the National Institute of Allergy and Infectious Diseases (NIAID), part of the National Institutes of Health, is the first large-scale study to show marked geographic differences in allergen exposure and sensitivity in inner-city children. Most homes in northeastern cities had high levels of cockroach allergens, while those in the south and northwest had dust mite allergen levels in ranges known to exacerbate asthma symptoms.

The study results are published in the March issue of the *Journal of Allergy and Clinical Immunology.*

"These data confirm that cockroach allergen is the primary contributor to childhood asthma in inner-city home environments," said NIEHS Director Kenneth Olden, Ph.D. "However, general cleaning practices, proven extermination techniques, and consistent maintenance methods can bring these allergen levels under control."

Cockroach allergens come from several sources such as saliva, fecal material, secretions, cast skins, and dead bodies. People can reduce their exposure to cockroach allergen by eating only in the kitchen and dining room, putting non-refrigerated items in plastic containers or sealable bags, and taking out the garbage on a daily basis. Other measures include repairing leaky faucets, frequent vacuuming of carpeted areas and damp-mopping of hard floors, and regular cleaning of countertops and other surfaces.

NIH provided $7.5 million to researchers at the University of Texas Southwestern Medical Center at Dallas and seven other research institutions, including the Data Coordinating Center at Rho, Inc., for the three-year study.

"We found that a majority of homes in Chicago, New York City, and the Bronx had cockroach allergen levels high enough to trigger asthma symptoms, while a majority of homes in Dallas and Seattle had dust mite allergen levels above the asthma symptom threshold," said Dr. Rebecca Gruchalla, associate professor of internal medicine and pediatrics at the University of Texas Southwestern Medical Center and lead author of the study.

"We also discovered that the levels of both of these allergens were influenced by housing type," noted Gruchalla. "Cockroach allergen levels were highest in high-rise apartments, while dust mite concentrations were greatest in detached homes."

While cockroach allergen exposure did produce an increase in asthma symptoms, researchers did not find an increase in asthma symptoms as a result of exposure to dust mite and pet dander. "Children who tested positive for, and were exposed to, cockroach allergen experienced a significant increase in the number of days with cough, wheezing and chest tightness, number of nights with interrupted sleep, number of missed school days, and number of times they had to slow down or discontinue their play activity," said Gruchalla.

While cockroaches are primarily attracted to water sources and food debris, house dust mites, microscopic spider-like creatures that feed on flakes of human skin, reside in bedding, carpets, upholstery, draperies, and other dust traps. Dust mite allergens are proteins that come from the digestive tracts of mites and are found in mite feces.

Researchers tested 937 inner-city children with moderate to severe asthma symptoms. The children, ages 5 to 11, were given skin tests for sensitivity to cockroach and dust mite allergens, pet dander, and mold. Bedroom dust samples were analyzed for the presence of each allergen type.

This study was part of the larger Inner-City Asthma Study, a cooperative multi-center project comprised of seven asthma study centers across the country. The goal of the study was to develop and implement a comprehensive, cost-effective intervention program aimed at reducing asthma incidence among children living in low socioeconomic areas.

The National Institute of Environmental Health Sciences is a federal agency that conducts and funds basic research on the health effects of exposure to environmental agents.

Chapter 33

Animal and Pet Dander

Chapter Contents

Section 33.1

Understanding Animal Allergy

Facts about Allergies

The tendency to develop allergies may be inherited. If you have allergic tendencies and are exposed to certain things in your environment (allergens), you may develop allergies to some of those things. Examples of allergy symptoms include itchy eyes, runny nose, asthma symptoms, eczema, and rash. The timing of the allergic response may be immediate or delayed. Allergy testing may be recommended to help identify your allergies.

What Are Allergies to Animals?

Animal dander (dead skin that is continually shed), urine, and saliva can cause an allergic reaction. Exposure to these allergens, especially breathing in particles that include dander, cause the allergic reaction to animals.

Feathered or furry animals such as cats, dogs, birds, and rodents (hamsters, gerbils, mice) can cause allergy symptoms. Unfortunately, there is no such thing as a hypoallergenic cat or dog, and short-haired breeds are no less of a problem than animals with long hair. Exposure to other warm-blooded animals such as livestock, or to products made with feathers or down, may also cause allergy symptoms. If you do not own a feathered or furry pet, do not get one because you can develop allergies with repeated exposure.

What about Environmental Control?

Once an allergy has been identified, the next step is to decrease or eliminate exposure to the allergen. This is called environmental control. Evidence shows that allergy and asthma symptoms may improve over time, if the recommended environmental control changes are made. Many of the changes are for the entire home. The bedroom is the most important, because the bedroom is where people usually spend one third to one half of their time.

Steps to Control Animal Allergens

- Remove the animal from your home.

- If you must have a pet, keep it out of the allergic person's bedroom at all times.

- If you have forced air heating and a pet, close the air ducts in the allergic person's bedroom. If necessary, use an electric heater instead.

- The pet should be washed weekly by a non-allergic person.

- Avoid visits to friends and relatives with feathered or furry pets.

Other Helpful Suggestions

- Choose a pet without feathers or fur (fish, reptiles, amphibians).

- A HEPA [high efficiency particulate air filter] air cleaner can remove dander from the air. However, the benefits may be limited because of the large reservoir of dander in furniture and carpet.

Your health care provider may recommend additional medications, therapies, or other environmental controls. Exposure to furry or feathered animals can make allergy, asthma, and/or eczema symptoms worse in some people. To avoid these problems follow the above steps to decrease or eliminate exposure.

371

Section 33.2

Myths and Facts about Allergies and Pets

"The Real Truth about Cats and Dogs," reprinted courtesy of Allergy &
Asthma Network Mothers of Asthmatics (AANMA), 800-878-4403, www
.breatherville.org, © 2000. Reviewed by David A. Cooke, M.D., January 5,
2007.

Can animal lovers with asthma and allergies learn to coexist with
their pet? Robert A. Wood, M.D., separates fact from fiction.

Fact or Fiction? Find a new home for your pet and your pet-related allergy symptoms will soon disappear.

Dr. Wood: Fact and fiction—There are no convincing studies demonstrating the direct clinical benefits of removing an animal from the
home. No research has focused on whether finding a new home for a
pet will eliminate the pet-related asthma or allergy symptoms.

However, there is compelling clinical experience to support the best
currently available advice: Finding a new home for the pet is likely
to reduce levels of pet-allergen exposure in the home. Avoidance of
allergens is always the most appropriate advice a physician can give.

Once the cat or dog has been removed from the home, symptoms may
not improve for weeks or even months, as allergen levels fall quite slowly.
In homes with cats, for example, the allergen load typically takes as long
as four to six months to reach that of non-cat homes. Levels may fall
much more quickly if the homeowner makes extensive environmental
changes, such as removing carpets, upholstered furniture, and other
allergen reservoirs. It has been shown that cat allergen may persist in
mattresses for years after a cat has been removed from a home, so new
bedding or impermeable encasements must also be recommended.

Fact or Fiction? Some breeds of cats and dogs are less likely to trigger allergy symptoms in people with pet allergies than others.

Dr. Wood: Fiction—While it is true that some breeds of cats or dogs
are said to produce much more allergen than others, there is absolutely

no breed that is hypoallergenic or can promise to be best for people with asthma or pet allergies. It is not possible to predict with any accuracy which animals are likely to be more or less allergenic based on a particular breed, size, hair length, or propensity to shed. There is no perfect furry pet for people with allergies to cats and dogs.

Fact or Fiction? People who have asthma and exhibit allergy symptoms when exposed to animals tend to have more severe disease.

Dr. Wood: Fact—A diagnosis of cat or dog allergy can be made by a skin test or blood (radioallergosorbent test [RAST]) test. If the test is negative, it is very unlikely that cat or dog exposure will affect the asthma in any way. However, if the test is positive, then it is very likely that animal exposure will lead to a worsening of asthma or allergic rhinitis.

Fact or Fiction? Washing the cat or dog frequently will reduce the level of allergens in the home.

Dr. Wood: Neither fact nor fiction—A number of studies have investigated measures that might help reduce the allergen load in a home. One study demonstrated significant reductions in airborne cat allergen with a combination of air filtration, cat washings, vacuum cleaning, and removal of furnishings. It was a small study and the purpose was to measure the ability to reduce the allergen load, not to establish any clinical improvement in symptoms. When cat washing was evaluated separately in that study, dramatic reductions in airborne cat allergen were seen after cat washes.

Subsequent studies have produced conflicting results demonstrating either no change or only a very transient improvement. The current opinion is that the benefits of cat washing are so transient that it is unlikely to be worth the effort or the trauma to the cat. Preliminary information regarding dogs looks very similar.

Fact or Fiction? Using a HEPA (high-efficiency particulate air) filter in the bedroom while the dog sleeps next to (not on) the bed makes it possible for man and beast to coexist happily.

Dr. Wood: Fiction—While using a HEPA filter helps to remove allergens flowing through the machine, the best advice is to keep the dog out of the bedroom at all times.

For pet-allergic families who insist on keeping pets, the following recommendations are the best available until pending studies are concluded:

- Restrict pets to one area of the home when inside.
- Keep pets out of the bedroom.
- Use HEPA or electrostatic air cleaners, especially in the room(s) of the person(s) with pet allergies.
- Remove carpets, upholstered furniture, heavy drapes (that cannot be washed), with a focus on the bedroom—even though the pet is not allowed in the room.
- Encase pillows, mattress, and box spring with allergen-proof encasings.

Although tannic acid (chemical product used to typically reduce dust mite allergens) has been shown to reduce cat allergen levels, the effects are modest and short-lived when a cat is present so this treatment should not be routinely recommended.

Fact or Fiction? Immunotherapy (allergy shots) makes it possible for pet lovers to keep their pets.

Dr. Wood: Neither fact nor fiction—Most studies over the last 20 years demonstrate a positive effect, particularly for cat allergen. However, the outcomes of these studies have been based largely on laboratory studies, so what this means for the average allergic pet owner remains a question. Based on available studies, it is most likely that immunotherapy will not allow allergic pet owners to live with a cat or dog more comfortably. More studies are needed to fully define the strategies, both immunologic and environmental, that will be most effective.

Although most asthma and allergies can be controlled by medication, it makes far more sense to begin treatment with allergy avoidance and then to use the least amount of medication possible to control the disease. This approach can have dramatic short-term effects in asthma control and potentially even more important long-term effects in improving the eventual outcome of the asthma.

In the meanwhile, it is best for patients with significant animal allergy, especially if they have asthma, to find new homes for their pets.

Dr. Wood is associate professor of pediatrics, Johns Hopkins University School of Medicine, and director, Pediatric Allergy Clinic, Johns Hopkins Hospital, Baltimore, MD.

Section 33.3

Dog and Cat Allergens Are Universally Present in U.S. Homes

"National Study Shows Dog and Cat Allergens Are Universally Present in U.S. Homes," National Institutes of Health (NIH, www.nih.gov) and National Institute of Environmental Health Sciences (NIEHS, www.niehs .nih.gov), July 6, 2004.

Scientists at the National Institute of Environmental Health Sciences (NIEHS), one of the National Institutes of Health, and the U.S. Department of Housing and Urban Development have found that detectable levels of dog and cat allergens are universally present in U.S. homes. Although allergen levels were considerably higher in homes with an indoor dog or cat, levels previously associated with an increased risk of allergic sensitization were common even in homes without the pets.

This report by Arbes et al., which appeared in the July 2004 issue of the *Journal of Allergy and Clinical Immunology,* is one of a series of allergen reports from the National Survey of Lead and Allergens in Housing. In that nationally representative survey of 831 homes, researchers collected dust samples, asked questions, and examined homes.

Interestingly, the researchers found that dog and cat allergen levels were higher among households belonging to demographic groups in which dog or cat ownership was more prevalent, regardless of whether or not the household had the indoor pet. Because dog and cat allergens can be transported on clothing, the researchers speculated that the community, particularly communities in which dog or cat ownership is high, may be an important source of these pet allergens. For pet-allergic patients in such communities, allergen avoidance may be a difficult challenge.

The survey was conducted using established sampling techniques to ensure that the surveyed homes were representative of U.S. homes. The homes were sampled from seventy-five randomly selected areas (generally counties or groups of counties) across the entire country.

The 831 homes included all regions of the country (northeast, southeast, midwest, southwest, northwest), all housing types, and all settings (urban, suburban, rural). For statistics derived from the 831 homes, the contribution from each home was weighted as necessary to ensure that the statistics were representative of the U.S. population. Until now, exposure to these allergens had not previously been studied in residential environments on a national scale.

Section 33.4

Multiple Pets May Decrease Children's Allergy Risk

From the National Institutes of Health (NIH, www.nih.gov) and the National Institute of Allergy and Infectious Diseases (NIAID, www.niaid.nih.gov), August 27, 2002.

Children raised in a house with two or more dogs or cats during the first year of life may be less likely to develop allergic diseases as compared with children raised without pets, according to a study in the August 28 issue of the *Journal of the American Medical Association*. The study was supported by the National Institute of Allergy and Infectious Diseases (NIAID) and the National Institute of Environmental Health Sciences (NIEHS).

"The striking finding here is that high pet exposure early in life appears to protect against not only pet allergy but also other types of common allergies, such as allergy to dust mites, ragweed, and grass," says Marshall Plaut, M.D., chief of the allergic mechanisms section at NIAID. "Other studies have suggested a protective effect of pet exposure on allergy and asthma symptoms, but generally have looked only at whether pet exposure reduced pet allergy. This new finding changes the way scientists think about pet exposure; scientists must now figure out how pet exposure causes a general shift of the immune system away from an allergic response."

In their paper, lead author Dennis R. Ownby, M.D., of the Medical College of Georgia, and colleagues suggest that bacteria carried by pets may be responsible for suppressing the immune system's allergic response. These bacteria release molecules called endotoxins, and endotoxins are believed to shift the developing immune system away from responding to allergens through a class of lymphocytes called Th-2 cells, which are associated with allergic reactions. Instead, endotoxins may stimulate the immune system to activate Th-1 cells, which may block allergic reactions.

The researchers followed 474 children from birth to six or seven years of age. When the children were one year old, the researchers contacted parents by telephone to find out how many pets were in the home. When the children were two years old, researchers measured the level of dust mite allergen in their bedrooms. When the children were six or seven, the researchers tested them for allergic antibodies to common allergens by two approaches—a skin prick test and a blood measurement.

After adjusting for factors such as dust mite allergen levels, parental smoking, and current dog or cat ownership, the researchers found that children exposed to two or more dogs or cats during the first year of life were on average 66 to 77 percent less likely to have any allergic antibodies to common allergens, as compared with children exposed to only one or no pets during their first year.

"Our findings suggest an area of research with many possibilities, one that could potentially bear fruit over the next decade or so," says Dr. Ownby. "If we could find out exactly what it is about pets or the bacteria they carry that prevents the allergic response, scientists might be able to develop a new allergy therapy based on that knowledge."

Reference: D.R. Ownby et al. Exposure to dogs and cats in the first year of life and risk of allergic sensitization at 6 to 7 years of age. *Journal of the American Medical Association* 288(8): 963–972 (2002).

Chapter 34

Chemicals, Pollution, and Other Irritants

Chapter Contents

Section 34.1

Understanding Chemical Sensitivity

A variety of vague and hard-to-pinpoint symptoms are experienced by an undetermined, but possibly sizable, number of adults and children. Occasionally, they may suggest allergy or asthma, but most often the symptoms are much wider in scope.

Not much is currently known about what is referred to as chemical sensitivity, but it is a subject that is often mentioned as a growing problem in the popular media. Since there are considered to be a variety of adverse health effects from so-called chemical sensitivities, the public and their health care providers are rightly confused about what it is all about.

Why are chemical sensitivities gaining so much interest?

There are several reasons, which include:

- a greater number of complex chemical compounds (polymers) in our natural environment than in the past;

- less indoor air exchange in more highly insulated houses and buildings; and

- greater media coverage of news and opinions about chemical sensitivities and their possible ill effects on our health.

A few physicians who refer to themselves as "ecologically oriented" have proposed diagnoses such as the "Twentieth Century Disease," "Chemical AIDS," "multiple chemical sensitivities," or "*Candida* hypersensitivity." Intriguing as these labels may be to some whose symptoms seem to frustrate the attempts of a medical diagnosis and treatment, no single test or combination of tests has yet to clearly identify the causes of these symptoms.

Nevertheless, caring physicians are sensitive to patients with vague complaints. They endeavor to keep them from seeking, in desperation, care and "cures" that lack a medical-scientific basis or require much more study.

What are considered chemical sensitivities?

There are four general ways that we can classify chemical sensitivity.

- **Annoyance Reactions:** These result from a heightened sensitivity to unpleasant odors, called olfactory awareness, in some susceptible individuals. Your ability to cope with offensive—but mostly nonirritating—odors has a lot to do with genetic or acquired factors, among which are infection and inflammation of the mucous membranes or polyps (growths of the nasal or sinus membranes) and abuse of tobacco and nasal decongestants.

- **Irritational Syndromes:** These are caused by significant exposure to irritating chemicals that are more likely than others to penetrate the mucous membranes. These types of reactions can affect certain nerve endings and cause burning sensations in the nose, eyes, and throat. They usually come and go and can be reversed.

- **Immune Hypersensitivity:** This is the basis of allergic diseases, such as allergic rhinitis (hay fever) and asthma. They are generally caused by naturally occurring organic chemicals found in pollens, molds, dust, and animals. At present, only a relatively few industrial chemicals are known to have the capability of provoking a true immune system response. Among them are acid anhydrides and isocyanates and other chemicals that are able to bond to human proteins.

- **Intoxication Syndrome:** In some cases, long-term exposure to noxious chemicals may cause serious illness or even death. Permanent damage to health may be the outcome of such reactions, which are dependent on the nature and extent of the chemical exposure. Toxic pollutants are given off by a number of building products, such as furniture, cleaning fluids, pesticides, and paints.

How does pollution affect my health?

Most people who believe they have symptoms from chemical sensitivity are concerned that their symptoms are related to their exposure to pollution, either outdoors or indoors. Outdoor pollution may result from natural causes (the eruption of volcanoes, dust storms, or forest fires) or manmade causes (vehicle exhaust, fossil fuel combustion, or petroleum refining). Other pollutants that may cause respiratory illness include sulfur dioxide, ozone and nitrogen dioxide, cigarette smoke, wood-burning stoves, and building-related illness.

Sulfur Dioxide: Substantial scientific evidence has linked specific air pollutants to increased respiratory illness and decreased pulmonary function, especially in children. People prone to allergy, especially those with allergic asthma, can be extremely sensitive to inhaled sulfur dioxide, for example. Symptoms may include bronchospasm, hives, gastrointestinal disorders, and inflammation of the blood vessels (vasculitis-related disorder).

Ozone and Nitrogen Dioxide: Temporary or perhaps permanent bronchial hypersensitivity has been connected to inhaled ozone and nitrogen dioxide. Long-term exposure to nitrogen dioxide has been associated with the increased occurrence of respiratory illness.

Significant exposure to airborne pollution occurs inside homes, offices, and non-industrial buildings. These settings have not received nearly the attention by pollution control agencies that they deserve.

Cigarette Smoke: One of the most disagreeable and potentially dangerous indoor pollutants is cigarette smoke. It is made up of a complex mixture of gases and particles that contain numerous chemicals. Indoor tobacco smoking substantially increases levels of carbon monoxide, formaldehyde, nitrogen dioxide, acrolein, polycyclic aromatic hydrocarbons, hydrogen cyanide, and many other substances and inhaled particles found in the air.

Formaldehyde is not only found indoors from cigarette smoke, but also outdoors from gasoline and diesel combustion. Data indicates that formaldehyde is capable of acting as a respiratory irritant. It also is known to cause an allergic skin rash. However, there is no convincing evidence that this pollutant is able to sensitize the respiratory system.

Wood-Burning Stoves: There are more than 11 million wood-burning units in American homes today. Wood burning usually occurs in cold, oxygen-poor conditions that heighten the emission of carbon monoxide and other inhaled chemicals and particles. Increased use of wood as a heating fuel has raised concern because of its ability to contaminate a home. Poorly ventilated stoves give off increased levels of carbon monoxide, nitrogen and sulfur oxides, formaldehyde, and benzopyrene.

Building-Related Illness: Poor air quality in today's tightly insulated homes and other buildings has been associated with a variety of syndromes, or group of symptoms. The term "building-related illness" or "sick-building syndrome" is applied to an office building in which one or more occupants develop a generally accepted, well-defined syndrome for which a specific cause related to the building is found.

There are a variety of illnesses broadly known as hypersensitivity pneumonitis—in which one or more organic dusts can create complex immune system reactions and symptoms, including mucous membrane irritation, coughing, chest tightness, headache, and fatigue. These are well defined, and there are validated tests for diagnosing these conditions. Building occupants with these symptoms have been identified as having "multiple chemical sensitivities" or other forms of environmental illness.

One study, however, showed that the majority of nonspecific complaints by office workers had developed before the worker began working in the building suspected of causing their symptoms. Collaboration between the physician, industrial hygienist, and building engineer may be necessary to clearly establish a cause-and-effect relationship between any indoor air quality level and disease.

How is chemical sensitivity diagnosed?

There are strategies that can produce reliable diagnoses with relatively low costs, reliable diagnoses at significant costs, or questionable diagnoses at great expense. Obviously, the first alternative is preferable. It includes:

- a careful patient medical history that includes a review of all previous medical records and, when symptoms may be related to potentially hazardous substances in the workplace, reviewing a Materials Safety Data Sheet supplied by the employer;

- upper respiratory tract and selective skin tests and a neurological examination;

- routine laboratory studies, including nasal smear; and

- lung function measurements (spirometry and peak flow monitoring).

If these diagnostic procedures do not produce a definite diagnosis, more expensive—but worthwhile—evaluations may help. They include an industrial hygiene evaluation of the workplace, an evaluation of the home environment, and psychiatric evaluations.

Diagnostic approaches are expensive and not effective in explaining suggested chemical sensitivity such as the RAST [radioallergosorbent test] and tests for the Epstein-Barr virus, autoimmune disease, food allergies, and evaluations to determine airborne molds and bacteria.

Section 34.2

Environmental Illness (Multiple Chemical Sensitivity Syndrome)

"Multiple Chemical Sensitivities Syndrome (MCSS)," National Institute of Environmental Health Sciences (NIEHS, www.niehs.nih.gov), January 2004. This document was contributed by Dan Nebert, with help from Steve Leeder, and Jonathan Bernstein.

What is it and what is known about MCSS?

Actually, the preferred medical term is idiopathic environmental intolerance (IEI), which can be defined as a "chronic, recurring disease caused by a person's inability to tolerate an environmental chemical or class of foreign chemicals."

IEI thus represents a complex gene-environment interaction, the true cause of which is currently unknown. There is almost always a precipitating event, usually associated with the smell of a chemical, and a response involving one or more organ systems. Once the imitating event has passed, the same response or even an exaggerated occurs each time the stimulus is encountered again. Often the initiating stimulus is a higher dose or an overwhelming dose, but subsequently much lower doses can trigger the symptoms. A number of unrelated chemicals (e.g., insecticides, antiseptic cleaning agents) might precipitate the same response. Because the syndrome is similar to certain allergic conditions and to certain organ-system responses caused by emotional disturbances, IEI has often been confused with allergy (atopy) or psychiatric illness. Disagreement among physicians and medical researchers—as to what IEI really is—has, of course, made research funding difficult ("is this a real syndrome, or is this a mental problem or a simple allergy?") In fact, in an environmental health sciences meeting in Brisbane, Australia, several years ago, there was an old-fashioned debate on MCSS, and the proponents who believed that it was simply a psychiatric disorder won the debate.

What are the six criteria for IEI?

Several years ago a committee of experts in their field decided upon a consensus as to what "qualifies" the patient as truly having IEI [*Arch Environ Health* 1999; 54: 147]. Six criteria were decided upon:

- Symptoms are reproducible with repeated (chemical) exposures.

- The condition is chronic.

- Low levels of exposure (lower than previously or commonly tolerated) result in manifestations of the syndrome (i.e., increased sensitivity).

- The symptoms improve, or resolve completely, when the triggering chemicals are removed.

- Responses often occur to multiple chemically unrelated substances.

- Symptoms involve multiple-organ symptoms (runny nose, itchy eyes, headache, scratchy throat, earache, scalp pain, mental confusion or sleepiness, palpitations of the heart, upset stomach, nausea and/or diarrhea, abdominal cramping, aching joints).

Several medical conditions appear to be related to, or overlap with, IEI—such as sick-building syndrome (SBS), food intolerance syndrome (FIS), and perhaps the Gulf War illness (GWI). In each of these, a chemical (smell usually, or taste) appears to precipitate one or more organ-system responses. The initiating culprit might be: chemicals in a new rug, cockroach dander, or Freon circulating in a closed-ventilation building (SBS); chemicals in wine, processed corn products, or sulfites consumed (FIS); or nerve gas, organophosphates, or pesticides to which soldiers were exposed during the brief 1991 was in the Middle East (GWI). Additional conditions (of discomfort, pain or dysfunction) that might have a genetic component but also seem to have an environmental stimulus include: chronic fatigue syndrome, fibromyalgia, irritable bowel syndrome, atypical connective tissue disease after silicone breast implants, chronic hypoglycemia (low blood sugar), drug-induced autoantibodies/hepatitis (liver toxicity), illness while living near a toxic waste dump site, dental amalgam disease, and MTBE (methyl-tert-butyl ether, a gasoline additive)-associated symptoms. Inflammation of the lungs caused by diesel exhaust particles (DEPs) is of particular interest, since it illustrates the potential for the drug-biotransformation and immune systems (which protect us from small and large foreign compounds, respectively) to interact and contribute to the disease process. In this situation, cellular processes regulated by the aryl hydrocarbon receptor (AHR) apparently activate an inflammatory response involving Th-2 helper cells, subsequently increasing immunoglobulin E (IgE) production.

How might we dissect this complex disease?

Frequently, individuals with IEI present with symptoms of rhinitis (runny nose), along with other diffuse systemic complaints. First, the physician must determine whether the patient has a runny nose due to an allergy problem (allergic rhinitis) or not an allergy problem (nonallergic rhinitis).

Seasonal allergic rhinitis refers to patients with allergy symptoms triggered by pollen or mold-spore allergens. "Triggering stimuli" occur when the patient is outdoors during the pollen seasons. Symptoms can include sneezing fits (i.e., 5 to 10 sneezes in succession), itching of the eyes/ears/nose/throat/roof of the mouth, runny nose, watery/puffy eyes, nasal stuffiness, postnasal drip, sinus pressure, and fatigue. Perennial allergic rhinitis refers to year-round hay fever symptoms that are triggered by indoor allergens such as dust mites, cockroaches, mold spores, feathers, and animal dander. Perennial allergens may be difficult to identify by history alone; skin testing is necessary to confirm sensitization to these allergens but does not indicate that the individual is currently being exposed.

A patient with nonallergic rhinitis is one who has had an allergic component ruled out by skin tests. Nonallergic rhinitis can be further divided into inflammatory (nonallergic rhinitis with eosinophilic syndrome [NARES]) and noninflammatory (vasomotor rhinitis [VMR]) subtypes. Nonallergic rhinitis is an organ-specific disorder of unknown etiology (cause not understood) that is aggravated by strange chemical smells and weather changes. The noninflammatory form of nonallergic rhinitis, VMR, satisfies the first five of the above criteria, suggesting that this disorder is a potential model (*Ann Allergy Asthma Immunol* 2001: 86;494] for investigating the genetic etiology of the more global disease, IEI.

Nonallergic VMR can mimic allergic rhinitis. Patients with nonallergic VMR experience nasal congestion, postnasal drip, headaches/sinus pressure, and ear plugging. Skin testing to seasonal and perennial allergens is negative (i.e., non-atopic). "Triggering stimuli" for nonallergic VMR include weather changes (temperature or barometric pressure changes), postural changes, and irritants such as smoke, perfumes, potpourris, solvents, cleaning agents, incense, and soaps and detergents (to name a few).

Is IEI associated with mutations in olfactory receptor (OR) genes?

The field of olfaction (ability to smell distinct classes of things) has recently exploded with the advent of genomics and the Human Genome Project. A superfamily of about 1000 odorant receptor (OR) genes has been discovered, located in multiple clusters on all but two of the 24 human chromosomes (22 autosomes, X Y chromosome). These OR clusters comprise 17 gene families, four of which contain more than 100 members each [*Genome Res* 2001; 11;685]. Interestingly, 64% of the human's OR genes are nonfunctional (pseudogenes). The fact that apes have a greater percentage of functional OR genes is strong evidence that the evolving human species has lost its need for maintaining a very keen sense of smell. The OR gene superfamily comprises 1% to 3% of the entire genomic complement of genes, and is likely to be the largest gene superfamily in the genome of any species.

Other clusters of human chemosensory genes include the vomeronasal receptors, related to an accessory olfactory organ thought to be largely inactive in primates. The OR genes are members of the 7-transmembrane domain G-protein-coupled receptor (GPCR) superfamily. In situ hybridization studies indicate that each OR gene is expressed in about 1 per 1,000 olfactory epithelial (OE) neurons, suggesting that each OE neuron expresses only one OR gene [*Cell* 2000; 100:611]. People clearly have very different abilities to sense smells. Polymorphisms in many of these genes have been reported, implying a mechanism for interindividual variation in olfactory responses [*Gene* 2000; 260:87]—and perhaps to diseases triggered by olfactory stimuli.

What are the conclusions?

IEI is a complex disease involving gene-environment interactions [*Environ Health Perspect* 2000; 108:1219]. Perhaps one place to begin, in dissecting this complex disease, would be to study nonallergic VMR because it can be more precisely defined. Would polymorphisms, in particular functional OR genes, be responsible for nonallergic VMR? Could nonallergic VMR be a sufficient phenotypic end-point such that it could be examined in a phenotype-genotype association study involving a candidate-gene approach, a candidate-gene-region approach, or a total genome scan?

It seems tempting to postulate that nonallergic VMR might be a sufficiently quantitative trait that it can be used first in attempting to dissect the very complex disease syndromes associated with IEI, SBS, FIS and GWI. Anyway, this is the approach that is being taken by three University of Cincinnati CEG [Center for Environmental Genetics] researchers—Jonathan Bernstein, Dan Nebert, and Li (Felix) Jin. Given the exploding advances in our knowledge about the human genome, it seems that the time to tackle this complicated (and very common) environmental disease is now.

Section 34.3

Diesel Emissions Can Trigger Allergic Symptoms

From "Scientists Identify Genes That Regulate Allergic Response to Diesel Fumes," a press release by the National Institutes of Health (NIH, www.nih.gov) and the National Institute of Allergy and Infectious Diseases (NIAID, www.niaid.nih.gov), January 8, 2004.

The risk of developing respiratory allergies from exposure to diesel emissions depends largely on genetics, according to a study funded by the National Institute of Allergy and Infectious Diseases (NIAID), part of the National Institutes of Health (NIH). Given their findings, researchers estimate that up to 50 percent of the United States population could be in jeopardy of experiencing health problems related to air pollution. The study is published in the January 10, 2005 issue of the British journal *The Lancet*.

"This important study adds to previous data that suggest how modern environmental factors interact with the body's defenses to produce 'airway' diseases considered rare before the advent of industrialized society," says Anthony S. Fauci, M.D., director of NIAID.

"The knowledge provided by this work will help us identify people who are susceptible to the deleterious effects of diesel emissions on the clinical course of asthma and hay fever," says Kenneth Adams, Ph.D., who oversees asthma research funded by NIAID. "It will also help accelerate development of drugs to treat and prevent these diseases."

This study also received support from the National Institute of Environmental Health Sciences, another NIH component.

The authors of the study examined how a family of antioxidant-related genes—GSTM1, GSTT1, and GSTP1—reacts to diesel exhaust particles, a common air pollutant. The body generates antioxidants to detoxify harmful particles and limit the corresponding allergic reaction.

Researchers sampled the DNA of volunteers who are allergic to ragweed to find which forms of the genes they had. The participants were then given doses of ragweed through the nose, followed by either a placebo or quantities of diesel exhaust particles equivalent to breathing the air in Los Angeles, California, for 40 hours.

The mix of ragweed and diesel exhaust triggered greater allergic responses than ragweed alone. Additionally, the diesel particles caused volunteers who lacked the antioxidant-producing form of the GSTM1 gene to have significantly greater allergic responses, compared to the other participants. Up to 50 percent of the U.S. population does not have this form of the GSTM1 gene. Within the group that lacked GSTM1, those who had a particular variant of the GSTP1 gene experienced even greater allergic reactions. Researchers estimate that 15 to 20 percent of the U.S. population falls into this category.

"Diesel emissions can trigger allergic symptoms, but the genetic factors involved in the process are quite complex," says David Diaz-Sanchez, Ph.D., assistant professor in the Division of Immunology and Allergy at the University of California Los Angeles, who coauthored the study with scientists from the University of Southern California. "Our findings suggest that people who lack the genes to make key antioxidants may have difficulty fighting the harmful effects of air pollution."

Dr. Diaz-Sanchez says that he and the other researchers will work to find other genes involved in pollution-related health problems such as asthma, lung cancer and heart disease, with the goal of discovering possible treatments and preventions. "We are focused on investigating ways we can overcome this genetic deficiency," he says. "This may be accomplished by either giving people drugs that replace the role of the genes or by boosting the body's natural defenses."

NIAID is a component of the National Institutes of Health (NIH), which is an agency of the Department of Health and Human Services. NIAID supports basic and applied research to prevent, diagnose and treat infectious and immune-mediated illnesses, including HIV/AIDS and other sexually transmitted diseases, illness from potential agents of bioterrorism, tuberculosis, malaria, autoimmune disorders, asthma and allergies.

Reference

F. Gilliland et al. Effect of glutathione-S-transferase M1 and P1 genotypes on xenobiotic enhancement of allergic responses: randomised, placebo-controlled crossover study. *The Lancet* 363 (9403): 119–125 (2004).

Chapter 35

Insect Venom Allergy

Chapter Contents

Section 35.1

Allergic Reactions to Insect Venom

Reprinted with permission. Dawna L. Cyr and Steven B. Johnson, "First Aid for Bee and Insect Stings," bulletin #2345 of the "Maine Farm Safety Program" (Orono, ME: University of Maine Cooperative Extension). © 1995, 2002.

Most bees and insects will not attack if left alone. If provoked, a bee will sting in defense of its nest or itself. Thousands of people are stung each year and as many as 40 to 50 people in the United States die each year as a result of allergic reactions.

Reducing the Risk of Being Stung

1. Wear light-colored, smooth-finished clothing.

2. Avoid perfumed soaps, shampoos, and deodorants. Don't wear cologne or perfume. Avoid bananas and banana-scented toiletries.

3. Wear clean clothing and bathe daily. Sweat angers bees.

4. Cover the body as much as possible with clothing.

5. Avoid flowering plants.

6. Check for new nests during the warmer hours of the day during July, August, and September. Bees are very active then.

7. Keep areas clean. Social wasps thrive in places where humans discard food, so clean up picnic tables, grills, and other outdoor eating areas.

8. If a single stinging insect is flying around, remain still or lie face down on the ground. The face is the most likely place for a bee or wasp to sting. Swinging or swatting at an insect may cause it to sting.

9. If you are attacked by several stinging insects at the same time, run to get away from them. Bees release a chemical when

they sting. This alerts other bees to the intruder. More bees often follow. If possible, get indoors when there are few, if any, bees around you. Outdoors, a shaded area is better than an open area to get away from the insects.

10. If a bee comes inside your vehicle, stop the car slowly, and open all the windows.

What to Do If a Person Is Stung

1. Have someone stay with the victim to be sure that they do not have an allergic reaction.

2. Wash the site with soap and water.

3. The stinger can be removed using a 4-inch x 4-inch gauze wiped over the area or by scraping a fingernail over the area. Never squeeze the stinger or use tweezers. It will cause more venom to go into the skin and injure the muscle.

4. Apply ice to reduce the swelling.

5. Do not scratch the sting. This will cause the site to swell and itch more and increase the chance of infection.

Allergic Reactions to Bee Stings

Allergic reactions to bee stings can be deadly. People with known allergies to insect stings should always carry an insect sting allergy kit and wear a medical ID bracelet or necklace stating their allergy. See a physician about getting either of these.

There are several signs of an allergic reaction to bee stings. Look for swelling that moves to other parts of the body, especially the face or neck. Check for difficulty in breathing, wheezing, dizziness, or a drop in blood pressure. Get the person immediate medical care if any of these signs are present. It is normal for the area that has been stung to hurt, have a hard swollen lump, get red, and itch. There are kits available to reduce the pain of an insect sting. They are a valuable addition to a first-aid kit.

Section 35.2

Insect Sting Allergies during Childhood Often Do Not Fade away during Adult Years

"UT Southwestern allergist recommends children with serious allergies to insect stings get shots to avoid life-threatening reactions," © 2004 University of Texas Southwestern Medical Center at Dallas. Reprinted with permission.

Children who have severe allergic reactions when stung by bees, wasps, and other insects should receive venom immunotherapy, or allergy shots, to reduce the chance of future life-threatening reactions if a repeat sting should occur, said an allergist at UT Southwestern Medical Center at Dallas.

In an editorial published in [the August 12, 2004] issue of *The New England Journal of Medicine,* Dr. Rebecca Gruchalla, chief of the allergy division of internal medicine and associate professor of pediatrics at UT Southwestern, recommends the shots for children who have had a serious systemic allergic reaction to an insect sting.

Systemic allergic reactions go beyond the expected swelling and pain at the sting site and could include low blood pressure, tightness in the chest, and swelling in the throat. These types of reactions require immediate medical care due to their life-threatening nature, she said.

"Claritin isn't going to be able to fix this," Dr. Gruchalla said of the over-the-counter medicine used for seasonal allergies. "Severe reactions to stings and the stuffiness caused by ragweed are mediated by the same 'allergy antibody,' immunoglobulin E, but the clinical manifestations are very different."

"It's similar to having a food allergy. The majority of kids with documented food allergies have only mild hive reactions when they eat the 'culprit' food, but for those with a severe allergy, the reaction could be deadly."

The article accompanies a study by researchers from the Johns Hopkins Asthma and Allergy Center in Baltimore. Researchers found that children who had severe allergic reactions to bee stings and who were given the venom allergy shots were significantly less likely to suffer life-threatening reactions when restung, even if the repeat sting happened years later.

"The common belief has been that children typically outgrow insect sting allergies and for this reason, venom immunotherapy may not be needed. This study sets the record straight," Dr. Gruchalla said, adding that the therapy is not necessary for kids who suffer from allergic skin reactions such as hives.

"Hopefully now, since hard data have been provided, physicians will be able to move beyond previous misconceptions and endorse venom immunotherapy for these children most at risk," she said.

The culprits responsible for most of the reactions include honeybees, bumblebees, yellow jackets, yellow hornets, white-faced hornets, paper wasps, and fire ants.

There are at least 40 fatal stings in the nation each year but it is likely that many deaths go unreported, Dr. Gruchalla said. Almost 1 percent of all children are reported to have a medical history of severe allergic reactions to insect stings, she said.

Chapter 36

Allergic Reactions to Medications and Ingredients in Medical Products

Chapter Contents

Section 36.1

Allergic Reactions to Medicines

"Drug Reactions," Copyright © 2000 American College of Allergy,
Asthma and Immunology. Reprinted with permission. Reviewed and
revised by David A. Cooke, M.D., January 5, 2007.

Most people have probably experienced an unwanted side effect to
a medicine at some time in their lives. Many drugs commonly cause
side effects, such as an upset stomach after taking aspirin or drowsiness after taking a cold medication. Adverse drug reactions also can
be quite serious; they account for an estimated 106,000 deaths each
year in the United States. As more medications are approved each
year, the problem is expected to grow.

An adverse drug reaction is any effect not intended by proper administration of a medication. Reactions also can occur between medications, even nonprescription ones. Most adverse drug reactions—more
than 90 percent—do not involve the immune system. When the immune system is involved, a person is said to have drug hypersensitivity. Allergy is one type of hypersensitivity reaction.

What Is Drug Hypersensitivity?

Medications can cause unwanted reactions in many ways. Sometimes,
it's a direct effect of the drug on the body. Drug hypersensitivity reactions occur when the immune system responds to a medication or to the
biologic products that result when the body breaks down a medication.
In some cases, the immune system tries to attack the substance, causing symptoms of the drug reaction. Drugs also can cause allergic reactions similar to those caused by bee stings or other allergenic substances.

People who have a family history of allergic diseases may be more
likely to have drug allergy, but are not at greater risk to develop
nonallergic types of reactions. Fortunately, a family history of allergy
to a particular drug does not increase a person's chance of being allergic to that same drug.

A person must have a previous exposure to a drug in order to have
a true allergic reaction to it. Such reactions most often occur when a

drug is administered intravenously or by injection, delivery methods that send the drug directly to the bloodstream. Reactions occur less frequently when drugs are taken by mouth. The chance of an allergic reaction increases when a medication is administered frequently or in large doses.

Certain medications are more likely to cause allergic reactions than others due to their chemical structure. Penicillin and other antibiotics are some of the most common culprits of allergic drug reactions. Penicillin, however, can also cause other types of immune reactions, as well as reactions that do not involve the immune system.

Symptoms

The most common types of allergic reactions to a drug are:

- skin rash or hives;
- itchy skin;
- wheezing or other breathing problems;
- swelling of body parts; and
- anaphylaxis, a life-threatening allergic reaction.

While these are the most common symptoms of drug allergy, adverse reactions can occur in any organ or system of the body.

Allergic reactions can occur within minutes or hours of exposure to a medication. Drug reactions can even occur some time after a medication has been stopped. For example, a person may develop a rash or hives a week after stopping a medication.

A "pseudoallergic," or anaphylactoid, reaction does not involve allergic antibodies and can occur without prior exposure. Symptoms are similar to a true allergic reaction: a person may develop a rash or hives, have difficulty breathing, and experience swelling of body parts. Common causes of pseudoallergic reactions include aspirin and x-ray dye.

Diagnosis

Adverse drug reactions can be difficult to diagnose, because they often can look like other conditions. Further, although many common reactions to certain drugs are known, others may not have been identified yet.

It is important to distinguish an allergic (hypersensitivity) reaction from a nonallergic reaction. If drug hypersensitivity is suspected, your doctor may send you to a specialist in allergy and immunology.

If you suspect you are having, or had, an adverse reaction to a medication, take note of the circumstances. Your doctor will want to know when the medication was taken, when the symptoms started, what the symptoms were and how long they lasted, and any other medications you were taking at the time, including nonprescription medications. Bring copies of any treatment records of the reaction with you to the doctor's office. This information is important for the diagnosis and treatment of your condition.

Be sure to have the name of the exact medications you took to help the doctor identify which drugs should be tested for hypersensitivity. It also will allow the allergist to determine if there are alternative medications that would be safe for you to take—and which additional medications you should avoid in the future. If possible, bring the suspected medications with you.

Next, an allergist will perform a physical examination. This is necessary to check for different problems that may occur as part of an allergic reaction and to determine if there are other, nonallergic causes of the symptoms. The allergist will pay special attention to any symptoms of a reaction that you still have, such as a skin rash.

Allergy skin testing is available to test for allergic reactions to only a few drugs. Many experts recommend that testing not be done until there is a future, compelling need to use the same medication again. In some cases, an allergist will perform blood tests to identify antibodies against a medication. Blood tests tend to be less sensitive than skin tests, so a skin test will be used whenever possible.

Treatment

If a drug reaction is mild, treatment may be limited to stopping the medication. In many cases, discontinuing the drug is all that is needed.

To relieve the symptoms of a more serious or persistent reaction, an allergist may administer antihistamines, corticosteroids, and other medications. Antihistamines work by counteracting the chemical histamine, which is released during the body's allergic response. Corticosteroids work by reducing inflammation.

In most cases, a person with drug hypersensitivity can safely be given other types of drugs, and the drug that caused the reaction is simply avoided. When no alternate medication exists, an allergist can undertake desensitization or graded challenge. These are methods of gradually introducing a medication into the body in small doses until a therapeutic dose is reached.

Anaphylaxis

Anaphylaxis is a severe, potentially life-threatening reaction that can occur within seconds or minutes of administration of a drug. Symptoms of anaphylaxis include swelling of body parts; shortness of breath or wheezing; a sudden drop in blood pressure, which may cause dizziness or loss of consciousness; and shock.

Anaphylaxis requires emergency treatment. Several drugs, including epinephrine, antihistamines, and corticosteroids, are often administered. The patient may also receive oxygen and intravenous fluids.

If you take a medication and develop any of the symptoms of anaphylaxis, immediately call your local emergency phone number (911 in most locations in the United States and Canada). Although antihistamines are sometimes given to patients with anaphylaxis, antihistamines alone are not likely to be adequate treatment. If you are with someone who develops any symptoms of anaphylaxis, call your local emergency number. If he or she loses consciousness, lay the person down and elevate the feet.

If you have had a reaction to a drug:

- Make sure all of your doctors know the medication you took and the reaction you had.

- Talk to your primary care doctor or allergist about other medications you should avoid and which medications are safe for you to take.

- If the reaction is severe, wear a medical alert tag or bracelet in case of emergency.

For more medical information, please contact an allergist in your area.

Section 36.2

Antibiotic-Related Allergic Reactions

"Antibiotic Can Cause Reaction in Penicillin-Sensitive Patients," September 2003. © 2003 Medical College of Wisconsin. Reprinted with permission of Medical College of Wisconsin HealthLink, www.healthlink .mcw.edu.

Even though the antibiotic cephalosporin can set off allergic reactions in penicillin-sensitive patients, one out of 10 non-allergist physicians said that they would prescribe it even for patients known to have had severe reactions to penicillin, according to a survey conducted by Medical College of Wisconsin researchers.

The survey results show a need for more continuing education among doctors in the area of penicillin allergy, said study co-author Michael C. Zacharisen, M.D., Associate Professor of Pediatrics and Medicine.

"I worked with Dr. Thomas Puchner, Jr., on the study while he was at the Medical College on a fellowship to train in allergy," said Dr. Zacharisen. "Prior to the fellowship he was a practicing internist for ten years, and what he was hearing about penicillin allergy and cephalosporin from the experts in lectures was not what he had seen in private practice. So the whole goal of the survey was to find out what people are really doing in practice. Are they following guidelines and expert opinion, or are they simply doing what they've always done?"

Students, residents, general internists, and allergists were among the 378 physicians surveyed. The researchers learned that all of the allergists said that they would not prescribe cephalosporin to someone who had once had a severe reaction to penicillin, but 11% of non-allergist doctors said that they would.

For patients who had had milder reactions to penicillin, such as a rash, more than half of the pediatricians and more than one third of the allergists surveyed said they would prescribe cephalosporin. And one out of three internists and pediatricians were unaware that standardized skin tests for penicillin allergy are readily available.

About the Allergies and Reactions

Penicillin was discovered in 1928, and the antibiotic Cephalosporin C was isolated in 1953. Penicillin-allergic patients might also be allergic to cephalosporin. The study noted, however, that while physicians routinely avoid prescribing penicillin to patients with penicillin allergy, the approach to prescribing cephalosporin is less clear.

"Any antibiotic—in fact almost any medication—has the potential to cause an allergic reaction," said Dr. Zacharisen. "Usually it's antibiotics, because they are frequently given, and usually it's penicillin or its derivatives because they're the most frequent used antibiotics."

"There are different types of cephalosporins," Dr. Zacharisen explained. "There have been three generations, and as the newer ones come out they have different aspects about them that are good. It appears that penicillin is more closely linked or similar to the first generation of cephalosporin. So if you have a reaction to penicillin you're more likely to have a reaction to the first generation of cephalosporin, less so to the second, and even less so to the third."

"The most common reactions are skin reactions—rash, hives, and swelling. Reactions can range from mild skin reactions to severe skin reactions to anaphylactic shock," said Dr. Zacharisen. Anaphylactic shock is often severe and sometimes fatal, with characteristics that include respiratory symptoms, fainting, itching, and raised patches of skin or mucous membrane.

"There are many people who have had allergic reactions as infants, children, or young adults," said Dr. Zacharisen, "and as time goes along that risk decreases. But you can have an allergic reaction at any point in your life, so your first penicillin or cephalosporin reaction may not be until you're an adult or even an elderly person. We don't know exactly why that is."

Simple Skin Test Aids Detection

Dr. Zacharisen said that there are about 50 deaths from penicillin anaphylaxis in the United States each year, while between 4% and 5% of all persons may be penicillin sensitive and exhibit the milder symptoms. "Here at the Medical College we generally see those patients with the more severe reactions who come to us from primary care physicians," he said, "hence the survey to find out what's really going on in practice."

"The symptoms of penicillin allergy can be similar to those of any other allergy, such as allergies to foods or other drugs. There are no specifically distinguishable symptoms for these antibiotic allergies. The most important thing is the temporal relationship. You take the medication and then the symptoms occur. When we're evaluating patients for a medication allergy, they may be on six medications and the question is, which one is it?"

"Unfortunately, we don't have any good allergy skin tests for any antibiotic other than penicillin," said Dr. Zacharisen. "If people want to know if they're allergic to cephalosporin, there's not a good, accurate way to tell that." The knowledge that a patient is sensitive to penicillin is a predictor of sensitivity to cephalosporin, though, which makes the standardized skin test for penicillin allergy a useful tool. One of the outcomes from the survey that Dr. Zacharisen hopes for is that more pediatricians and internists will be made aware of the availability of the skin test.

"Generalists have to take care of all groups of patients and all diseases, but when it comes to drug allergies there have been some recent advances. It's difficult for doctors to keep up with everything in the field, especially knowing what skin tests are available. For a period of time even the penicillin skin test was not available on the market but then it came back. I think the biggest thing is education. What are we teaching students and residents? And what are the allergy education needs of community physicians?"

Section 36.3

Latex Allergy

From the Centers for Disease Control and Prevention (CDC, www.cdc.gov), updated December 1997. Reviewed by David A. Cooke, M.D., October 27, 2006.

What Is Latex Allergy?

Latex allergy can result from repeated exposures to proteins in natural rubber latex through skin contact or inhalation. Reactions usually begin within minutes of exposure to latex, but they can occur hours later and can produce various symptoms. These include skin rash and inflammation, respiratory irritation, asthma, and in rare cases shock. In some instances, sensitized employees have experienced reactions so severe that they impeded the worker's ability to continue working in their current job.

The amount of exposure needed to sensitize individuals to natural rubber latex is not known, but reductions in exposure to latex proteins have been reported to be associated with decreased sensitization and symptoms. People at increased risk for developing latex allergy include workers with ongoing latex exposure, persons with a tendency to have multiple allergic conditions, and persons with spina bifida. Latex allergy is also associated with allergies to certain foods such as avocados, potatoes, bananas, tomatoes, chestnuts, kiwifruit, and papaya.

How Large a Problem Is Latex Allergy?

Reports of work-related allergic reactions to latex have increased in recent years, especially among employees in the health care industry, where latex gloves are widely used to prevent exposure to infectious agents. Once sensitized, workers may go on to experience the effects of latex allergy.

Studies indicate that 8% to 12% of health care workers regularly exposed to latex are sensitized, compared with 1% to 6% of the general population, although total numbers of exposed workers are not

405

known. In the health care industry, workers at risk of latex allergy from ongoing latex exposure include physicians, nurses, aides, dentists, dental hygienists, operating room employees, laboratory technicians, and housekeeping personnel.

Workers who use gloves less frequently, such as law enforcement personnel, ambulance attendants, firefighters, food service employees, painters, gardeners, housekeeping personnel outside the health care industry, and funeral home employees, also may develop latex allergy. Workers in factories where natural rubber latex products are manufactured or used also may be affected.

Prevention

The National Institute for Occupational Safety and Health (NIOSH) recommends wherever feasible the selection of products and implementation of work practices that reduce the risk of allergic reactions. These recommendations include:

- Use nonlatex gloves for activities that are not likely to involve contact with infectious materials (food preparation, routine housekeeping, maintenance, etc.).

- Appropriate barrier protection is necessary when handling infectious materials. If you choose latex gloves, use powder-free gloves with reduced protein content.

- When wearing latex gloves, do not use oil-based hand creams or lotions unless they have been shown to reduce latex-related problems.

- Frequently clean work areas contaminated with latex dust (upholstery, carpets, ventilation ducts, and plenums).

- Frequently change the ventilation filters and vacuum bags used in latex-contaminated areas.

- Learn to recognize the symptoms of latex allergy: skin rashes; hives; flushing; itching; nasal, eye, or sinus symptoms; asthma; and shock.

- If you develop symptoms of latex allergy, avoid direct contact with latex gloves and products until you can see a physician experienced in treating latex allergy.

- If you have latex allergy, consult your physician regarding the following precautions:

- Avoid contact with latex gloves and products.
- Avoid areas where you might inhale the powder from latex gloves worn by others.
- Tell your employers, physicians, nurses, and dentists that you have latex allergy.
- Wear a medical alert bracelet.

- Take advantage of latex allergy education and training provided by your employer.

Part Five

Diagnosing and Treating Allergies

Chapter 37

When Should I See an Allergist?

Asthma and other allergic diseases are two of the most common health problems. Approximately 50 million Americans have asthma, hay fever, or other allergy-related conditions.

Some allergy problems—such as a mild case of hay fever—may not need any treatment. Sometimes allergies can be controlled with the occasional use of an over-the-counter medication. However, sometimes allergies can interfere with day-to-day activities or decrease the quality of life. Allergies can even be life threatening.

The Allergist Treats Asthma and Allergies

An allergist is a physician who specializes in the diagnosis and treatment of asthma and other allergic diseases. The allergist is specially trained to identify the factors that trigger asthma or allergies. Allergists help people treat or prevent their allergy problems. After earning a medical degree, the allergist completes a three-year residency-training program in either internal medicine or pediatrics. Next the allergist completes two or three more years of study in the field of allergy and immunology. You can be certain that your doctor has met these requirements if he or she is certified by the American Board of Allergy and Immunology.

What Is an Allergy?

One of the marvels of the human body is that it can defend itself against harmful invaders such as viruses or bacteria. But sometimes the defenses are too aggressive and harmless substances such as dust, molds, or pollen are mistakenly identified as dangerous. The immune system then rallies its defenses, which include several chemicals to attack and destroy the supposed enemy. In the process, some unpleasant and, in extreme cases, life-threatening symptoms may be experienced in the allergy-prone individual.

The Cause of Allergic Reactions

There are hundreds of ordinary substances that can trigger allergic reactions. Among the most common are plant pollens, molds, household dust (dust mites), cockroaches, pets, industrial chemicals, foods, medicines, feathers, and insect stings. These triggers are called allergens.

Who Develops Asthma or Allergies?

Asthma and allergies can affect anyone, regardless of age, gender, race, or socioeconomic factors. While it's true that asthma and allergies are more common in children, they can occur for the first time at any age. Sometimes allergy symptoms start in childhood, disappear for many years, and then start up again during adult life.

Although the exact genetic factors are not yet understood, there is a hereditary tendency to asthma and allergies. In susceptible people, factors such as hormones, stress, smoke, perfume, or other environmental irritants also may play a role.

Types of Allergy Problems

An allergic reaction may occur anywhere in the body but usually appears in the nose, eyes, lungs, lining of the stomach, sinuses, throat, and skin. These are places where special immune system cells are stationed to fight off invaders that are inhaled, swallowed, or come in contact with the skin.

Allergic Rhinitis (Hay Fever)

Allergic rhinitis is a general term used to describe the allergic reactions that take place in the nose. Symptoms may include sneezing, congestion, runny nose, and itching of the nose, the eyes, and/or the roof of the mouth. When this problem is triggered by pollens or outdoor molds, during the spring, summer, or fall, the condition is often called hay fever. When the problem is year-round, it might be caused by exposure to house dust mites, household pets, indoor molds, or allergens at school or in the workplace.

Asthma

Asthma symptoms occur when airway muscle spasms block the flow of air to the lungs and/or the linings of the bronchial tubes become inflamed. Excess mucus may clog the airways. An asthma attack is characterized by labored or restricted breathing, a tight feeling in the chest, coughing, and/or wheezing. Sometimes a chronic cough is the only symptom. Asthma trouble can cause only mild discomfort or it can cause life-threatening attacks in which breathing stops altogether.

Contact Dermatitis/Skin Allergies

Contact dermatitis, eczema, and hives are skin conditions that can be caused by allergens and other irritants. Often the reaction may take hours or days to develop, as in the case of poison ivy. The most common allergic causes of rashes are medicines, insect stings, foods, animals, and chemicals used at home or work. Allergies may be aggravated by emotional stress.

Anaphylaxis

Anaphylaxis is a rare, potentially fatal allergic reaction that affects many parts of the body at the same time. The trigger may be an insect sting, a food (such as peanuts), or a medication. Symptoms may include:

- vomiting or diarrhea;
- a dangerous drop in blood pressure;
- redness of the skin and/or hives;
- difficulty breathing;
- swelling of the throat and/or tongue; and
- loss of consciousness.

Frequently these symptoms start without warning and get worse rapidly. At the first sign of an anaphylactic reaction, the affected person must go immediately to the closest emergency room or call 911.

When to See an Allergist

Often, the symptoms of asthma or allergies develop gradually over time.

Allergy sufferers may become used to frequent symptoms such as sneezing, nasal congestion, or wheezing. With the help of an allergist, these symptoms usually can be prevented or controlled with major improvement in quality of life.

Effectively controlling asthma and allergies requires planning, skill, and patience. The allergist, with his or her specialized training, can develop a treatment plan for your individual condition. The goal will be to enable you to lead a life that is as normal and symptom-free as possible.

A visit to the allergist might include:

- **Allergy testing:** The allergist will usually perform tests to determine what allergens are involved.

- **Prevention education:** The most effective approach to treating asthma or allergies is to avoid the factors that trigger the condition in the first place. Even when it is not possible to completely avoid allergens, an allergist can help you decrease exposure to allergens.

- **Medication prescriptions:** A number of new and effective medications are available to treat both asthma and allergies.

- **Immunotherapy (allergy shots):** In this treatment, patients are given injections every week or two of some or all of the allergens that cause their allergy problems. Gradually the injections get stronger and stronger. In most cases, the allergy problems diminish over time.

You should see an allergist if:

- your allergies are causing symptoms such as chronic sinus infections, nasal congestion, or difficulty breathing;

- you experience hay fever or other allergy symptoms several months out of the year;

- antihistamines and over-the-counter medications do not control your allergy symptoms or create unacceptable side effects, such as drowsiness;

- your asthma or allergies are interfering with your ability to carry on day-to-day activities;

- your asthma or allergies decrease the quality of your life; or

- you are experiencing warning signs of serious asthma such as:

  - you sometimes have to struggle to catch your breath;

  - you often wheeze or cough, especially at night or after exercise;

  - you are frequently short of breath or feel tightness in your chest; or

  - you have previously been diagnosed with asthma, and you have frequent asthma attacks even though you are taking asthma medication.

Chapter 38

Overview of Allergy Tests

A wide variety of substances may cause allergic reactions in some people. Allergy testing is the procedure used to determine which particular substances (allergens) are responsible for provoking an allergic reaction. The procedure used depends on the type of allergy, but may include skin and blood tests or special diets.

Symptoms Associated with Allergies

Symptoms associated with allergies can include:

- skin rashes—such as eczema (atopic dermatitis) or hives (urticaria);
- swelling—or angioedema;
- sneezing and running nose—or allergic rhinitis (hay fever);
- teary, red, itchy eyes—or allergic conjunctivitis;
- asthma;
- nausea and vomiting; and
- anaphylaxis—this is a severe allergic reaction that causes serious breathing problems. Anaphylaxis can be fatal.

Medical Issues to Consider

Before undergoing allergy testing, you need to discuss a range of issues with your doctor, including:

- your medical history;
- clinical symptoms and when they occur;
- possible allergen triggers; and
- any medicines you take that may interfere with skin prick test reactions, such as antihistamines.

The Procedures

Specific tests are needed to determine which substance or substances are causing an allergy. These tests can include:

- **Skin prick tests**—Selected allergens are applied to the forearm or the back with a dropper, and the skin is gently pricked with a needle. A positive result shows as a red wheal or flare on the skin within 20 minutes.

- **Allergen-specific IgE blood tests (RAST [radioallergosorbent test])**—These tests are useful when skin testing is not possible or is inconclusive. A blood sample is taken and the level of an immunoglobulin associated with allergic reaction (allergen-specific IgE) is measured in a laboratory.

- **Elimination diets and challenge testing**—An elimination diet is used to isolate foods that may be causing an allergic reaction. This usually takes a number of weeks and involves avoiding foods identified as common causes of food allergy. No foods or fluids may be consumed other than those specified. If symptoms improve, foods are added one at a time until symptoms recur (this is known as 'challenge testing'). Usually, a diary is kept to record any symptoms so they can be linked to the correct food. This procedure must only be performed under medical supervision.

- **Patch tests**—Are most commonly used to investigate contact dermatitis. Common triggers include fragrances (for example, in soaps), nickel (in jewelry, watch buckles, and coins) and chrome (in leathers and bricklayers' cement). Patches are applied to the back in adhesive strips. The area is examined after two and four days. A positive result shows as redness or blisters at the site of a particular substance.

After a Test

After the test, you can expect:

- If you have a skin prick test, your doctor will examine you for signs of an allergic reaction after 20 minutes.

- Patch tests require further visits at two and four days after they are applied.

- The results of blood tests may take up to a week to be known.

- An elimination and challenge diet may take many weeks to provide results.

False reactions can occur with any test, so results need to be assessed in conjunction with your clinical symptoms. Once the offending allergen or allergens are identified, you should try to avoid or reduce exposure to them in future.

Possible Complications

Some people with allergies experience severe reactions when exposed to particular allergens. For example, the red wheals associated with skin prick tests can be painful, inflamed, and irritated.

Some reactions, such as anaphylaxis, are potentially life threatening. It is important that allergy tests are performed by a qualified health professional who can anticipate and treat any allergic reactions you may have.

Seek Medical Help to Diagnose Allergies

A number of other tests have been misleadingly promoted to diagnose allergies. Such tests include the cytotoxic food test, the Vega test, bioelectrical testing, hair analysis, pulse test, and kinesiology. These tests have not been scientifically validated and the results should not be used for diagnosis or treatment.

Remember, reactions to allergens can be life threatening. Allergy testing should always be conducted under medical supervision.

Taking Care of Yourself at Home

Be guided by your health care professional, but general suggestions for care after allergy tests include:

419

- If you had skin tests, follow all recommendations given by your doctor.

- If you are following an elimination diet, be careful not to consume any foods or fluids that are not allowed. This may affect the results of the test and you may need to start all over again.

Long-Term Outlook

Allergy testing can help a person suffering from allergies to discover which allergens trigger their symptoms.

In some cases, an experienced allergist can offer immunotherapy. This exposes a person to increasing amounts of a particular allergen, to a point where they no longer have symptoms when exposed to 'normal' amounts of that allergen or they experience reduced symptoms. Immunotherapy should be conducted only under strict medical supervision.

Other Forms of Treatment

Other forms of treatment for allergies include:

- avoiding the allergens;

- taking medications to treat the symptoms, including over-the-counter medications available from your chemist (such as corticosteroid nasal sprays or antihistamines); and

- using corticosteroids and other medications that may be prescribed by your doctor to help manage your symptoms.

Where to Get Help

- In an emergency, dial 911
- Your doctor

Things to Remember

- Allergy testing is used to find out which substances provoke an allergic reaction.

- Tests can include skin and blood tests or special diets.

- Allergy tests must be performed by a qualified health professional who can anticipate and treat any allergic reactions.

420

Chapter 39

Skin Testing to Diagnose Allergies

Many common types of allergies can be confirmed with the use of skin testing. But many people may not realize how and why skin testing is used or think that this procedure is painful and inconvenient. In truth, skin testing is now more accurate than ever, and it need not be painful or an ordeal.

Skin testing is used to diagnose immediate-type hypersensitivity allergy. This is the most common type of allergic reaction. In this type of allergy, symptoms occur very quickly after you are exposed to certain allergens. The body responds to allergens by producing certain kinds of proteins, called immunoglobulin E (IgE) antibodies. Antibodies are proteins that the body produces to fight off foreign invaders. One way to test a person for allergies is to measure the level of IgE antibodies in the blood. A simpler, more definitive way is to see whether exposure to certain allergens provokes a local response. This is the purpose of skin testing.

How is skin testing done?

Skin testing involves the use of allergens—substances that provoke an allergic response. These might be types of pollen found in your area, as well as dust mites, mold, cockroach debris, animal hair, and food. Extracts are made of common allergens such as these and are placed just beneath the surface of the skin. After a certain amount of time has elapsed, a person who is sensitive to a substance will have a red, raised bump appear on their skin where certain extracts were placed. This positive result as well as the findings of the physical examination and medical history are used by your doctor to identify whether you are allergic to that substance. A positive skin test by itself does not confirm whether the substance is causing your symptoms. Skin testing may be done by one of the two methods described below.

The Percutaneous Method: In one method of skin testing, a drop of each allergen extract is placed on the skin. Then the topmost layer of skin under the drops is lightly broken by pricking, puncturing, or scratching. This allows the extract to seep into the skin. Sometimes the drops are placed directly on one or more needles or clusters of needles. This method, called the percutaneous method, is usually done on the patient's lower arm or back.

The Intracutaneous Method: The second method of skin testing involves injecting the allergen extract under the first few layers of skin. This is done with a syringe and a very fine needle.

One of the advantages of this method over the percutaneous method is that it is more sensitive—more often positive. It has the drawback, though, of yielding more false-positive results than the percutaneous method. A false-positive result is one that shows a reaction to an extract when the patient does not develop any symptoms on exposure to that allergen.

What do the results show?

Once the allergen extracts have been placed on the skin, the doctor or nurse looks for signs of an allergic response. This appears in the form of a red, raised lump, or wheal, surrounded by a red, inflamed area, or flare. The exact size of the wheal and flare shows how allergic you are to that allergen. Usually, with a percutaneous test, the raised area must be at least 3 mm (about one-tenth of an inch) across to indicate a positive reaction. With an intracutaneous test, an even larger reaction is required.

A positive test only shows that you are allergic to the allergen. It does not necessarily mean that you will have symptoms on exposure to that allergen, or that allergen is a cause of your symptoms. Indeed, you may have positive skin tests, and your disease may be non-allergenic.

Since they are less sensitive, positive percutaneous skin tests are more closely related with your actually having symptoms (clinical sensitivity) than are the more sensitive intracutaneous tests. That is why it is important to have a physician with training in allergy performing and interpreting your skin tests.

Is skin testing accurate?

Skin testing methods are more reliable now than in the past. At one time, it was found that the extracts used in skin testing varied greatly in how active they were in producing an allergic response. Even extract samples labeled as having the same strength were found to have different levels of activity. This finding greatly reduced the usefulness of skin testing in the opinion of many doctors.

Today, these problems have been corrected to a large extent. Now, standardized extracts have been developed for many allergens. Efforts are still underway to improve the standardization of food allergen extracts. Extracts made from these allergens tend to be less stable than other types of extracts.

How can skin testing help me?

There is no reason to dread skin testing. This is an easy method to find out what specific substances are causing your allergies. It takes little time and causes only minor discomfort.

By pinpointing the specific allergens causing your allergy symptoms, your doctor can tailor your treatment to your particular case. For instance, if you have allergies only during a certain time of year, you may have an allergy to a specific kind of grass pollen. You may be able to use a medication to control your symptoms during the season when this grass is blooming. If you are allergic to substances that are present year round, such as dust or animal hair, you can take steps to limit your exposure to those allergens.

In other cases, your doctor may advise immunotherapy, or allergy shots. This treatment uses a serum containing minute amounts of the specific substances to which you are known to be allergic. Over time, your immune system's response to these allergens can be lessened by getting injections at regular intervals.

Whatever course of action you and your doctor decide to take, skin testing can provide valuable information about how your body responds to allergens. Armed with this knowledge, together you and your doctor can work out a treatment plan to keep your allergies under control.

Chapter 40

Blood Test to Screen for Allergies

The Test Sample

What is being tested?

Immunoglobulin E (IgE) is a protein associated with allergic reactions; it is normally found in very small amounts in the blood. IgE is an antibody that functions as part of the body's immune system, its defense against "intruders." When someone with a predisposition to allergies is exposed to a potential allergen (such as food, grass, or animal dander) for the first time, they become sensitized. Their body perceives the potential allergen as a foreign substance and produces a specific IgE antibody that binds to mast cells (specialized cells in your tissues) and basophils (a type of white blood cell) in your bloodstream. The mast cells are found in tissues throughout your body but are highest in concentration in your skin, respiratory system, and gastrointestinal tract. With the next exposure, these attached IgE antibodies recognize the allergen and cause the mast and basophil cells to release histamine and other chemicals, resulting in an allergic reaction that begins at the exposure site.

The allergen-specific IgE antibody test is used to screen for an allergy to a specific allergen. It measures the amount of that suspected IgE antibody in the blood. Each selection is one separate test, and the

"Allergy Tests," © 2006 American Association for Clinical Chemistry. Reprinted with permission. For additional information about clinical lab testing, visit the Lab Tests Online website at www.labtestsonline.org.

425

tests are very specific: honeybee versus bumblebee, egg white versus egg yolk, giant ragweed versus western ragweed. Groupings of these tests, such as food panels or regional weed, grass, and mold panels, can be done. Alternatively, you and your doctor may pick and choose selectively from a long list of individual allergens suspected of causing your allergies.

The allergen-specific IgE test can be done using a variety of methods. The traditional method that has been used is the RAST (radioallergosorbent test), but it has been largely replaced in most laboratories with the newer IgE-specific immunoassay method. Some doctors refer to all IgE allergy tests as RAST even though this is a specific methodology and may not be the exact assay that the testing lab is using.

How is the sample collected for testing?

A blood sample is obtained by inserting a needle into a vein in the arm.

The Test

How is it used?

The allergen-specific IgE antibody test is done to screen for an allergy (a type I hypersensitivity) to a specific substance or substances when a patient presents with acute or chronic allergy-like symptoms.

The allergen-specific IgE antibody test may be done (instead of other medically supervised allergy testing) when the patient has significant dermatitis or eczema (also a sign of allergies), is taking necessary histamines or antidepressants that would make other testing more difficult, or if a dangerous allergic reaction could be expected to follow another test.

The allergen-specific IgE antibody test may also be done to monitor immunotherapy or to see if a child has outgrown an allergy, although it can only be used in a general way; the level of IgE present does not correlate to the severity of an allergic reaction, and someone who has outgrown an allergy may have a positive IgE for many years afterward.

When is it ordered?

The allergen-specific IgE antibody test is usually ordered when you have signs or symptoms that suggest that you have an allergy to one or more substances.

What does the test result mean?

Normal negative results indicate that you probably do not have a "true allergy," an IgE-mediated response to that specific allergen, but the results of allergen-specific IgE antibody tests must always be interpreted and used with caution and the advice of your doctor. Even if your IgE test is negative, there is still a small chance that you do have an allergy.

Elevated results usually indicate an allergy, but even if your specific IgE test was positive, you may or may not ever have an actual physical allergic reaction when exposed to that substance. And the amount of specific IgE present does not necessarily predict the potential severity of a reaction. Your clinical history and other allergy tests, done under close medical supervision, may be necessary to confirm an allergy diagnosis.

Is there anything else I should know?

Sometimes your doctor will look at other blood tests for an indirect indication of an ongoing allergic process, including your total IgE level or your complete blood count (CBC) and white blood cell differential (specifically at your eosinophils and basophils). Elevations in these tests may suggest an allergy, but they may also be elevated for other reasons.

Common Questions

What other tests are available for allergy testing?

Skin prick or scratch tests, patch tests, and oral food challenges are usually done by an allergist or dermatologist. Your doctor may also try eliminating foods from your diet and then reintroducing them to find out what you are allergic to. It is important that these tests be done under close medical supervision, as a life-threatening anaphylactic reaction is possible.

My allergy test was negative, but I am having symptoms. What else could it be?

You could have a genetic hypersensitivity problem, like Celiac disease's sensitivity to gluten, or an enzyme deficiency, such as lactase deficiency causing lactose intolerance. It could also be an allergy-like condition that is not mediated by IgE for which there are no

427

specific laboratory tests. Or it could be another disease that is causing allergy-like symptoms. It is important to investigate your individual situation with your doctor's assistance.

My allergy symptoms are generally mild. How serious is this really?

Allergic reactions are very individual. They can be mild or severe, vary from exposure to exposure, get worse over time (or may not), involve the whole body, and can sometimes be fatal.

Will my allergies ever go away?

Although children do outgrow some allergies, adults usually do not. Allergies that cause the worst reactions, such as anaphylaxis caused by peanuts, do not usually go away. Avoidance of the allergen and advance preparation for accidental exposure, in the form of medications such as antihistamines and portable epinephrine injections, is the safest course. Immunotherapy can help decrease symptoms for some unavoidable allergies, but they won't work for food and the treatment, which usually consists of years of regular injections, may need to be continued indefinitely.

Why am I told to avoid fresh fruit when my allergy is to tree pollen?

There are cross-reactions between some airborne allergens and fruit proteins. Your body thinks it is detecting tree pollen and creates an allergic reaction to the fruit. It is, however, a relatively rare occurrence.

Chapter 41

Testing for Food Allergies: Food Challenge Tests

Chapter Contents

Section 41.1

What Is a Food Challenge?

A food challenge consists of having a patient eat a food suspected of previously causing symptoms in a controlled fashion under medical supervision. This is done by feeding gradually increasing doses of the suspected food at predetermined time intervals (such as every half hour) until a reaction occurs or a normal amount of the food is eaten without causing symptoms. Food challenges can be performed in a variety of ways.

In an open food challenge (OFC), both the patient and medical staff are aware that the patient is eating the suspected food. For example, a child receiving an OFC to egg might be given increasing doses of scrambled egg every 30 minutes until a whole egg is ingested.

In a single-blind placebo-controlled food challenge (SBPCFC) the medical staff is aware of what the patient is being fed, but the patient is not. A child receiving a SBPCFC to egg receives egg masked by concealing it in another food. The medical staff knows if and how much egg is contained in each challenge dose, but the patient and the patient's family do not. Each dose could either contain concealed egg, or a placebo. However, the final dose of any food challenge is the open ingestion of a normal portion of the suspected food. SBPCFCs are performed to eliminate bias on the part of the patient and/or the patient's family.

In a double-blind placebo-controlled food challenge (DBPCFC) neither the patient nor the medical team involved in administering the challenge is aware of what the patient is being fed. The DBPCFC is performed to eliminate both patient and observer bias. For the safety of the patient at least one medical care provider not directly involved in the challenge must be aware of the challenge contents even in a DBPCFC. The final dose of the DBPCFC is a normal portion of the suspected food ingested openly.

A food challenge is completed when the patient has an obvious reaction to the food or when a normal portion of the food has been ingested openly without symptoms. The length of time a patient is kept for observation after completion of the challenge depends upon several factors including the timing and severity of previous reactions. The results of the challenge are thoroughly reviewed with the patient and his or her family and all questions are addressed in light of the results of the challenge.

Section 41.2

The Importance of a Food Challenge

"Food Challenges: Why Bother?" © Copyright 2006 National Jewish Medical and Research Center. All rights reserved. For additional information, visit http://www.nationaljewish.org or call 1-800-222-LUNG.

Few procedures in medicine answer a posed clinical question as directly as a properly performed food challenge. The information obtained can be life-altering. Food challenges are performed to answer a variety of questions and play a vital role in the evaluation and management of patients with histories suggestive of food allergy. Indeed, their necessity is supported by studies revealing that more than half of patients with histories of adverse reactions to a food fail to react during blinded challenges to that food. There are a number of reasonable explanations for this that underscore the importance of food challenges.

- Sometimes the wrong food is suspected as the cause of symptoms.

- Some food challenges are performed to prove that a food is not the cause of symptoms.

- Discovering the degree of sensitivity is another reason for performing food challenges.

- Some patients outgrow their food allergies.

Sometimes the wrong food is suspected as the cause of symptoms. Inaccurate or misleading assumptions about which specific food is to blame can be based on history, skin testing, and lab testing results.

431

Contamination of a food by other allergens is one way history may lead to inaccurate conclusions. For example, a child having reacted to a french fry might be suspected of being allergic to peanut when the actual cause of the reaction was fish protein from fish fried in the same oil. Or, sometimes the reaction is caused by a nonfood contaminant such as latex proteins deposited on foods by handlers wearing latex gloves. Reactions to dust mites in mite-contaminated baked goods are another example.

Differences between how patients react to allergens in a testing environment compared to how they react in "real life" may lead to inaccurate conclusions as well. Sometimes the food responsible for the reaction is not apparent from skin testing or laboratory testing. For example, a patient may have a positive skin test to several suspected foods and food challenges may be necessary to determine which, if any, of the foods is the culprit. Determining which food actually caused the reaction is necessary to aid in preventing future reactions and to avoid needlessly eliminating foods from the diet.

Some food challenges are performed to prove that a food is not the cause of symptoms. An example is the patient who has been mislabeled as allergic to one or more foods despite an unconvincing history or suspicious skin test or laboratory test results. Giving the food under medical supervision reassures patients that they can eat the food safely.

Furthermore, sometimes the reactions are not related to food at all, but are brought on by other things such as medications, toxins, parasites, allergen exposures by inhalation or contact, viral illness, exercise, or panic, to list just a few potential causes.

Discovering the degree of sensitivity is another reason for performing food challenges. Some patients or their families become concerned that exposure to even tiny amounts of a food might cause a life-threatening reaction. These concerns occasionally interfere with participation in normal activities and can lead to social isolation.

Although some patients are indeed exquisitely sensitive, others find that more of the food than was expected can be tolerated without a severe reaction—even though large positive skin tests and histories may suggest otherwise. This can be a relief for patients who have avoided activities out of concern about the possibility of exquisite sensitivity. Alternatively, some patients are found to be more sensitive than was previously suspected. In this case, the importance of strict avoidance, as well as being thoroughly prepared to treat severe reactions, is reinforced.

Some patients outgrow their food allergies. Most children born allergic to milk, egg, wheat, or soy outgrow their food allergies by their third to sixth birthday. Studies over the past few years have even suggested that about 20% of children with allergic reactions to peanut in the first years of life may outgrow their sensitivity. A carefully performed food challenge can safely document when the food can be returned to the diet, or at least when the likelihood of a significant reaction is drastically diminished.

Given the possibility of severe reactions, food challenges should be performed in a medical setting with the necessary medications, equipment, and personnel experienced in the treatment of severe allergic reactions (anaphylaxis). Decisions about who should be challenged are reached only after a thorough evaluation and discussion of the risks and benefits with the patient or his or her family. However, few procedures in medicine answer a posed clinical question as directly as a properly performed food challenge. The information obtained can be life-altering.

Chapter 42

An Overview of
Allergy Medications

Antihistamines

Is there a major difference between Claritin and Clarinex?

Dr. Rosenwasser's answer: Clarinex is a bit more pure, so a lower dose causes the same effect. Other than that, it is very similar to Claritin.

I take Claritin and it works. Should I switch to Clarinex? Are there any advantages?

Dr. Rosenwasser's answer: They are very similar. If Claritin works well for you, it is fine to stay with it.

Why do I get sleepy from Clarinex? I never got sleepy on Claritin. I tried immunotherapy, but had to quit because I had severe reactions. Is there something else that I can try or look forward to?

Dr. Rosenwasser's answer: At certain doses, both Claritin and Clarinex can cause sleepiness. If Claritin worked well without sleepiness, you should go back to it. Allegra is an alternative, as sleepiness is not a side effect.

"Frequently Asked Questions about Allergy Treatments and Medications," © Copyright 2006 National Jewish Medical and Research Center. All rights reserved. For additional information, visit http://www.nationaljewish.org or call 1-800-222-LUNG. Questions in this document answered by Henry Milgrom, M.D., and Lanny J. Rosenwasser, M.D.

Are any over-the-counter allergy medications effective at reducing mild allergy/hay fever symptoms? In my experience, I haven't found one that helps at all.

Dr. Milgrom's answer: Over-the-counter antihistamines are effective. Benadryl works well but can make you drowsy. Claritin is a non-sedating antihistamine and is now sold over-the-counter. Antihistamine/decongestant combinations are also effective. Their effectiveness can be increased by not using a single preparation for longer than a couple of weeks. Cromolyn is available over-the-counter under the name of NasalCrom and is highly effective but must be used four times a day or more.

Steroids

What are the long-term effects of nasal steroid use?

Dr. Rosenwasser's answer: Nasal steroids—in the usual doses—can be tolerated for long periods of time by most people. Some of the side effects of steroids in general are higher in people who use nasal steroids than people who don't take any steroids. These effects may range from cracking and minor bleeding in the nose to a very small but measurable increased risk of diabetes, osteoporosis, and cataracts.

Question: Can nasal steroids cause thrush?

Dr. Rosenwasser's answer: Yes, if the medicine is swallowed into the throat. This is rare with a nasal steroid but the treatment is the same as with an inhaled steroid. Rinse your mouth after use with the nasal steroid. If you use an inhaled steroid, make sure you use a spacer.

If one is using a nasal steroid spray, such as Nasonex or Flonase, is it okay or even desirable to use concomitantly an oral antihistamine such as Zyrtec or Claritin?

Dr. Rosenwasser's answer: Yes, both antihistamines and nasal steroids can be used, depending on the clinical symptoms and the response to treatment. Many patients use both.

I used to live in Denver, but now I live in Lima, Peru. Since moving, my allergies have gotten really bad. It seems weird, but they seem to be related to the weather—it's very humid here. Maybe it's the pollution, too. I take Clarinex but it makes me sleepy. When I take Zyrtec D it makes me shaky and nervous. What do you recommend I take?

Dr. Rosenwasser's answer: It's difficult to tell what's causing your allergies without taking a complete history and allergy tests. However, weather can cause hay fever symptoms in some people. Nasal steroids are probably the best treatment for vasomotor rhinitis, but I'm not sure of that diagnosis based on your question. Talk to your doctor in Lima about trying a nasal steroid.

I have always had normal rhinitis symptoms, but this year I have also developed asthma and food allergies. Now, in the last three weeks, as trees are budding, I have developed severe skin "itchiness." I am very sensitive to various fabrics— cotton seems to be the only thing I can tolerate. My questions: Is this a typical allergic response? What can I do to stop the itching?

Dr. Rosenwasser's answer: Many people with allergic rhinitis and spring-time allergies develop significant symptoms such as itchy skin, as you are experiencing. Another phenomenon known as oral allergy syndrome occurs when cross-reactions between allergy pollen and food allergens cause itchiness and swelling in the mouth and throat after eating the food. Antihistamines are a good treatment for this. If you develop hives, or urticaria, topical steroids (used on the skin) could be used to help control the itching. However, you should see an allergist and use all prescription medications in conjunction with a physician's consultation and proper monitoring.

My allergy goes to my eyes and the doctor here in Lima, Peru, told me not to use drops with steroids. What do you recommend for me to use?

Dr. Rosenwasser's answer: Patanol eye drops are not steroids and may help.

Other Medications for Allergies

How does Singulair help with allergies? Why is it suggested to take it in the evening?

Dr. Rosenwasser's answer: Singulair is a prescription medicine approved to help control asthma in adults and children as young as

12 months and to help relieve the symptoms of seasonal allergies in adults and children as young as 2 years. The reason why it works with both conditions is because the mediators present in asthma are also present in allergic rhinitis. In all of its studies, Singulair has only been tested with a single dose in the evening, so that is how it has been approved for use (it was originally formulated for relief of nighttime asthma symptoms). However, it is a once-a-day medication so its effects should last 24 hours. Singulair has no side effects such as drowsiness or dryness, like antihistamines. Singulair is a leukotriene antagonist, different than antihistamines.

My respiratory allergies result in recurrent development of polyps in my nose and sinuses. I've recently had a fifth operation on my sinuses, just to remove the polyps this time. My ENT [ear, nose, and throat] physician has suggested that I use Singulair to inhibit the growth of polyps. (I regularly take either Allegra or Claritin, and I also have asthma that is fully controlled by four inhalations of Vanceril and four inhalations of Intal each day.) Do you think that Singulair or other medications might reduce the recurrence of polyps?

Dr. Rosenwasser's answer: Yes, it is not published yet but Singulair and Accolate can help sinusitis and polyps.

I've heard that work is in progress on a new drug that will inhibit the action of IL-4, specifically an IL-4 receptor blocker. Do you know the status of such a drug?

Dr. Rosenwasser's answer: The IL-4 work with the receptor antagonist by Immunex is on hold because of equivocal results in helping asthma. Other companies are going ahead with trials of an anti-IL-4 humanized monoclonal antibody. The results are too preliminary to comment on at this point.

I would appreciate some information on the upcoming IgE medication and the effects on spring allergies—how does it relate to allergy? When will it be available? Who would benefit from it? How would it benefit a person who has asthma—like myself? Where can I read more about it?

Dr. Rosenwasser's answer: The new anti-IgE medication is called Xolair. It is indicated for the treatment of moderate to severe allergic asthma and has not been approved for allergic rhinitis. However, it has been shown in studies that it can relieve hay fever and/or rhinitis symptoms, but it must be injected and is far too expensive to justify its use for rhinitis only. Most people can treat their hay fever with much cheaper medication that doesn't require injections. You can check the website for Genentech or Novartis for more information on Xolair.

What is the cause(s) and how do I get relief for watery eyes? I am a 70-year-old male with asthma. My eyes water constantly, so much so that tears run down my face. This occurs when I go outside—e.g., grocery shopping, walking, etc.

Dr. Rosenwasser's answer: Watery, itchy eyes are usually related to allergic conjunctivitis, although other eye conditions can cause these same symptoms. Patanol eye drops can relieve the symptoms of itchy, watery eyes that you describe. Patanol uses a combination of antihistamines and mast-cell stabilizers. Check with your doctor about trying this.

I have hay fever really bad in the spring and the fall; how soon before my bad season starts should I take my allergy meds?

Dr. Milgrom's answer: Most medications are effective within a matter of days. Cromolyn takes a full month to be completely effective. Allergy shots may take as long as 2 years.

What is the best precaution to take knowing that I have severe reactions to insect bites (like swelling and blisters)? Are there certain over-the-counter medications that I should always carry?

Dr. Milgrom's answer: Patients who have had systemic reactions to stings by vespids (honey bee, wasp, hornet, yellow jacket) or ants are at risk for allergic reactions that may be life threatening. Systemic reactions are those that cause low blood pressure, shortness of breath, gastrointestinal symptoms, or swelling or rash distant from the site of the sting. Individuals who have experienced such reactions should carry injectable adrenaline that comes in preloaded syringes under the names Ana-Kit or EpiPen. These preparations are available by prescription only but can be life saving and should be carried by all patients with a history of systemic responses to these insects. It is especially important to carry one of these preparations if one is going to be participating in activities in remote areas. Antihistamines can be helpful but are not adequate for a life-threatening situation. Some hikers have found that applying Adolph's Meat Tenderizer, a preparation that contains the enzyme papain, can make their stings less painful.

Frequently Asked Questions about Allergy Drug Interactions and Other Concurrent Respiratory and Sinus Diseases

Can people with COPD [chronic obstructive pulmonary disease] take Allegra? I know Sudafed and others are not recommended for COPD patients.

Dr. Rosenwasser's answer: People who have allergies as well as COPD can take antihistamines for their allergies. Sudafed is a decongestant and a different type of medicine.

I have COPD and problems with my sinuses. I currently use Claritin-D. Is there another medicine that will work better to clear up the drainage? I am also on Serevent, Atrovent, Proventil, and Uniphyl. I rarely take Proventil.

Dr. Rosenwasser's answer: Claritin-D can help sinus drainage for people with allergy and sinus drainage problems. Other antihistamines and decongestants can work including Allegra-D and Zyrtec. There are also over-the-counter antihistamine and decongestant combinations that help with sinus drainage. These medicines, however, would have no direct effect on COPD—the medicines you are already taking are treatment for COPD.

Are there new medications for allergy out that are safe for those with COPD?

Dr. Rosenwasser's answer: New treatments are being tested all the time for COPD. It would be best to check with your pulmonary specialist.

I moved to New Mexico three years ago after 45 years in Michigan—I started having almost constant sinusitis, especially in spring and fall. Once it became so bad—after three courses of 10 days of antibiotics, which obviously didn't do the job—I landed in the emergency room with severe bronchitis, hardly able to breathe. I had a CT scan, was put on 21 days of antibiotics, and given Flonase to use daily, which I do. I have had three serious sinus infections in last four months and am now on 7-day course of 500 mg Levaquin (and antibiotic eyedrops). My doctor has recommended switching to Nasonex. I am in normal good health, weight, etc. and am 53 years old. Should I be taking an oral drug daily as well as the nasal spray? These infections are depressing me, in terms of the amount of time and energy (not to mention cost) they are taking up. I am also worried about how much antibiotic I've pumped through my system.

Dr. Rosenwasser's answer: Significant sinus disease may require long-term treatment with nasal washes, antihistamines, nasal steroids, and occasionally antibiotics for adequate control. The decision to do any of these things depends on the clinical circumstances and the risk/benefit of any of the interventions. It sounds as though your sinusitis is complicated and requires significant medication. It would be good to be checked by a specialist to make sure there are no immune or other complicating problems for your sinus condition.

Frequently Asked Questions about Allergy Medications, Pediatrics, and Pregnancy

Is Claritin dangerous if I am pregnant? I heard something about Claritin and hypospadias last week in the news.

Dr. Rosenwasser's answer: All medications should be used cautiously in pregnancy. Older antihistamines, such as pyribenzamine and Benadryl, are probably the safest to use in pregnancy.

Can you suggest a safe medicine for a nursing mother with allergic rhinitis and itchy eyes and skin?

Dr. Rosenwasser's answer: First of all, every pregnant or nursing mother and her doctor must carefully weigh the benefits to the woman against the risks to her fetus or infant when using any medication. Always inform your doctor if you are pregnant, planning a pregnancy, or breastfeeding before using any medicine. That being said, nasal steroids are generally well tolerated during pregnancy and by nursing mothers. Benadryl is probably the safest antihistamine to use because it's been around the longest although it can cause drowsiness. Many of the newer antihistamines have either not been tested or have been found to be present in breast milk. Great caution should be used with all of these medications, and they certainly should not be used before a thorough consultation with your doctor.

I have a 6-month old baby with eczema who is sneezy all the time. His eyes are not red or watery, but at night he has trouble breathing from congestion. His nose is not runny, though. Do you have treatment suggestions? Is he too young for seasonal allergies? We are getting ready to try Triaminic based on our pediatrician's suggestion.

Dr. Rosenwasser's answer: You are correct—your baby is too young for seasonal allergies. However, food allergy may play a role, especially with eczema and the sneeziness. Pediatric Triaminic as a decongestant is OK.

What would you recommend for treating a severe allergy to Timothy grass for a child under the age of 12?

Dr. Rosenwasser's answer: The standard treatments for a child under the age of 12 would be in place, including Allegra, Claritin, Zyrtec and immunotherapy. The antihistamines are approved at least to age 6 and above and some forms of antihistamine medication, such as Claritin Redi-Tab and Zyrtec syrup, can be given to children as young as 2. Allegra, at a dose of 30 mg, is approved for children age 6 and older.

Frequently Asked Questions about Immunotherapy (Allergy Shots)

I have been reading about a 6-week program for allergic rhinitis. Will allergists soon be able to offer this to their patients?

Dr. Rosenwasser's answer: Immunotherapy can be given in a rush pattern that is completed in six weeks. Other, more experimental treatments can be given within a season, but they are not yet approved. If you experience only one allergy season, then standard treatment with antihistamines and nasal steroids can work well.

If you have allergies to oak, grass, weeds, mold, etc. would you recommend taking Claritin all year? This is what has been recommended to me and I wanted your thought on this.

Dr. Rosenwasser's answer: Immunotherapy is an alternative to antihistamine therapy in patients with multiple allergies and rhinitis. Otherwise, use of antihistamines—like Claritin—and nasal steroids may be required for both perennial (year-round) and seasonal allergic rhinitis.

I am extremely allergic to grass, tree, and weed pollen, mold, and mites, dogs, and cats. I avoid the latter animals but this season is so intense with pollen nothing I take lasts for more than 4 or 5 hours. I can't even go outside of my house without a mask—and that doesn't help much. Within minutes my eyes, nose and asthma kick up. I've tried taking lots of different antihistamines in high doses, but they tend to make me very drowsy. Also, I don't like having to take so much medicine all of the time. Any ideas?

Dr. Rosenwasser's answer: Immunotherapy may help with such numerous and severe allergies. It may avoid some of the side effects that you describe from the medicines.

I am 30 years old and have been suffering from allergies for 10 years. All the medicines I have tried over the years have failed to control it. Are there any alternatives?

Dr. Rosenwasser's answer: Besides medication, allergic hay fever and rhinitis can also be effectively treated with allergy shots or allergy immunotherapy, as it is known. This kind of treatment is very often effective but requires initially a weekly commitment for shots followed by a monthly shot. However, this mode of treatment is the only one available that potentially could cure allergies.

I am considering allergy shots for my daughter and was wondering if this will lead to her taking less medicine (Advair, Clarinex, Flonase, Singular).

Dr. Rosenwasser's answer: Hopefully, if the allergy immunotherapy is selected the proper way, use of less asthma medicines should be a result. This works especially well in children and young adults.

Is immunotherapy relatively safe? This is one of the reasons I have held off giving it to my daughter (14). Her doctor has recommended it but the anaphylactic thing scares me.

Dr. Rosenwasser's answer: There is some risk to immunotherapy when done with proper dosing of allergens. These risks are minimized by proper observation after injections (in the doctor's office). If immunotherapy is truly indicated for a 14-year-old, adolescents usually respond well.

Can you tell me if more allergists will offer the sublingual drops to put under the tongue instead of allergy shots?

Dr. Rosenwasser's answer: The sublingual allergy immunotherapy treatments are still controversial as to how effective they are. Proper studies to monitor the immune reactions have not been done. This form of treatment has become very popular in Europe, especially Italy. It is not considered an accepted treatment by allergists in the United States.

I have numerous allergies: outdoor pollens and other airborne particulates, as well as indoor exposure to dust, mildews, etc. and particularly animal dander. I am forced to take antihistamines year-round in the form of pills (currently over-the counter Tavist), eye drops (Visine A), and nose spray (NasalCrom) daily. My symptoms include itchy, swollen eyes; itchy, runny nose; sneezing; and also asthmatic shortness of breath. This combination of antihistamines, as well as my daily asthma prescriptions, do keep my symptoms under control. However, I worry about long-term use of all of these products. Allergy shots, with the extent and nature of my allergies, are not a viable option.

Dr. Rosenwasser's answer: The extent of your allergies and nature of your symptoms are not contraindications to immunotherapy per se. Immunotherapy may be difficult to give if you are so sensitive, but it may significantly reduce requirements for the medicines you worry about taking so frequently.

Chapter 43

Antihistamines, Decongestants, and Cold Remedies for Allergies

Drugs for stuffy nose, sinus trouble, congestion, and the common cold constitute the largest segment of the over-the-counter market for America's pharmaceutical industry. When used wisely, they provide welcome relief for at least some of the discomforts that affect almost everyone occasionally and that affect many people chronically. Drugs in these categories are useful for relief of symptoms from allergies, upper respiratory infections (i.e., sinusitis, colds, flu), and vasomotor rhinitis (a chronic stuffy nose caused by such unrelated conditions as emotional stress, thyroid disease, pregnancy, and others). These drugs do not cure the allergies and infections; they only relieve the symptoms, thereby making the patient more comfortable.

Antihistamines

Histamine is an important body chemical that is responsible for the congestion, sneezing, and runny nose that a patient suffers with an allergic attack or an infection. Antihistamine drugs block the action of histamine, therefore reducing the allergy symptoms. For the best result, antihistamines should be taken before allergic symptoms get well established.

The most annoying side effect that antihistamines produce is drowsiness. Though desirable at bedtime, it is a nuisance to many people who need to use antihistamines in the daytime. To some people, it is even hazardous. These drugs are not recommended for daytime use for people who may be driving an automobile or operating equipment that could be dangerous. Newer non-sedating antihistamines, available by prescription only, do not have this effect. The first few doses cause the most sleepiness; subsequent doses are usually less troublesome.

Typical antihistamines include Allegra®, Benadryl®, Chlor-Trimeton®, Claritin®, Clarinex®, Teldrin®, and Zyrtec®.

Decongestants

Congestion in the nose, sinuses, and chest is due to swollen, expanded, or dilated blood vessels in the membranes of the nose and air passages. These membranes have an abundant supply of blood vessels with a great capacity for expansion (swelling and congestion). Histamine stimulates these blood vessels to expand as described previously.

Decongestants, on the other hand, cause constriction or tightening of the blood vessels in those membranes, which then forces much of the blood out of the membranes so that they shrink, and the air passages open up again.

Decongestants are chemically related to adrenalin, the natural decongestant, which is also a type of stimulant. Therefore, the side effect of decongestants is a jittery or nervous feeling. They can cause difficulty in going to sleep, and they can elevate blood pressure and pulse rate. Decongestants should not be used by a patient who has an irregular heart rhythm (pulse), high blood pressure, heart disease, or glaucoma. Some patients taking decongestants experience difficulty with urination. Furthermore, decongestants are often used as ingredients in diet pills. To avoid excessively stimulating effects, patients taking diet pills should not take decongestants.

Typical decongestants are phenylephrine (Neo-Synephrine®*) and pseudoephedrine (Sudafed®).

*May be available over-the-counter without a prescription. Read labels carefully, and use only as directed.

Combination Remedies

Theoretically, if the side effects could be properly balanced, the sleepiness sometimes caused by antihistamines could be canceled by the stimulation of decongestants. Numerous combinations of antihistamines with decongestants are available: Actifed®,* Allegra-D®, Chlor-Trimeton D®,* Claritin D®, Contac®,* Co-Pyronil 2®,* Deconamine®,

446

Demazin®,* Dimetapp®,* Drixoral®,* Isoclor®,* Nolamine®, Novafed A®, Ornade®, Sudafed Plus®, Tavist D®,* Triaminic®,* and Trinalin® to name just a few.

A patient may find one preparation quite helpful for several months or years but may need to switch to another one when the first loses its effectiveness. Since no one reacts exactly the same as another to the side effects of these drugs, a patient may wish to try his own ideas on adjusting the dosages. One might take the antihistamine only at night and take the decongestant alone in the daytime. Or take them together, increasing the dosage of antihistamine at night (while decreasing the decongestant dose) and then doing the opposite for daytime use.

For example: Antihistamine (Chlor-Trimeton®,* 4 mg)—one tablet three times daily and two tablets at bedtime **Plus** Decongestant (Sudafed®,* 30 mg)—two tablets three times daily and one tablet at bedtime.

Cold Remedies

Decongestants and/or antihistamines are the principal ingredients in cold remedies, but drying agents, aspirin (or aspirin substitutes), and cough suppressants may also be added. The patient should choose the remedy with ingredients best suited to combat his or her own symptoms. If the label does not clearly state the ingredients and their functions, the consumer should ask the pharmacist to explain them.

Nose Sprays

The types of nose sprays that can be purchased without a prescription usually contain decongestants for direct application to nasal membranes. They can give prompt relief from congestion by constricting blood

Table 43.1. Symptom Relief and Side Effects of Allergy Medications

Medicine	Symptoms Relieved	Possible Side Effects
Antihistamines	Sneezing, runny nose, stuffy nose, itchy eyes, and congestion	Drowsiness and dry mouth and nose
Decongestants	Stuffy nose and congestion	Stimulation, insomnia, and rapid heartbeat
Combinations of above	All of above	Any of above (more or less)

447

vessels. However, direct application creates a stronger stimulation than decongestants taken by mouth. It also impairs the circulation in the nose, which after a few hours, stimulates the vessels to expand to improve the blood flow again. This results in a "bounce-back" effect. The congestion recurs. If the patient uses the spray again, it starts the cycle again. Spray—decongestion—rebound—and more congestion.

In infants, this rebound rhinitis can develop in two days, whereas in adults, it often takes several more days to become established. An infant taken off the drops for 12 to 24 hours is cured, but well-established cases in adults often require more than a simple cold turkey withdrawal. They need decongestants by mouth, sometimes corticosteroids, and possibly (in patients who continuously have used the sprays for months and years) a surgical procedure to the inside of the nose. For this reason, the labels on these types of nose sprays contain the warning "Do not use this product for more than three days." Nose sprays should be reserved for emergency and short-term use.

The above description and advice does not apply to the type of prescription antiallergy nose sprays that may be ordered by your physician.

Chapter 44

Corticosteroids for Allergic Conditions

In 1935, the Mayo Clinic reported a research breakthrough that would affect millions of lives. Doctors had isolated the hormone cortisone from the adrenal glands, the walnut-sized glands sitting on top of the kidneys. Cortisone produced by the adrenal glands reduces inflammation in the body.

The Mayo Clinic physicians first used cortisone to treat people with severe rheumatoid arthritis. Improvements were so dramatic in soothing swollen joints that patients crippled from the disease were actually able to walk again.

Pharmaceutical companies have since produced corticosteroid medications that mimic the hormone cortisone. For people with asthma, corticosteroids literally can be lifesavers by preventing or reversing inflammation in the airways, making them less sensitive to triggers. The drugs, sometimes referred to as preventive or long-term control medicines, work effectively to keep asthma episodes in check. They are not the same as anabolic steroids, which some athletes take illegally to build muscle mass.

Are Corticosteroids Safe?

Oral, or systemic, corticosteroids quickly help out-of-control asthma, but more than two weeks of daily use may sometimes lead to serious side effects. Inhaled corticosteroids are considered much safer for lengthier treatment. Unlike the oral forms that must travel throughout your body to reach your lungs, inhaled corticosteroids are delivered directly to the airways in small doses with less chance of reaching other parts of the body. The National Institutes of Health (NIH) calls inhaled corticosteroids "the most effective long-term therapy available for patients with persistent asthma. In general [they] are well tolerated and safe at the recommended dosages."

You have probably read or heard varying reports about the risks of corticosteroid use. The bottom line is that the relatively few side effects are usually balanced by the good they do for your asthma. Steroids are definitely safe when used in the lower dosage range. Problems generally arise with high doses over long periods of time. As consumers and patients, it's important to know what specific side effects may occur and how we can work with our physicians to control them and our asthma.

Localized Risks

Oral Candidiasis (Thrush)

Only 10 percent to 30 percent of inhaled steroid doses actually reach the lungs. The remainder is left in the mouth or throat or is swallowed, sometimes resulting in thrush, a fungal infection that produces milky white lesions in the mouth. Clinical thrush is far less common in lower dosages and affects more adults than children.

Physicians recommend using a spacer or holding chamber with your inhaler and rinsing your mouth with water after each treatment to reduce the amount of the inhaled steroid deposited in the mouth and throat. If you develop thrush, your doctor may also prescribe a less frequent dose and/or topical or oral antifungal medication.

Dysphonia (Hoarseness)

This condition is associated with increasing dosages of inhaled corticosteroids and vocal stress. Treatment may include using a spacer/holding chamber, less frequent dosing, and/or temporarily decreasing medication.

Systemic Risks

Slowed Growth in Children

Some studies have shown that medium-dose inhaled corticosteroids may affect a child's growth. It is not certain that this results in shorter stature in adulthood, but in general, the higher the dose, the greater the risk.

In a 1995 study of 7- to 9-year-olds treated daily with 400 mcg of beclomethasone for seven months, growth was significantly decreased in both boys and girls. There was no evidence of catchup growth after a five-month period without medication. Yet a 1994 study of inhaled beclomethasone found no significant adverse effects on achieving adult height.

The National Institutes of Health (NIH) advises physicians to carefully monitor a young patient's height and to "step down" therapy when possible. NIH notes that even high doses of inhaled corticosteroids with children experiencing severe, persistent asthma create less risk of delayed growth than treatment with oral systemic corticosteroids (pills or capsules).

Osteoporosis (Bone Disease)

In some people, high corticosteroid usage can reduce bone mineral density, leading to osteoporosis. Links have been found between steroid use and inhibiting bone formation, calcium absorption, and the production of sex hormones that help keep bones vital. Brief courses of systemic corticosteroids or low-dose inhaled steroids are not dangerous, but inhaling 1500 mcg of beclomethasone per day can lead to bone loss. The doses of other inhaled steroids, which may constitute a risk for osteoporosis, have not been studied.

Even if you need to take steroids for your asthma, you can take measures to protect yourself against osteoporosis. Here are some recommendations:

- Take the lowest dose possible and use inhaled steroids rather than oral preparations.

- Get about 1,500 mg of calcium daily through nutrition or supplements. Because vitamin D helps the body absorb calcium, it may help to take 800 international units (IU) daily of vitamin D.

- Receive replacement female hormone therapy unless prohibited for medical reasons. There are non-hormonal drugs available (bisphosphonates or calcitonin) that work similarly.

Disseminated Varicella (Chickenpox)

The U.S. Food and Drug Administration (FDA) reported that long-term or high-dose oral corticosteroid treatment might place people exposed to chickenpox or measles at increased risk of unusually severe infections or even death. That's because some doses suppress the immune system. "Children who are on immunosuppressant drugs are more susceptible to infections than healthy children," said the FDA. Yet the NIH Guidelines said there is no evidence that recommended doses of inhaled corticosteroids suppress the immune system.

NIH advises that children who have not had chickenpox and periodically take oral corticosteroids should receive the varicella vaccine after they've been steroid-free for at least one month. Kids who have finished a short course of prednisone may receive the vaccine immediately. Unimmunized adults and children who are exposed to chickenpox while being treated with immunosuppressive levels of steroids may take immunoglobulin and acyclovir.

Cataracts

The risk of cataracts in patients taking systemic corticosteroids has been well identified, but reports among those taking inhaled steroids are rare. In a notable exception, the *New England Journal of Medicine* published findings of a recent Australian study of inhaled corticosteroid users between the ages of 49 and 97. The authors concluded that the use of inhaled steroids is associated with an increased risk for development of cataracts. Patients taking moderate to high doses of inhaled corticosteroids especially should have regular eye exams.

Other Risks

The NIH Guidelines also list a few other rare but potential risks of high-dose corticosteroid use. In some cases, oral steroid use has been linked with adrenal suppression, effects on glucose metabolism, and hypertension. Serious medical complications have also been recorded in people on high doses of oral steroids with tuberculosis.

None of the above risks have been reported with inhaled corticosteroids. However, their use in moderate to high doses has been found to contribute to thinning and bruising of the skin, especially among women.

Oral (Systemic) Corticosteroids

- Generally for short-term use
- Quickly control persistent asthma

- Forms: pills, tablets, or liquid (for children)
- Medications: Methylprednisolone, prednisolone, prednisone

Inhaled Corticosteroids

- For long-term asthma prevention; suppress, control and reverse inflammation
- Forms: dry powder or aerosol
- Medications: Beclomethasone dipropionate, budesonide, flunisolide, fluticasone propionate, triamcinolone acetonide

Table 44.1. Low, Medium, and High Corticosteroid Dosages for Children and Adults

Note: A = adult; C = child. All dosages are daily, in micrograms (mcg).

Drug	Low	Medium	High
Beclomethasone	A 168-504	504-840	840+
dipropionate	C 84-336	336-672	672+
Budesonide	A 200-400	400-600	600+
Turbuhaler	C 100-200	200-400	400+
Flunisolide	A 500-1000	1000-2000	2000+
	C 500-750	1000-1250	1250
Fluticasone	A 88-264	264-660	660+
	C 88-176	176-440	440+
Triamcinolone	A 400-1000	1000-2000	2000
acetonide	C 400-800	800-1200	1200

Source: NIH Guidelines of the Diagnosis and Management of Asthma, April 1997.

Chapter 45

Allergy Shots and Immunotherapy

Asthma and allergies are two quite personal conditions in the sense that they can work so differently from one person to another. Treatment plans don't come in a one-size-fits-all formula. Lifestyle choices and/or demands can make it easier or more difficult to avoid allergens. Sometimes medications that once worked have become ineffective. When medications aren't helping and you're having a hard time avoiding your allergens, it might be time to consider allergen immunotherapy, or allergy shots.

What is immunotherapy?

With immunotherapy treatment, you receive increasingly higher doses of your allergens over time, gradually becoming less sensitive to them. Allergy shots have been proven effective for symptoms caused by grass, tree and weed pollens, dust mites, cat dander, certain molds, and stinging insects.

To date, allergen immunotherapy is the only treatment that has the potential to provide long-term prevention of allergic asthma or rhinitis symptoms. Allergy shots may have a lasting effect after they are stopped, whereas medications do not.

"Immunotherapy," reprinted with permission from the Asthma and Allergy Foundation of America, © 2005. All rights reserved.

Who is eligible?

To help determine if you will be a good candidate for allergy shots, your physician will look at two key factors: how long you experience allergy symptoms each year and how well other treatments are controlling them. People with perennial or prolonged allergies are generally the best match, as well as those needing multiple medications for their symptoms. A switch to allergy shots is usually not cost-effective for patients whose seasons last only a few months and who are achieving good control with cromolyn sodium inhalers, topical corticosteroids, or non-sedating antihistamines.

Additional considerations include your age and health. Patients into their 60s can be good candidates for treatment. However, the younger the patient, not only the better the chances for relief, but also the more years of potential benefit. Your body must also be able to respond to epinephrine, which would be used in the rare event that you should have a severe reaction from the injections. Arrhythmia or other heart problems would make you ineligible in this case.

How does the process work?

Once your doctor has verified that immunotherapy is a good option for you, he or she will conduct tests that will determine what allergens should be in your allergy extract. Skin testing is one of the most common, accurate, and inexpensive ways to do this.

In prick/scratch testing, a small drop of a possible allergen is placed on the skin, followed by lightly pricking or scratching through the drop with a needle. In intradermal (under the skin) testing, a very small amount of allergen is injected into the outer layer of skin. With either test, if you are allergic to the substance, you will develop redness, swelling, and itching at the test site within 20 minutes. You may also see a raised, round area that looks like a hive. Usually, the larger the area, or wheal, the more sensitive you are to the allergen. Most people are tested for about five to 25 allergens at a time, depending on whether sensitivity is being tested for indoor allergens only or for both indoor and outdoor allergens.

After allergen identification comes the actual treatment. You'll begin with shots once or twice a week, until you start to feel relief (this process usually takes four to six months). Monthly maintenance doses are then given to help keep your "allergen resistance level" steady. You can expect your symptoms to be reduced after your first year of immunotherapy. If not, the use of allergy shots for your condition should be reconsidered. After you've been taking allergy shots for three to five years, it's time to stop for a reevaluation of treatment and symptoms. If the result is a return of symptoms, another course of therapy may be recommended, as a gradual relapse has been known to occur in some patients.

Is there a quicker alternative?

Because of time, cost, and convenience issues, rush immunotherapy has reemerged as a viable option to conventional allergy shots. First suggested 65 years ago by British physician John Freeman, this accelerated version of the traditional course of shots brings patients to maintenance dosing levels within several weeks instead of months.

A typical rush regimen at National Jewish Medical and Research Center schedules four daily injections at one-hour intervals on five consecutive days. Maintenance doses are reached in five to 10 days. After maintenance is achieved, injections move to a weekly, then biweekly, and finally, a monthly schedule.

In one recent study, 44 patients, ages 2 to 50, successfully achieved full maintenance dosing in one day. Diagnosed with a variety of conditions including asthma, allergic rhinoconjunctivitis, and chronic sinusitis, all were able to complete the therapy and showed no signs of blood pressure changes. Peak flow meter readings also remained stable. Participants had been premedicated with prednisone and various antihistamines for two days prior to the study as well as on the morning it began. Two patients developed and were treated for generalized itching.

Chapter 46

Alternative Medicine Treatments for Allergies

Chapter Contents

Section 46.1

All about Alternative Therapies for Allergies

What is alternative medicine?

Any unproven treatment for an illness or disease is considered an alternative medical approach by most American medical doctors. "Unproven" means there is not enough acceptable scientific evidence to show that the treatment works. The term alternative medicine refers to a wide variety of treatments considered outside "mainstream" or "usual" medical approaches in the United States today.

Many people turn to alternative medicine to help alleviate their asthma or allergy symptoms. These treatment approaches may include, but are not limited to, one or more of the following:

- Acupuncture
- Ayurvedic medicine
- Biofeedback, mental imaging, stress reduction, and relaxation techniques
- Chiropractic spinal manipulation
- Diet, exercise, yoga, and lifestyle changes
- Herbal medicine and vitamin supplements
- Folk medicine from various cultures
- Laser therapy
- Massage
- Hypnosis
- Art or music therapy

Why do people use alternative medicine?

Recent statistics show that nearly 40 percent of Americans try some form of alternative medicine. Medical and scientific experts do believe that some remedies may be worth a try, providing they are not harmful. In some cases, specific alternative medical treatment may improve or relieve symptoms of a specific illness or disease. Risks should not outweigh the potential benefits.

If you believe a particular alternative medical approach might help reduce your asthma or allergy symptoms, talk with your doctor about it, and how you could integrate that treatment into your overall asthma/allergy management plan.

No one should use alternative medicine without first consulting a board-certified physician. Any alternative medical approach should be used in addition to your normal asthma or allergy management plan.

You should not substitute an alternative medical treatment for your regular medications or treatments. Be especially careful about use of alternative medicine on children. Approaches that are harmless for adults may not be harmless for children.

Does health insurance cover alternative medical treatment?

Health plans vary in what alternative medicine expenses they will pay. Many plans provide coverage for some but not all alternative therapies. If your doctor writes you a prescription for a specific treatment such as acupuncture or massage, you may be more likely to get partial or full reimbursement of the expense. Always check with your insurance provider before assuming the coverage is available.

What are cautions or considerations for people who use alternative medicine?

Beware the placebo effect:. If you really want an alternative medical treatment to work, you may think it is working, even if it really isn't. This placebo effect often occurs for people using alternative medicine. Symptoms of asthma or allergy also may improve on their own as an illness (like a cold or flu) runs its course. If you use prescribed medications for your allergy or asthma symptoms, it may take time for them to kick in. So you may simply be feeling better because your medications started working—not because the alternative medicine is working.

Read between the label lines: The federal government requires labels to state how an herb or vitamin may affect the body but labels are not required to carry health warnings. Labels also cannot claim any medical or health benefit. Products often are not properly labeled, especially those imported from other countries. Many people experience toxic—and sometimes deadly—effects from improperly using labeled herbs. Some products contain unnamed medicines such as steroids, anti-inflammatories, or sedatives that act to reduce your symptoms. Other hidden ingredients in various products can be dangerous or even lethal. Use products tested for safety and effectiveness.

Follow directions: Never increase the amount or frequency of a dose or use a treatment or device in a different way than recommended. Do not use herbs in combinations. Do not take herbs if you are pregnant or breastfeeding.

Beware of developing allergy symptoms: Allergies to specific plants and other substances (such as latex or nickel) can build up over time. Products you've used for years may suddenly cause mild to serious allergy symptoms, especially if you already are allergic to something. Check to see if new herbs, foods, or other products you plan to use are in the same "family" as your known allergens.

Use quality products and services: Lack of quality standards is a serious problem for people who use various alternative medical treatments. Look for products that list the amount of the active ingredient(s). Make sure people giving you any kind of treatment are properly certified. Ask your pharmacist or health product store manager for recommendations. Research the product or service before you use it.

Consult with your physician before starting any new treatment: This point cannot be stressed enough. If you have symptoms of asthma or allergy, but you have not been diagnosed, consult a board-certified doctor for a proper diagnosis. Do not rely on health product store personnel to help treat undiagnosed symptoms. If you know you have asthma or allergies, again, talk with your doctor about the alternative medicine you want to use—before you try it.

Are there useful alternative therapies for people who have asthma or allergies?

Keep in mind: alternative therapy is medical treatment for which there is no conclusive, supporting scientific evidence. This does not necessarily mean the treatment is useless or ineffective. You simply must be careful in what you choose and how you use it.

Acupuncture: A technique that involves inserting needles into key points of the body. Evidence suggests that acupuncture may signal the brain to release endorphins. These are hormones made by the body. When released, endorphins can help reduce pain and create a sense of well-being. People with asthma or allergy may experience more relaxed or calmer breathing. Users should be aware of the risk of contaminated needles or punctured organs.

Biofeedback: A technique that helps people control involuntary physical responses. Results are mixed, with children and teenagers showing the greatest benefit.

Chiropractic spinal manipulation: A technique that emphasizes manipulation of the spine in order to help the body heal itself. People who get chiropractic treatment for allergies or asthma may find it easier to breathe after treatment. There is no evidence that this treatment impairs the underlying disease or pulmonary function.

Hypnosis: An artificially induced dream state that leaves the person open to suggestion, hypnosis is a legitimate technique to help people manage various conditions. Hypnosis might give people with asthma or allergies more self-discipline to follow good health practices.

Laser treatment: A technique that uses high intensity light to shrink swollen tissue or unblock sinuses. Laser therapy may provide temporary relief, but it may also cause scarring or other long-term physical problems.

Massage, relaxation techniques, art/music therapy, and yoga: Stress and anxiety may cause your airways to constrict more if you have asthma or allergies. Various techniques can help you relax, reduce anxiety, or control your breathing. The results may provide some benefit in helping you cope with asthma or allergy symptoms. However, evidence is not conclusive that these techniques improve lung function.

Section 46.2

Antibiotic Desensitization Useful for Allergy to Life-Saving Drug

When patients with life-threatening bacterial infections are allergic to antibiotics, drug desensitization may be an option when no other alternative exists, according to a report published [in the April 2004 issue of the] *Annals of Allergy, Asthma & Immunology,* the scientific journal of the American College of Allergy, Asthma and Immunology (ACAAI).

Stuart E. Turvey, MB, BS, DPhil, and colleagues at Children's Hospital in Boston, retrospectively reviewed the medical records of all patients undergoing antibiotic desensitization at their institution during a five-year period between 1996 to 2001, in what they describe is the largest combined series of antibiotic desensitization outcomes published to date.

The investigators compiled and analyzed data on 57 desensitizations performed in 21 patients, 19 of whom had been diagnosed as having cystic fibrosis. Patients with cystic fibrosis, who during their lifetime receive multiple courses of antibiotics, may be predisposed to allergic sensitization against a range of antibiotics.

Desensitization allows safe delivery of an antibiotic to a patient who has an IgE-mediated sensitivity to that drug by administering it in small doses until a full therapeutic dose is clinically tolerated. The procedure entails risk of acute allergic reactions, including death, and authors recommend it be performed only in a controlled inpatient setting.

Dr. Turvey and his team reported that desensitizations were performed to 12 different antibiotics, with successful outcomes in 75 percent. Of the 11 cases that were terminated due to an allergic reaction, there were no fatalities, intubations, or other aggressive interventions besides the use of epinephrine, antihistamines, and corticosteroids.

In seven of 11 unsuccessful desensitizations, a non-IgE mechanism appeared to be responsible for the allergic reaction.

The report outlines the process involved in selecting a candidate for antibiotic desensitization and presents standard protocols for desensitization for a range of common antibiotics used in cystic fibrosis patients.

Section 46.3

Stopping Symptoms before They Start: Anti-IgE Therapy

"Anti-IgE Therapy: A revolutionary approach to controlling allergy and asthma," by William Berger, M.D. Reprinted courtesy of Allergy & Asthma Network Mothers of Asthmatics (AANMA), 800-878-4403, www .breatherville.org, © 2004.

To understand anti-IgE therapy and its role in treating allergies and asthma, it is first important to understand the relationship between allergies and the body's immune system.

IgE antibodies are key players in allergic reactions. IgE antibodies prompt other cells (mast and basophil cells, among others) to begin the complex chain reaction that culminates in allergy and asthma symptoms such as coughing, sneezing, watery eyes, and shortness of breath.

Traditionally, allergies and allergy-induced asthma are managed using medications that treat IgE-mediated symptoms once they have already begun in the body. While each treatment has its use, none of the available therapies provides a preventive measure against the binding of IgE to mast cells.

A novel, more targeted approach to the treatment of allergies and allergy-induced asthma is called anti-IgE therapy. This new class of medications holds great promise for people with moderate-to-severe allergies and asthma because it is specifically designed to block IgE from initiating the allergic response, potentially preventing the onset of symptoms before they start.

The first medication in this class, called Xolair® (omalizumab), has been approved by the U.S. Food and Drug Administration (FDA) for the treatment of moderate-to-severe persistent asthma in patients age 12 and older whose symptoms do not respond to standard treatment.

Xolair® is the first biologic treatment that targets allergic asthma. "Biologic" means it uses genetically engineered mammalian proteins, rather than chemicals. Physicians say it breaks the "allergy cascade"— the chain of events that lead to asthma. Specifically, it stops the allergic reaction before it begins, by attaching itself to IgE antibodies and preventing them from causing the allergic reactions that set off asthma symptoms.

Xolair is not a medicine you swallow or inhale; it is an injection given two to four times a month. The effects last as long as you continue the injections. For some of those who have taken it, Xolair offers a way to control allergies and asthma when other options have not worked.

Candidates for Xolair must be 12 years of age or older with moderate-to-severe allergic asthma triggered by year-round allergens in the air as confirmed by a doctor using a skin or blood test, whose symptoms persist even when using inhaled corticosteroids. Frequently, such patients will have the following characteristics:

- Daily asthma symptoms
- Need for a bronchodilator every day
- Two or more times a week when asthma symptoms worsen, either quickly or gradually
- Asthma symptoms that disturb sleep one or more nights a week
- Below-normal peak flow meter readings (less than 80%)

Researchers are testing Xolair in patients, both children and adult, who have food and pollen allergies, but the product is not yet approved for treating these disorders.

Despite its potential, it's important to note that anti-IgE therapy is not a cure for asthma or allergies, and that in some cases other medications may still be needed. Additionally, while many people who have taken Xolair have been exposed to allergens without experiencing symptoms, it is advised that people still continue to maintain their allergen avoidance program.

Chapter 47

Using Allergy Medications during Pregnancy

Asthma is the most common potentially serious medical condition to complicate pregnancy. In fact, asthma affects almost 7 percent of women in their childbearing years. Well-controlled asthma is not associated with significant risk to mother or fetus. Although uncontrolled asthma is rarely fatal, it can cause serious complications to the mother, including high blood pressure, toxemia, and premature delivery. For the baby, complications of uncontrolled asthma include increased risk of stillbirth, fetal growth retardation, premature birth, low birth weight, and a low APGAR score at birth.

Asthma can be controlled by careful medical management and avoidance of known triggers, so asthma need not be a reason for avoiding pregnancy. Most measures used to control asthma are not harmful to the developing fetus and do not appear to contribute to either miscarriage or birth defects.

Although the outcome of any pregnancy can never be guaranteed, most women with asthma and allergies do well with proper medical management by physicians familiar with these disorders and the changes that occur during pregnancy.

What is asthma and what are its symptoms?

Asthma is a condition characterized by obstruction in the airways of the lungs caused by spasm of surrounding muscles, accumulation of mucus, and swelling of the airway walls due to the gathering of inflammatory cells. Unlike individuals with emphysema who have irreversible destruction of their lung cells, asthmatic patients usually have a condition that can be reversed with vigorous treatment.

Individuals with asthma most often describe what they feel in their airways as a tightness. They also describe wheezing, shortness of breath, chest pain, and cough. Symptoms of asthma can be triggered by allergens (including pollen, mold, animals, feathers, house dust mites, and cockroaches), environmental factors, exercise, infections, and stress.

What are the effects of pregnancy on asthma?

When women with asthma become pregnant, a third of the patients improve, one third worsen, and the last third remain unchanged. Although studies vary widely on the overall effect of pregnancy on asthma, several reviews find the following similar trends:

- Women with severe asthma are more likely to worsen, while those with mild asthma are more likely to improve.

- The change in the course of asthma in an individual woman during pregnancy tends to be similar on successive pregnancies.

- Asthma exacerbations are most likely to appear during weeks 24 to 36 of gestation, with only occasional patients (10 percent or fewer) becoming symptomatic during labor and delivery.

- The changes in asthma noted during pregnancy usually return to prepregnancy status within three months of delivery.

Pregnancy may affect asthmatic patients in several ways. Hormonal changes that occur during pregnancy may affect both the nose and sinuses, as well as the lungs. An increase in the hormone estrogen contributes to congestion of the capillaries (tiny blood vessels) in the lining of the nose, which in turn leads to a stuffy nose in pregnancy (especially during the third trimester). A rise in progesterone causes increased respiratory drive, and a feeling of shortness of breath may be experienced as a result of this hormonal increase. These events may be confused with or add to allergic or other triggers of asthma.

Spirometry and peak flow are measurements of airflow obstruction (a marker of asthma) that help your physician determine if asthma is the cause of shortness of breath during pregnancy.

How is fetal monitoring used for pregnant women with asthma?

For pregnant women with asthma, the type and frequency of fetal evaluation is based on gestational age and maternal risk factors. Ultrasound can be performed before 12 weeks if there is concern about the accuracy of an estimated due date and repeated later if a slowing of fetal growth is suspected. Electronic heart rate monitoring, called "non-stress testing" or "contraction stress testing" and ultrasonic determinations in the third trimester may be used to assess fetal well-being. For third trimester patients with significant asthma symptoms, the frequency of fetal assessment should be increased if problems are suspected. Asthma patients should record fetal activity or kick counts daily to help monitor their baby according to their physician's instructions.

During a severe asthma attack in which symptoms do not quickly improve, there is risk for significant maternal hypoxemia, a low oxygen state. This is an important time for fetal assessment; continuous electronic fetal heart rate monitoring may be necessary along with measurements of the mother's lung function.

Fortunately during labor and delivery, the majority of asthma patients do well, although careful fetal monitoring remains very important. In low risk patients whose asthma is well-controlled, fetal assessment can be accomplished by 20 minutes of electronic monitoring (the admission test). Intensive fetal monitoring with careful observation is recommended for patients who enter labor and delivery with severe asthma, have a nonreassuring admission test, or other risk factors.

How can pregnant women with asthma avoid and control exposure to allergens?

The connection between asthma and allergies is common. Most asthmatic patients (75 to 85 percent) will be allergic to one or more substances such as: pollens, molds, animals, house dust mites, and cockroaches. Pet allergies are caused by protein found in animal dander, urine, and saliva. These allergens may trigger asthma symptoms or make existing symptoms worse.

469

Other nonallergic substances may also worsen asthma and allergies. These include tobacco smoke, paint and chemical fumes, strong odors, environmental pollutants (including ozone and smog), and drugs, such as aspirin or beta-blockers (used to treat high blood pressure, migraine headache, and heart disorders).

Avoidance of specific triggers should lessen the frequency and intensity of asthmatic and allergic symptoms. Allergist/immunologists recommend the following methods:

- Remove allergy-causing pets from the house or at the least keep them out of the bedroom at all times.

- Seal pillows, mattresses, and box springs in special dust mite-proof casings (your allergist should be able to give you information regarding comfortable cases).

- If possible, wash bedding weekly in 130 degree Fahrenheit water (comforters may be dry cleaned periodically) to kill dust mites. However, keeping the hot water tank at this temperature may not be advisable if there are small children or others at risk of scalding at home.

- Keep home humidity under 50 percent to control dust mite and mold growth.

- Use filtering vacuums or "filter vacuum bags" to control airborne dust when cleaning.

- Close windows, use air conditioning, and limit outdoor activity between 5 and 10 a.m. when pollen and pollution are at their highest.

- Limit exposure to chemical fumes and, most importantly, tobacco smoke.

Can asthma medications safely be used during pregnancy?

Though no medication has been proven entirely safe for use during pregnancy, your doctor will carefully balance medication use and symptom control. Your treatment plan will be individualized so that potential benefits of medications outweigh the potential risks of these medications or of uncontrolled asthma.

Asthma is a disease in which intensity of symptoms can vary from day to day, month to month, or season to season regardless of pregnancy. Therefore, a treatment plan should be chosen based both on asthma severity and experience during pregnancy with those medications. Remember that the use of medications should not replace avoidance of allergens or irritants, as avoidance will potentially reduce medication needs.

In general, asthma medications used in pregnancy are chosen based on the following criteria:

- Inhaled medications are generally preferred because they have a more localized effect with only small amounts entering the bloodstream.

- When appropriate, time-tested older medications are preferred since there is more experience with their use during pregnancy.

- Medication use is limited in the first trimester as much as possible when the fetus is forming. Birth defects from medications are rare (no more than one percent of all birth defects are attributable to all medications).

In general, the same medications used during pregnancy are appropriate during labor and delivery and when nursing.

Bronchodilator Medication: Inhaled beta2-agonists, often called "asthma relievers" or "rescue medications," are used as necessary to control acute symptoms. Any of the short-acting beta agonists, including metaproterenol (Metaprel, Alupent), albuterol (Proventil, Ventolin), isoetharine (Bronkometer), bitolterol (Tornalate), pirbuterol (Maxair), and terbutaline (Brethaire) are considered safe in pregnancy. Albuterol, metaproterenol, and terbutaline have been studied in humans. Injections of terbutaline are sometimes used to control premature labor.

A long-acting inhaled beta agonist, salmeterol (Serevent), as well as oral forms of albuterol (Proventil Repetabs, Volmax) are available. No trials of these medications in pregnancy have been performed, and careful consideration is advised with use during pregnancy. These medications may be especially helpful for control of nighttime symptoms to ensure uninterrupted sleep.

Theophylline has extensive human experience without evidence of significant abnormalities. Newborns can have jitteriness, vomiting, and fast pulse if the maternal blood level is too high. Therefore, patients who receive theophylline should have blood levels checked during pregnancy.

Ipratropium (Atrovent), an anticholinergic bronchodilator medication, does not cause problems in animals; however, there is no published experience in humans. Ipratropium is absorbed less than similar medications in this class, such as atropine.

Anti-Inflammatory Medication: The anti-inflammatory medications are preventive, or "asthma controllers," and include inhaled cromolyn (Intal), nedocromil (Tilade), corticosteroids, and antileukotrienes. Patients requiring the use of beta2-agonists more often than three times a week, or have reduced peak flow readings or spirometry (lung function studies), usually need daily anti-inflammatory medication. Inhaled cromolyn sodium is virtually devoid of side effects, but is less effective than inhaled corticosteroids. Nedocromil is a newer medication, similar to cromolyn. Although there is no reported experience with nedocromil during human pregnancy, animal data are reassuring.

Beclomethasone (Beclovent, Vanceril) is generally considered the inhaled corticosteroid of choice because of its length of time in clinical use and good safety profile in humans. However, this medication in recommended doses does not control asthma symptoms in all pregnant patients. Other drugs in this class, which have been available for a number of years, are triamcinolone (Azmacort) and flunisolide (AeroBid). There are limited data during human pregnancy for these drugs. Experience with the newer inhaled corticosteroids, fluticasone (Flovent) and budesonide (Pulmicort), is even more limited. Maximum benefits of all these inhalers may not be evident for several weeks.

In some cases oral or injectable corticosteroids, prednisone, prednisolone, or methylprednisolone, may be necessary for a few days in moderately severe patients, or throughout pregnancy in severe cases. Some studies have demonstrated a slight increase in the incidence of preeclampsia, premature deliveries, or low-birth-weight infants with chronic use of corticosteroids. However, they are the most effective drugs for the treatment of patients with more severe asthma and other allergic disorders. Therefore, their significant benefit usually far exceeds their minimal risk.

Three antileukotrienes, zafirlukast (Accolate), zileuton (Zyflo), and montelukast (Singulair), are available. Results of animal studies are reassuring for zafirlukast and montelukast, but there are no data in human pregnancy with this new class of anti-inflammatory drugs.

Can allergy medications safely be used during pregnancy?

Antihistamines may be useful during pregnancy to treat the nasal and eye symptoms of seasonal or perennial allergic rhinitis, allergic conjunctivitis, the itching of urticaria (hives) or eczema, and as an adjunct to the treatment of serious allergic reactions including anaphylaxis (allergic shock). With the exception of life-threatening anaphylaxis, the benefits from their use must be weighed against any risk to the fetus. Because symptoms may be of such severity to affect maternal eating, sleeping, or emotional well-being, and because uncontrolled rhinitis may predispose a person to sinusitis or may worsen asthma, antihistamines may provide definite benefit during pregnancy.

Chlorpheniramine (Chlor-Trimeton), tripelennamine (Pyribenzamine), and diphenhydramine (Benadryl) have been used for many years during pregnancy with reassuring animal studies. Generally, chlorpheniramine would be the preferred choice, but a major drawback of these medications is drowsiness and performance impairment in some patients. Although there have been no reports of harm with the newer nonsedating drugs including astemizole (Hismanal), fexofenadine (Allegra), loratadine (Claritin), cetirizine (Zyrtec), or the nasal spray azelastine (Astelin), human data are very limited. Loratadine and cetirizine have reassuring animal study data and may be useful if older drugs cause performance impairment or excessive sleepiness.

The use of decongestants is more problematic. The nasal spray oxymetazoline (Afrin, Neo-Synephrine Long-Acting, etc.) appears to be the safest product because there is minimal, if any, absorption into the bloodstream. However, these and other over-the-counter nasal sprays can cause rebound congestion and actually worsen the condition for which they are used. Their use is generally limited to very intermittent use or regular use for only three consecutive days.

Although pseudoephedrine (Sudafed) has been used for years, and studies have been reassuring, there have been recent reports of a slight increase in abdominal wall defects in newborns. Use of decongestants during the first trimester should only be entertained after consideration of the severity of maternal symptoms unrelieved by other medications. Phenylephrine and phenylpropanolamine are less desirable than pseudoephedrine based on the information available.

An anti-inflammatory nasal spray, such as cromolyn (NasalCrom), or beclomethasone (Beconase, Vancenase), a corticosteroid, should be considered in any patient whose allergic nasal symptoms last for more than a few days. These medications prevent symptoms and lessen the need for oral medications. They have a record of use for many years. Newer corticosteroid sprays including triamcinolone (Nasacort, Tri-Nasal), fluticasone (Flonase), budesonide (Rhinocort), flunisolide (Nasarel), and mometasone (Nasonex) lack pregnancy data, although their absorption into the bloodstream is so minimal as to be of doubtful risk.

Can pregnant women with asthma receive immunotherapy and influenza vaccines?

Allergen immunotherapy (allergy shots) is often effective for those patients in whom symptoms persist despite optimal environmental control and proper drug therapy. Allergen immunotherapy can be carefully continued during pregnancy in patients who are benefiting and not experiencing adverse reactions. Due to the greater risk of anaphylaxis with increasing doses of immunotherapy and a delay of several months before it becomes effective, it is generally recommended that this therapy not be started during pregnancy.

Patients receiving immunotherapy during pregnancy should be carefully evaluated. It may be appropriate to lower the dosage in order to further reduce the chance of an allergic reaction to the injections.

Influenza (flu) vaccine is recommended for all patients with moderate and severe asthma. There is no evidence of associated risk to the mother or fetus.

Can asthma medications safely be used while nursing?

Nearly all medications enter breast milk, though infants are generally exposed to very low concentrations of the drugs. Hence, the medications described above rarely present problems for the infant during breastfeeding. Specifically, very little of the inhaled beta agonists, inhaled or oral steroids, and theophylline will appear in mother's milk. Some infants can have irritability and insomnia if exposed to higher doses of medication or to theophylline. Use of zafirlukast and zileuton while breastfeeding is not recommended because of lack of data regarding safety. In general the lowest drug concentration in mother's milk can be obtained by taking the necessary medications 15 minutes after nursing or three to four hours before the next feeding.

Summary

It is important to remember that the risks of asthma medications are lower than the risks of uncontrolled asthma, which can be harmful to both mother and child. The use of asthma or allergy medication needs to be discussed with your doctor, ideally before pregnancy. Therefore, the doctor should be notified whenever you are planning to discontinue birth control methods or as soon as you know that you are pregnant. Regular followup for evaluation of asthma symptoms and medications is necessary throughout the pregnancy to maximize asthma control and to minimize medication risks.

This text has been prepared by members of the Pregnancy Committee of the American College of Allergy, Asthma and Immunology, an organization whose members are dedicated to providing optimal care to all patients with asthma, including those who are pregnant.

For more medical information, please contact an allergist in your area.

Chapter 48

Treating Allergies at School

Chapter Contents

Section 48.1

Treating Allergic Reactions at School

This information was provided by KidsHealth, one of the largest resources online for medically reviewed health information written for parents, kids, and teens. For more articles like this one, visit www.KidsHealth.org, or www.TeensHealth.org. © 2005 The Nemours Foundation. This information was reviewed by Steven Dowshen, M.D., November 2005.

Severe, life-threatening allergic reactions sometimes require treatment at school, and parents may neglect to inform school officials of kids' severe allergies, say researchers from Harvard Medical School and Boston Children's Hospital in Massachusetts.

Between September 2001 and August 2003, nurses in 109 Massachusetts school districts provided information about their use of epinephrine, a medicine used to treat life-threatening allergic reactions. They answered questions about:

- the cause or trigger of each student's allergic symptoms

- where the student was when the allergic symptoms developed

- who administered the epinephrine

- whether the student received further medical care after receiving epinephrine

The results? Most of the students who received epinephrine were in elementary school, and a quarter of the reactions occurred in students who had allergies to peanuts or tree nuts. More than a third of the allergic reactions occurred in students who had allergies to more than one substance. Most of the time, students suffered reactions after eating some type of food that contained an allergen, such as a cookie or an item from the lunch menu. In some cases, though, students experienced reactions after inhaling or touching food containing the allergen. The students' symptoms ranged from itching, swelling, and hives to loss of consciousness, and three quarters of students developed symptoms that affected breathing.

The school staff didn't know students had potentially life-threatening allergies about a quarter of the time, so no health care plan or doctor's order for epinephrine was on file. And although most of the time allergic reactions occurred in the classroom, they also occurred on the playground, at home before the child got to school, traveling to or from school, or on field trips. In almost all cases, nurses gave the students epinephrine within about 10 minutes after symptoms developed. Most of the time (92% of cases), students rode to a medical facility in an ambulance after receiving epinephrine at school to be monitored and receive additional treatment, if needed.

What This Means to You

The results of this study provide a picture of how life-threatening allergic reactions are treated in schools. In many cases, schools aren't informed of children's severe allergies ahead of time, which may delay treatment if the child has a reaction. If your child has an allergy that can cause life-threatening reactions, work with your child's doctor to come up with a treatment plan and inform the school of how to respond if your child develops a reaction. Your child's plan should also stipulate that your child receive treatment at a medical facility after receiving epinephrine, because additional problems can develop even hours after the initial exposure to the allergen.

Source: C. Lynne McIntyre, RN, PhD; Anne H. Sheetz, RN, MPH; Constance R. Carroll, RN, MPH; Michael C. Young, MD; *Pediatrics,* November 2005.

Section 48.2

Injectable Epinephrine and Medic-Alert Bracelets

"Epi Pen and Anaphylaxis," © 2006 AllergicChild.com.
Reprinted with permission.

What Is an EpiPen? Advice from the Parent of an Allergic Child

Your allergist will likely prescribe an EpiPen® Jr for your child if your child has experienced anaphylaxis or has scored very high (4+) on a skin prick allergy test or RAST [radioallergosorbent test] blood test to a specific substance.

EpiPen® Jr is a prescription of epinephrine in a lightweight pen. The pen contains one dose (.15 mg) of epinephrine for a child. The EpiPen® is the prescription for older children and adults. Once your child is approximately 60 pounds, you will probably receive a prescription for an EpiPen® rather than the Jr. The pen contains the same amount of fluid at a higher concentration of epinephrine.

The EpiPen® Jr is an auto-injector for allergic emergencies (anaphylaxis) only. Before an emergency occurs, you and anyone else who takes care of your child should practice on a tester. A tester is available with the dual kit of EpiPens®.

There is a new product on the market called a Twinject, which has two injections of epinephrine available. I have received a sample of this product and have found it to be cumbersome and confusing, especially if I have to ensure that I can perform the operation correctly in an emergency. Some physicians may prefer to carry a Twinject in case of an emergency, and with their familiarity with shots the cumbersome aspect may not be an issue.

Keep the pen out of direct sunlight, and it should not be refrigerated. It should also not be left in a car due to temperature extremes. Additionally, once a pen has expired we dispose of it by practicing administering the shot on an orange. This is good practice so that you know the amount of time it will take to administer the medicine, the strength with which you need to push, and the sound of the 'click' upon injection.

You must keep the pen in close proximity to your child at all times. (However, be careful of curious siblings. You will need to explain to them the seriousness of the epinephrine kit.) The highest incidence of death from anaphylaxis occurs when a child having a reaction doesn't have the prescribed epinephrine with him/her.

Some children are mature enough to carry their own EpiPen® Jr with them in a lightweight fanny pack or other carrying device. The child must understand the medicine he or she is carrying and that showing it off or playing with it is not appropriate. Some states do not allow a child to carry his or her own medicine to school, and therefore the EpiPen® Jr would have to be stored with a teacher or school nurse.

Other states, such as Colorado, have recently passed legislation allowing children old enough to self-administer the EpiPen® to carry it with them at school. Inhalers would fall into this category also. For most children, this would be at the age of middle school.

The only way to obtain an EpiPen® Jr is through a pharmacist with a prescription. You will want to get several prescriptions for an EpiPen® Jr. We have one in my son's classroom at school and two in the school office so that one EpiPen® travels with the playground monitor to recess. He also has two EpiPens® in his fanny pack for nights and weekends. You may even want two in every location that your child goes, just in case one EpiPen® Jr fails or there is a misfire.

When you pick up the prescription at your pharmacy, check the expiration date. Some pharmacies have older EpiPen® Jr's on the shelf. In other words, they expire within 6 months. You should be able to obtain a kit that has an expiration date 12 to 14 months out. Once the expiration month has been hit, you will need to obtain a new one. Of course, if you should use one, you will need to replace it with a new one also.

In 1998 there was a massive recall of EpiPen® and EpiPen® Jr products due to a potential malfunction. Some people were left without one functioning product, which is a scary place to be. If you purchase your prescription from different pharmacies at different periods of time, you are less likely to have the EpiPen® Jr's expiring on the same date and to have them from the same lot. Keep a calendar of expiration dates and watch for recalls of any EpiPen® product to check the lot number of your various prescriptions.

You might want to comparison shop for the best price on an EpiPen® Jr. The internet offers various sites to purchase prescription drugs. However, we've found that mail order pharmacies are not careful as to keeping the EpiPen® heat/cold protected. We therefore purchase our EpiPens® from a local pharmacy. The pharmacies in your area may vary widely in their prices charged for this product, so it's worth shopping around.

Using an EpiPen®

If your child suffers a severe allergic reaction, it will necessitate using your EpiPen® Jr. Your child will be suffering more than just hives, more than just vomiting, but rather a combination of several factors, such as:

- hives;
- swelling of the throat continuing down to the lungs;
- vomiting/diarrhea; and
- difficulty breathing.

What can then follow is a dangerous lowering of blood pressure and loss of consciousness. All of this can occur within 2 minutes. The optimum time to administer the EpiPen® Jr is within 15 minutes, however, allergic reactions can progress much more quickly.

If your child is experiencing only hives, for example, a dose of antihistamine may be sufficient to curtail the allergic reaction. If you aren't sure whether to give an antihistamine or an epinephrine shot, our allergist has told us to err on the side of caution and administer the shot. There is no harm done if the shot is given and it wasn't necessary. There could be real harm done if the opposite occurs.

If, however, your child is experiencing anaphylaxis, administer the EpiPen® Jr., followed with 1 teaspoon of liquid Benadryl®. Call 911 and tell them your child is having an anaphylactic reaction and more epinephrine needs to be brought in the ambulance.

Some paramedics do not carry enough epinephrine to safely transport your child to the nearest hospital without the shock returning. Some states do not allow paramedics to carry epinephrine. Check your local laws to determine what precautions you need to take to keep your child safe. Your child will need to remain at the hospital for observation following an anaphylactic shock for 4 to 8 hours. The shock can return after an initial dose of epinephrine—called a biphasic reaction. It is always best to have a medical doctor observe your child, and to have additional doses of epinephrine when you leave the hospital.

We have a listing of written steps to take should an anaphylactic reaction occur. These steps were also given to my son's school and are outlined for any caregiver.

Why Should Your Child Wear a Medic Alert® Bracelet?

If your child's allergy to a specific food, several foods, a drug, or bee sting is life threatening, your doctor will probably suggest that your child wear a Medic Alert® bracelet. In other words, your child is at risk for anaphylaxis.

We have found that the bracelet creates a conversation that allows people to ask, "Why do you wear that bracelet?" My son then gets practice acknowledging what his allergies are in conversation. People who are meeting him for the first time sometimes share stories about someone else they know who has severe allergies. They generally remember his allergies when they meet him again, and that is the intent of the bracelet.

Our purpose for the bracelet is to let everyone know about his severe allergies. If people are aware of it, there is less chance for an offending food to enter his world. When my son has gone to the emergency room (for stitches, for example), our experience is that the nurses and doctors immediately check the Medic Alert bracelet.

Should your child be anywhere without you and have a reaction, any person can read the bracelet and pass this information on to a 911 operator. Also, there is a 1-800 number on the bracelet for people to contact Medic Alert and find out the complete medical information on your child. Your child should have an EpiPen® with them, in this case, and hopefully be able to self-administer it or be with someone who can administer it for him or her.

The bracelets can be ordered from Medic Alert in appropriate sizes to fit your child's wrist. We have the bracelet on my son's non-dominant hand. We ordered the stainless steel model because it is more durable. I have heard of children having reactions to stainless steel in the bracelet itself. The bracelet does come in silver and gold also if you're willing to pay a higher price for it.

There are necklaces available also. For a child, we felt the risk of catching a necklace on a piece of playground equipment was too dangerous. We therefore opted for the bracelet.

Should the red on the Medic Alert emblem wear off, they will replace the bracelet. Our son had this happen after a summer in the swimming pool. It is possible for your child to lose the bracelet, although this is unlikely with the clasp. My son has lost his, however. In that case, a new bracelet will need to be purchased.

If you find out your child has more allergies than what was originally indicated on the bracelet, you can order a new bracelet (at a charge). We have only my son's life-threatening allergies listed on the bracelet because of the small amount of space.

Section 48.3

The Americans with Disabilities Act: How It Affects Children with Allergies

Has your child been rejected by a preschool or excluded from a field trip because a teacher was afraid to use his or her EpiPen? Does a moldy carpet at work or school make you sick? Does stale smoke in offices, hotel rooms, or conference centers make it hard for you to take part in routine business activities?

The Americans with Disabilities Act (ADA) is a civil rights law that gives you the right to ask for changes where policies, practices, or conditions exclude or disadvantage you. As of January 26, 1992, public entities and public accommodations must ensure that individuals with disabilities have full access to and equal enjoyment of all facilities, programs, goods, and services.

The ADA borrows from Section 504 of the Rehabilitation Act of 1973. Section 504 prohibits discrimination on the basis of disability in employment and education in agencies, programs, and services that receive federal money. The ADA extends many of the rights and duties of Section 504 to public accommodations such as restaurants, hotels, theaters, stores, doctors' offices, museums, private schools, and child care programs. They must be readily accessible to and usable by individuals with disabilities. No one can be excluded or denied services just because he/she is disabled or based on ignorance, attitudes, or stereotypes.

Does the ADA Apply to People with Asthma and Allergies?

Yes. In both the ADA and Section 504, a person with a disability is described as someone who has a physical or mental impairment that substantially limits one or more major life activities, or is regarded as having such impairments. Breathing, eating, working, and going to school are "major life activities." Asthma and allergies are still considered disabilities under the ADA, even if symptoms are controlled by medication.

The ADA can help people with asthma and allergies obtain safer, healthier environments where they work, shop, eat, and go to school. The ADA also affects employment policies. For example, a private preschool cannot refuse to enroll children because giving medication to or adapting snacks for students with allergies requires special staff training or because insurance rates might go up. A firm cannot refuse to hire an otherwise qualified person solely because of the potential time or insurance needs of a family member.

In public schools where policies and practices do not comply with Section 504, the ADA should stimulate significant changes. In contrast, the ADA will cause few changes in schools where students have reliable access to medication, options for physical education, and classrooms that are free of allergens and irritants.

How Will the ADA Work?

In most cases, employees and employers, consumers and businesses, and administrators and students will work together to improve conditions and remove barriers to promote equal access and full inclusion.

Marie Trottier, Harvard University's Administrator of Disability Services, explains that her role includes educating nonallergic managers, colleagues, and coworkers about the needs of people with environmental sensitivities. She also trains staff in education and employment policies, benefits, and procedures.

"Changes depend as much on interpersonal consideration as they do on legal rights," she says. "It shouldn't be uncommon for people with asthma and allergies to get the same respect for their needs as people with more visible disabilities."

485

When Ms. Trottier arranges for accommodations in offices, classrooms, and student housing, she considers the nature of the disability and the specifics of each situation. She might install an air conditioner or arrange for an office with a window that opens. She has relocated a microwave oven and reorganized office spaces to help people with allergies avoid cooking odors.

Employees might need prior notice of renovation or lawn care projects so they can modify their schedules to avoid the irritants and allergens.

Professors may ask students not to wear scented products to class. Students affected by dust, paper fibers, or ink can have someone borrow library materials for them or they can use an on-line computer system. Ms. Trottier says that "all of these options for students and employees require time and energy, flexibility and creativity, more so than money." A sign in her office underscores her point, "Attitudes are the real disabilities."

Making the ADA Work for You

If you or your child would like consideration due to asthma or allergies, speak with a school administrator, manager, employer, human specialist, or disabilities service coordinator. He or she should know the procedure for collecting necessary information and planning appropriate changes, aids, or services. You can call on a variety of sources for advice and creative practical ideas.

Under Section 504, public schools and programs cannot avoid their responsibility by claiming to have limited funds or resources. Nor can they impose a "disparate impact" on people with disabilities. The ADA requires public accommodations to make changes, except in cases where an "undue burden" would result.

The law does not define "undue burden." It depends on the organization's size and the real costs of the changes. The business or program must show that it properly assessed the individual's needs and tried to find the necessary accommodations.

Don't Be Afraid to Speak Up

The ADA prohibits retaliation, harassment, or coercion against individuals who exercise their rights or assist others in doing so. If you feel you have been treated unfairly, you may file a complaint with the U.S. Attorney General who refers complaints to the appropriate agency. The Attorney General can bring lawsuits to seek money damages and civil penalties in cases of general public importance, or where there is a "pattern or practice" of discrimination.

Individuals can also file a private suit to get a court order requiring a business or program to make necessary changes and to pay attorney's fees. Other remedies may include reinstatement in your job and back pay.

The ADA Is Evolving

Court decisions and rulings will slowly define how the ADA will affect us. The real momentum for change will come as we work creatively together to promote the inclusive attitudes and environments that fulfill the promise of the ADA for ourselves and our children.

Part Six

Avoiding Triggers and Preventing Allergy Symptoms

Chapter 49

Managing Your Home Environment

Chapter Contents

Section 49.1

Controlling Allergy Triggers at Home

"Home Control of Asthma and Allergies," © 2006 American Lung Association. Reprinted with permission. For more information about the American Lung Association or to support the work it does, call 1-800-LUNG-USA (1-800-586-4872) or log on to http://www.lungusa.org.

Air Particles We Breathe

Many particles of different types and sizes are carried in the air we breathe. Some large particles may settle on the walls and furniture in your home. Other large particles are removed by your nose and mouth when you inhale. Smaller particles are breathed deep into the lungs.

Asthma may be triggered by both the large and small particles. Some air particles come from the indoors. Others are carried in the outdoor air. Outdoor particles come into your home through windows, doors, and heating systems.

For most people, the indoor air particles cause no problems. But people with allergic symptoms including asthma can have problems, right in their own home.

Asthma and Allergy Triggers

If you or someone you know have allergic symptoms or asthma, you are sensitive to triggers, including particles carried in the air. These triggers can set off a reaction in your lungs and other parts of your body. Triggers can be found indoors or outdoors. They can be simple things like:

- cold air;

- tobacco smoke and wood smoke;

- perfume, paint, hair spray, or any strong odors or fumes;

- allergens (particles that cause allergies) such as dust mites, pollen, molds, pollution, and animal dander—tiny scales or particles that fall off hair, feathers, or skin—and saliva from any pets; and

- common cold, influenza, and other respiratory illnesses.

You may be able to add more triggers to this list. Other things may also trigger your asthma or allergies. It's important to learn which triggers are a problem for you. Ask your doctor to help. Your doctor may suggest:

- keeping an asthma diary and/or
- skin testing to test for allergies.

Finding triggers isn't always easy. If you do know your triggers, cutting down exposure to them may help avoid asthma and allergy attacks.

If you don't know your triggers, try to limit your exposure to one suspected trigger at a time. Watch to see if you get better. This may show you if the trigger was a problem for you.

Outdoor Air, Indoor Air, and Air Conditioning

Controlling your exposure to triggers outdoors is hard. You may have to avoid outdoor air pollution, pollen, and mold spores. Any time air pollution and pollen levels are high, it's a good idea to stay indoors.

The air at home is easier to control. Some people with asthma and allergies notice that their symptoms get worse at night. Trigger controls in the bedroom or wherever you sleep need the most care.

Air conditioning can help. It allows windows and doors to stay closed. This keeps some pollen and mold spores outside. It also lowers indoor humidity. Low humidity helps to control mold and dust mites.

Avoid too much air conditioning or too much heat. Room air temperature should be comfortable for someone with allergies or asthma. Some people can't tolerate a big change in temperature, particularly from warm to cold air.

There are some devices that effectively remove particles from air. Their usefulness in reducing allergy symptoms is under study.

Trigger Controls

Here are some common triggers and some ways to help control them at home:

Tobacco Smoke

Smoke should not be allowed in the home of someone with asthma or allergies. Ask family members and friends to smoke outdoors. Suggest that they quit smoking. Your local American Lung Association can help. Ask your Lung Association how you can help a family member or friend quit smoking.

Wood Smoke

Wood smoke is a problem for children and adults with asthma and allergies. Avoid wood stoves and fireplaces.

Pets

Almost all pets can cause allergies, including dogs, cats, and especially small animals like birds, hamsters, and guinea pigs. All pets should be removed from the home if pets trigger asthma and allergy symptoms.

Pet allergen may stay in the home for months after the pet is gone because it remains in house dust. Allergy and asthma symptoms may take some time to get better.

If the pet stays in the home, keep it out of the bedroom of anyone with asthma or allergies. Weekly pet baths may help cut down the amount of pet saliva and dander in the home.

Sometimes you hear that certain cats or dogs are "non-allergenic." There really is no such thing as a "non-allergenic" cat or dog, especially if the pet leaves dander and saliva in the home. Goldfish and other tropical fish may be a good substitute.

Cockroaches

Even cockroaches can cause problems, so it's important to get rid of roaches in your home. Small pieces of dead roaches and roach droppings settle in house dust and can end up in the air you breathe.

Like humans, roaches need food and water and a place to live. Help keep your home roach free by storing food in sealable containers and keeping crumbs, dirty dishes, and other sources of food waste cleaned up; fixing leaks and wiping up standing water; and cleaning up clutter where roaches find shelter.

If you still have problems and you have to choose a pesticide, be sure to use it safely, and as directed on the label. Baits are less likely than sprays or foggers to harm your lungs.

Indoor Mold

When humidity is high, molds can be a problem in bathrooms, kitchens, and basements. Make sure these areas have good air circulation and are cleaned often. The basement in particular may need a dehumidifier. And remember, the water in the dehumidifier must be emptied and the container cleaned often to prevent forming mildew.

Molds may form on foam pillows when you perspire. To prevent mold, wash the pillow every week, dry thoroughly and make sure to change it every year.

Molds also form in houseplants, so check them often. You may have to keep all plants outdoors.

Strong Odors or Fumes

Perfume, room deodorizers, cleaning chemicals, paint, and talcum powder are examples of triggers that must be avoided or kept to very low levels.

Dust Mites

Dust mites are tiny, microscopic spiders usually found in house dust. Several thousand mites can be found in a pinch of dust. Mites are one of the major triggers for people with allergies and asthma. They need the most work to remove.

Following these rules can also help get rid of dust mites:

- Put mattresses in allergen-impermeable covers. Tape over the length of the zipper.

- Put pillows in allergen-permeable covers. Tape over the length of the zipper. Or wash the pillow every week.

- Wash all bedding every week in water that is at least 130 degrees Fahrenheit. Removing the bedspread at night may help.

- Don't sleep or lie down on upholstered (stuffed) furniture.

- Remove carpeting in the bedroom.

- Clean up surface dust as often as possible. Use a damp mop or damp cloth when you clean. Don't use aerosols or spray cleaners in the bedroom. And don't clean the room when someone with asthma or allergies is present.

- Window coverings attract dust. Use window shades or curtains made of plastic or other washable material for easy cleaning.

- Remove stuffed furniture and stuffed animals (unless the animals can be washed), and anything under the bed.

- Closets need extra care. They should hold only needed clothing. Putting clothes pin a plastic garment bag may help. (Do not use the plastic bag that covers dry cleaning).

- Dust mites like moisture and high humidity. Cutting down the humidity in your home can cut down the number of mites. A dehumidifier may help.

- Air cleaning devices, including portable units and central filtration systems, may be helpful in reducing some indoor air pollutants when used with effective source control and ventilation. Ask your doctor for advice about air cleaning devices. If you decide to use one, make sure it removes particles efficiently over an extended period of time and does not produce ozone.

General Rules to Help Control the Home Environment

Controlling the home environment is a very important part of asthma and allergy care. Some general rules for home control for all members of the family are:

- Reduce or remove as many asthma and allergy triggers from your home as possible.

- If possible, use air filters and air conditioners—and properly maintain them—to make your home cleaner and more comfortable.

- Pay attention to the problem of dust mites. Work hard to control this problem in the bedroom.

- Vacuum cleaners with poor filtration and design characteristics release and stir up dust and allergens.

Select a unit with high-efficiency filters such as micro filter or HEPA [high efficiency particulate air] media, good suction, and sealed construction. Ask for test data from manufacturers to determine the quantity and size of dust particles captured (e.g., 96% at 1.0 micron or 99.97% at 0.3 micron). Alternately, consider a central vacuum that exhausts particulate outside the home.

Anyone with asthma or allergies may want to avoid vacuuming.

Section 49.2

Bleach Found to Neutralize Mold Allergens

Researchers at National Jewish Medical and Research Center have demonstrated that dilute bleach not only kills common household mold, but may also neutralize the mold allergens that cause most mold-related health complaints. The study, published in the September [2005] issue of *The Journal of Allergy and Clinical Immunology*, is the first to test the effect on allergic individuals of mold spores treated with common household bleach.

"It has long been known that bleach can kill mold. However, dead mold may remain allergenic," said lead author John Martyny , Ph.D., associate professor of medicine at National Jewish. "We found that, under laboratory conditions, treating mold with bleach lowered allergic reactions to the mold in allergic patients."

The need for denaturing or neutralizing mold allergens is a critical step in mold treatment that has not been fully understood. Currently, most recommendations for mold remediation call for removal since dead mold retains its ability to trigger allergic reactions, according to Dr. Martyny.

The researchers grew the common fungus *Aspergillus fumigatus* on building materials for two weeks, and then sprayed some with a dilute household bleach solution (1:16 bleach to water), some with Tilex® Mold & Mildew Remover, a cleaning product containing both bleach and detergent, and others only with distilled water as a control. They then compared the viability and the allergenicity of the treated and untreated mold.

The researchers found that the use of the dilute bleach solution killed the *A. fumigatus* spores. When viewed using an electron microscope, the treated fungal spores appeared smaller, and lacked the surface structures present on healthy spores. In addition, surface allergens were no longer detected by ELISA [enzyme-linked immunosorbent assay] antibody-binding assays, suggesting that the spores were no longer allergenic.

The National Jewish researchers then allergy-tested eight *Aspergillus*-allergic individuals with solutions from the bleach and Tilex®-treated building materials. Seven of the eight allergic individuals did not react to the bleach-treated building materials, and six did not react to the Tilex®-treated building materials. This evidence suggests that, under laboratory conditions, fungal-contaminated building materials treated with dilute bleach or Tilex® may have significantly reduced allergic health effects.

"This study was conducted under controlled laboratory conditions. In order to assure that the bleach solutions will function similarly under actual field conditions, additional experiments will need to be conducted," said Dr. Martyny.

"We do believe, however, that there is good evidence that bleach does have the ability to significantly reduce the allergenic properties of common household mold under some conditions."

This study was partially funded by a grant from The Clorox Company.

National Jewish is the only medical and research center in the United Stated devoted entirely to respiratory, allergic, and immune-system diseases, including asthma, allergies, and chronic obstructive pulmonary disease. It is a non-profit, non-sectarian institution dedicated to enhancing prevention, treatment, and cures through research, and to developing and providing innovative clinical programs for patients regardless of age, religion, race, or ability to pay.

Section 49.3

How to Create a Dust-Free Bedroom

"How to Create a Dust-Free Bedroom" is a fact sheet from the National
Institute of Allergy and Infectious Diseases (NIAID, www.niaid.nih.gov),
part of the National Institutes of Health, August 2004.

If you are dust-sensitive, especially if you have allergies and/or
asthma, you can reduce some of your misery by creating a "dust-free"
bedroom. Dust may contain molds, fibers, and dander from dogs, cats,
and other animals, as well as tiny dust mites. These mites, which live
in bedding, upholstered furniture, and carpets, thrive in the summer
and die in the winter. They will, however, continue to thrive in the
winter if the house is warm and humid. The particles seen floating in
a shaft of sunlight include dead mites and their waste products. The
waste products actually provoke the allergic reaction.

The routine cleaning necessary to maintain a dust-free bedroom
also can help reduce exposure to cockroaches, another important cause
of asthma in some allergic people.

You probably cannot control dust conditions under which you work
or spend your daylight hours. To a large extent, however, you can eliminate dust from your bedroom. To create a dust-free bedroom, you must
reduce the number of surfaces on which dust can collect.

In addition to getting medical care for your dust allergy and/or
asthma, the National Institute of Allergy and Infectious Diseases
suggests the following guidelines.

Preparation

- Completely empty the room, just as if you were moving.

- Empty and clean all closets and, if possible, store contents elsewhere and seal closets.

- Keep clothing in zippered plastic bags and shoes in boxes off the
floor, if you cannot store them elsewhere.

- Remove carpeting, if possible.

- Clean and scrub the woodwork and floors thoroughly to remove all traces of dust.

- Wipe wood, tile, or linoleum floors with water, wax, or oil.

- Cement any linoleum to the floor.

- Close the doors and windows until the dust-sensitive person is ready to use the room.

Maintenance

- Wear a filter mask when cleaning.

- Clean the room thoroughly and completely once a week.

- Clean floors, furniture, tops of doors, window frames and sills, etc., with a damp cloth or oil mop.

- Carefully vacuum carpet and upholstery regularly.

- Use a special filter in the vacuum.

- Wash curtains often in water that's been heated to 130 degrees Fahrenheit.

- Air the room thoroughly.

Carpeting and Flooring

Carpeting makes dust control impossible. Although shag carpets are the worst type to have if you are dust sensitive, all carpets trap dust. Therefore, health care experts recommend hardwood, tile, or linoleum floors. Treating carpets with tannic acid eliminates some dust mite allergen. Tannic acid, however, is:

- not as effective as removing the carpet;

- is irritating to some people; and

- must be applied repeatedly.

Beds and Bedding

Keep only one bed in the bedroom. Most importantly, encase box springs and mattress in a zippered dust-proof or allergen-proof cover. Scrub bed springs outside the room. If you must have a second bed in the room, prepare it in the same manner.

Use only washable materials on the bed. Sheets, blankets, and other bedclothes should be washed frequently in water that is at least 130 degrees Fahrenheit.

- Lower temperatures will not kill dust mites.

- If you set your hot water temperature lower (commonly done to prevent children from scalding themselves), wash items at a Laundromat which uses high wash temperatures.

Use a synthetic, such as Dacron, mattress pad and pillow. Avoid fuzzy wool blankets or feather- or wool-stuffed comforters and mattress pads.

Furniture and Furnishings

- Keep furniture and furnishings to a minimum.

- Avoid upholstered furniture and blinds.

- Use only a wooden or metal chair that you can scrub.

- Use only plain, lightweight curtains on the windows.

Air Control

Air filters—either added to a furnace or a room unit—can reduce the levels of allergens. Electrostatic and HEPA (high-efficiency particulate absorption) filters can effectively remove many allergens from the air. If they don't function properly, however, electrostatic filters may give off ozone, which can be harmful to your lungs if you have asthma.

A dehumidifier may help because house mites need high humidity to live and grow. You should take special care to clean the unit frequently with a weak bleach solution (1 cup bleach in 1 gallon water) or a commercial product to prevent mold growth. Although low humidity may reduce dust mite levels, it might irritate your nose and lungs.

Children

In addition to the above guidelines, if you are caring for a child who is dust-sensitive, you should:

- Keep toys that will accumulate dust out of the child's bedroom.

501

- Avoid stuffed toys.
- Use only washable toys of wood, rubber, metal, or plastic.
- Store toys in a closed toy box or chest.

Pets

Keep all animals with fur or feathers out of the bedroom. If you are allergic to dust mites, you could also be allergic or develop an allergy to cats, dogs, or other animals.

Although these steps may seem difficult at first, experience plus habit will make them easier. The results—better breathing, fewer medicines, and greater freedom from allergy and asthma attacks will be well worth your effort.

Section 49.4

Air Filters: What Do I Need to Know?

What do I need to know about air filters?

When we think of air pollution, we usually associate it with outdoor air. But with the growing epidemic of asthma in the United States in the last 20 years, especially among infants and children who spend most of their time inside, much attention has been given to indoor air. In fact, in 1990 the United States Environmental Protection Agency (EPA) ranked indoor air pollution as "a high priority public health risk."

The EPA recommends three strategies for reducing indoor air pollution:

- controlling sources of pollution;
- ventilating adequately; and
- cleaning indoor air.

Before you make any changes to your indoor home environment or purchase any air filtration products, make sure to speak with a doctor who knows your personal medical history and current condition.

Will air filters really help my asthma or allergies?

Although the EPA recommends air filtration, controlling the sources of allergy-causing pollution and ventilation are more important. Air filters are worth considering, but not as a solution to your asthma or allergy problems by themselves. In fact, research studies disagree on whether filters give much added relief in a clean and well-ventilated home.

While many allergens and irritants are suspended in household air, there are far more resting on surfaces like rugs, furniture, and countertops. Keeping these areas clean is an important step in controlling your allergy and asthma triggers. However, the most effective step is to eliminate the source of these allergens and irritants in the first place.

Can air filters protect me from secondhand smoke?

The only effective way to eliminate environmental tobacco smoke (ETS)—also called secondhand smoke—is to eliminate the source of smoke: get smokers in your family to quit smoking. Some air cleaners may help to reduce secondhand smoke to a limited degree, but no air filtration or air purification system can completely eliminate all the harmful constituents of secondhand smoke. The U.S. Surgeon General has determined secondhand smoke to cause heart disease, lung cancer, and respiratory illness. Also, a simple reduction of secondhand smoke does not protect against the disease and death caused by exposure to secondhand smoke.

Are there national health standards for air filter performance?

No. The Food and Drug Administration (FDA) has asked groups of experts to recommend national standards, but no Federal standards have yet been adopted. So far they have concluded there isn't enough research data on the relationship between air filtration and actual health improvement to recommend national standards.

When you shop for air filters, you will find several rating systems that compare filters. But these are not health-related rating systems.

They are standards used by manufacturers or manufacturers' organizations, and provide little guidance for the health-conscious shopper.

How can I find a quality air filter?

Although the FDA has no health-related standards, it does consider some portable air filtration systems to be Class II medical devices. In the United States, nothing can claim this status without FDA approval. To get approval, a manufacturer must show two things: (1) that the device is safe, usually indicated by the Underwriters Laboratory (UL) seal, and (2) that it has a medical benefit. Look for both the UL seal and a statement of the FDA's Class II approval. If no FDA statement is available with the device, check the FDA's medical device listing before buying and always ask your doctor for guidance.

What is ozone versus ozone byproduct?

Most air filters have a normal ozone byproduct. In fact, many of products already in your home make an ozone byproduct—kitchen mixers, ceiling fans, hair dryers, computers, TVs, copiers, and more. An acceptable level for ozone byproduct for certain household devices has been set in the Code of Federal Regulations (CFR) at a maximum 50 parts per billion (ppb), or lower. [This standard for acceptable levels of ozone byproduct are found in section 21:801.415 of the Code of Federal Regulations (CFR) and Underwriters Laboratory (UL) standard 867.] This maximum has also been voluntarily adopted by most air filter manufacturers and makers of other household electronics.

However, machines called ozone generators directly produce ozone (O_3) molecules—not as a byproduct, but as a direct product—and blows it into the room to "clean" the air. Unfortunately these ozone generator machines can produce ozone up to 10-times more than the acceptable standard shown above. Therefore, AAFA [Asthma and Allergy Foundation of America] and other groups recommend that you do not use ozone generator machines in your home.

Are there different kinds of air filters?

Yes. Many homes have whole-house air filtration, but there are also several types of single-room air filters on the market. Here are five basic types of room air filters:

- **Mechanical filters (fan-driven HEPA filters, for example):** These force air through a special mesh that traps particles including allergens like pollen, pet dander, and dust mites. They also capture irritant particles like tobacco smoke. The fans in these types of devices produce ozone byproduct and are usually within the acceptable level. Make sure to ask for proof from the manufacturer that their product is within the acceptable level of ozone byproduct.

- **Electronic filters (ion-type cleaners, for example):** These use electrical charges to attract and deposit allergens and irritants. If the device contains collecting plates, the particles are captured within the system. The ion-chargers in these types of filters produce ozone byproduct, more than fans in mechanical filters but may still be within the acceptable level. Make sure to ask for proof from the manufacturer that their product is within the acceptable level of ozone byproduct.

- **Hybrid filters:** These contain the elements of both mechanical and electronic filters.

- **Gas phase filters:** These remove odors and non-particulate pollution like cooking gas, gasses given off by paint or building materials, and perfume. They cannot remove allergenic particles.

- **Ozone generators** [not recommended—these types of "filters" are not reliable since their ozone levels usually exceed acceptable levels]. Although ozone technically clears the air of some particles, most groups do not recommend these. (Note: these are not ion-type filters; see "Electronic Filters" above.) These devices all exceed the acceptable level for ozone.

If you have concerns about any air filter you own or are planning to buy, remember to talk to your doctor first, to find out if air filtration—and what type—is best for you.

What is a HEPA filter?

A HEPA filter is a kind of mechanical filter that means it's a high-efficiency particulate air filter. HEPA was invented during World War II to prevent the escape of radioactive particles from laboratories. To qualify as a true HEPA filter, it must be able to capture at least 99.97% percent of all particles 0.3 microns in diameter, or larger, that enter it.

What else should I consider before buying an air filtration system?

If your home is heated or air conditioned through ducts, it may be possible to build filters into your air handling system. This has the advantage of the great force with which air will pass through the filter. And it eliminates a space-consuming appliance and an additional sound in your home. On the other hand, the filters may be more expensive and more difficult to handle; they may also need to be changed more often. Consult your doctor and your heating service on this alternative to a portable system.

What questions should I ask before purchasing an air filter?

- What substances will the cleaner remove from the air in my home? What substances will it not?

- What is the efficiency rating of the cleaner in relation to the "true HEPA" standard?

- Will the unit clean the air in a room the size of my bedroom?

- How easy/difficult is it to change the filter? (Ask for a demonstration.) How often does it have to be changed? How much do filters cost? Are they readily available throughout the year?

- How much noise does the unit make? Is it quiet enough to run while I sleep? (Turn it on and try it, even though you will probably be in a noisy place.)

Chapter 50

Controlling Outdoor Triggers

Chapter Contents

Section 50.1

Checking Pollen and Mold Counts in Your Area

A sure sign of spring (or summer or fall) in many regions of the United States is news media reports of pollen counts. These counts are of interest to some 35 million Americans who get hay fever because they are allergic to pollen.

People also look for counts of mold or fungus spores. These are another major cause of seasonal allergic reactions. Pollen and mold counts are important in helping many people with allergies plan their day.

What is the pollen count?

The pollen count tells us how many grains of plant pollen were in a certain amount of air (often one cubic meter) during a set period of time (usually 24 hours). Pollen is a very fine powder released by trees, weeds, and grasses. It is carried to another plant of the same kind, to fertilize the forerunner of new seeds. This is called pollination.

The pollen of some plants is carried from plant to plant by bees and other insects. These plants usually have brightly colored flowers and sweet scents to attract insects. They seldom cause allergic reactions. Other plants rely on the wind to carry pollen from plant to plant. These plants have small, drab flowers and little scent. These are the plants that cause most allergic reactions, or hay fever.

When conditions are right, a plant starts to pollinate. Weather affects how much pollen is carried in the air each year, but it has less effect on when pollination occurs. As a rule, weeds pollinate in late summer and fall. The weed that causes 75 percent of all hay fever is ragweed, which has numerous species. One ragweed plant is estimated to produce up to 1 billion pollen grains. Other weeds that cause allergic reactions are cocklebur, lamb's quarters, plantain, pigweed, tumbleweed or Russian thistle, and sagebrush.

- Trees pollinate in late winter and spring. Ash, beech, birch, cedar, cottonwood, box, elder, elm, hickory, maple, and oak pollen can trigger allergies.

- Grasses pollinate in late spring and summer. Those that cause allergic reactions include Kentucky bluegrass, timothy, Johnson, Bermuda, redtop, orchard, rye, and sweet vernal grasses.

Much pollen is released early in the morning, shortly after dawn. This results in high counts near the source plants. Pollen travels best on warm, dry, breezy days and peaks in urban areas midday. Pollen counts are lowest during chilly, wet periods.

What is the mold count?

Mold and mildew are fungi. They differ from plants or animals in how they reproduce and grow. The seeds, called spores, are spread by the wind. Allergic reactions to mold are most common from July to late summer.

Although there are many types of molds, only a few dozen cause allergic reactions. *Alternaria, Cladosporium* (Hormodendrum), *Aspergillus, Penicillium, Helminthosporium, Epicoccum, Fusarium, Mucor, Rhizopus,* and *Aure basidium* (pullularia) are the major culprits. Some common spores can be identified when viewed under a microscope. Some form recognizable growth patterns, or colonies.

Many molds grow on rotting logs and fallen leaves, in compost piles, and on grasses and grains. Unlike pollens, molds do not die with the first killing frost. Most outdoor molds become dormant during the winter. In the spring they grow on vegetation killed by the cold.

Mold counts are likely to change quickly, depending on the weather. Certain spore types reach peak levels in dry, breezy weather. Some need high humidity, fog, or dew to release spores. This group is abundant at night and during rainy periods.

What are the symptoms for hay fever?

Pollen allergies cause sneezing, runny or stuffy nose, coughing, postnasal drip, itchy nose and throat, dark circles under the eyes, and swollen, watery and itchy eyes. For people with severe allergies, asthma attacks can occur.

Mold spores can contact the lining of the nose and cause hay fever symptoms. They also can reach the lungs, to cause asthma or another serious illness called allergic bronchopulmonary aspergillosis.

How are pollen and mold measured?

To collect a sample of particulates in the air, a plastic rod or similar device is covered with a greasy substance. The device spins in the air at a controlled speed for a set amount of time—usually over a 24-hour period. At the end of that time, a trained analyst studies the surface under a microscope. Pollen and mold that have collected on the surface are identified by size and shape as well as other characteristics. A formula is then used to calculate that day's particle count.

The counts reported are always for a past time period and may not describe what is currently in the air. Some counts reflect poorly collected samples and poor analytical skills. Some monitoring services give "total pollen" counts. They may not break out the particular pollen or mold that causes your allergies. This means that allergy symptoms may not relate closely to the published count. But knowing the count can help you decide when to stay indoors.

How can I prevent a reaction to pollen or mold?

Allergies cannot be cured. But the symptoms of the allergy can be reduced by avoiding contact with the allergen.

- Limit outdoor activity during pollination periods when the pollen or mold count is high. This will lessen the amount you inhale. The National Allergy Bureau (NAB) tracks pollen counts for different regions of the country. Contact the NAB through the American Academy of Allergy, Asthma and Immunology website [www.aaaai.org]. Pollen.com is also a reliable source of "pollen forecasts" in your zip code area, maintained by Surveillance Data Inc., a national monitor of medical and environmental statistics.

- Use central air conditioning set on "recirculate," which excludes much of the pollen and mold from the air in your home.

- Vacationing away from an area with a high concentration of the plants that cause your allergies may clear up symptoms. However, if you move to such an area, within a few years you are prone to develop allergies to plants and other offenders in the new location.

Section 50.2

Exercising Tips for People with Allergies

Exercise is an important activity for everyone. Exercise will help people with asthma and other allergy problems.

Is exercise recommended for patients with allergies and asthma?

In general, a person with allergies or asthma is usually able to exercise. However, exercise should not be done during times of sickness. Also, no person should push beyond his or her capabilities.

An exercise program should begin carefully. It is a good idea to discuss such a program with your physician before starting.

How can symptoms during exercise be prevented?

Patients can often prevent symptoms by taking medication prior to exercising. The type of medication used depends on several factors. For example, people with hay fever might take an antihistamine tablet before exercise.

For people with asthma, an inhaler can be used before exercise to prevent asthma problems. Your physician can recommend the best medication for you to use before exercise.

If you have dust mite allergy, you may want to exercise outdoors to avoid breathing indoor dust. If you are allergic to grasses and weeds, you may want to exercise in an indoor location during certain seasons.

Exercising should be avoided in areas where there are large amounts of chemicals. For example, you should not exercise outdoors near heavy traffic areas with high levels of exhaust fumes from cars and trucks. Indoor areas with irritating odors or fumes, also, should be avoided.

What form of exercise is best for people with asthma?

For people with asthma, exercise that has stop-and-go activity tends to cause less trouble than exercise involving long periods of running. Swimming seems to be the easiest form of exercise for people with asthma.

Weather conditions also are important. Cold air and very dry air can be quite irritating to the bronchial tubes. Warm, moist air generally allows people with asthma to exercise successfully.

Special Precautions

Special precautions should be taken by people with allergy problems from insect stings. If exercising is done outdoors, people with bee-sting allergy should not wear bright-colored clothing, cologne, perfume, or lotion. They should avoid areas such as flower beds and trash cans where bees and wasps like to hide.

In addition, people with severe bee-sting allergy should:

• wear a medical warning bracelet;

• carry a syringe filled with adrenaline for emergency treatment; and

• avoid exercise locations far away from hospitals and doctors.

Section 50.3

Gardening Tips for People with Allergies

"Allergies and Gardening," Leonard P. Perry.
© 2002 University of Vermont Extension.

If you're like one in six Americans, you get some sort of seasonal allergies each year. If you're a gardener, this doesn't mean you have to suffer. Or you don't have to give up gardening during part of the season. Or you don't have to convert your landscape into silk flowers, gravel beds, and garden gnomes or plastic flamingos! Perhaps changing some gardening practices or some of your plants may be all that's needed to lessen the grief.

Most see the yellow pollen on their car in spring or summer and think, that's it. But this relatively big, showy pollen you see from trees and flowers really isn't the culprit. It's the microscopic pollen you don't see that causes allergies. This can be from deciduous trees in the spring such as oak, elm, birch, maple, ash, alder, some pines, box elder, and willow. The hardwoods especially are the culprits. Other trees, especially in warmer parts of the country (whether you live there or may be traveling there to visit gardens) include cedar, cottonwood, hickory, mulberry, olive, palm, and pecan.

Trees with showy flowers, just as with flowers, tend to be pollinated by bees, butterflies, or similar, so have larger pollen which doesn't blow around and cause allergies. Examples of low- or no-allergen trees include many of the fruit trees such as apples, crabapples, cherries, pear, plum, and others in warmer climates such as dogwoods and magnolias.

Shrubs to avoid include many junipers and in warmer climates cypress and privet. Hydrangea, azaleas, and viburnum are okay, as are the boxwood and hibiscus in warmer climates.

In his book *Allergy-free Gardening,* author Thomas Ogren attributes many of our allergies to recent changes in our landscapes, particularly the planting of male trees and shrubs. We often do this to avoid messy fruit from female trees, but end up, as a result, with

513

more pollen. He even advocates sex-changes in trees—grafting a female top onto existing trunks of male trees. He has also developed and advocates using the Ogren Plant Allergy Scale, rating plants from 1 (low) to 10 (high) for pollen and allergies.

As with the woody plants, those herbaceous plants with showy flowers are generally okay and include many such as daffodil, tulip, daisies, geranium, impatiens, iris, lilies, pansies, petunias, roses, sunflowers, zinnias, and many more. Some flowers with strong scents may also aggravate allergies, even if they normally have larger pollen.

Most lawn grasses don't cause problems as they are mowed often and not allowed to set seed. But some can cause problems if allowed to go to seed, including perennial rye, fescue, and Bermuda in warmer climates.

Of course weeds are often the most allergenic plants. One ragweed plant can produce up to one billion pollen grains, and they have been tracked over 400 miles away. Others include pigweed and Russian thistle. A couple perennials are falsely accused of allergies, as they bloom at the same time as ragweed. You see the goldenrod and Helen's flower (alias "sneezeweed") and think these are the enemy, while it is really the ragweed lurking in the background.

Plants and pollen are the only allergy producers in the garden. Molds cause allergies in some people and children and can be produced from composts and decomposing bark mulch. If you or family members are allergic to molds, consider buying finished compost, not making it at home. And you may want to replace bark mulch, shredded leaves, cocoa hulls, or similar organic material with pebbles or even just clean cultivation. I prefer to quickly get plants established, so they cover the bed and leave no room or light for weed seeds to germinate (well, at least fewer seeds).

Here are 13 gardening practices you might change to reduce sneezing and itchy and runny noses—and still be able to garden:

- Limit gardening in the afternoon in spring, and early mornings in fall, when pollen counts tend to be highest.

- Remain indoors during windy days and during allergic pollen times, as pollen can blow in from far away (even though it is otherwise quite local in nature, such as from a tree in your yard).

- Once done working outdoors, wash well or shower and wash clothes.

- Don't hang laundry on the line during high pollen periods. (I learned this last year, hanging bed sheets on the line to dry, then wondering why I keep sneezing all night even indoors with the windows closed.)

- Use an air conditioner if you have one, particularly at night or while driving, and set on recirculate if possible.

- Beware of, and wash, pets that might pick up pollen outdoors and share with you.

- Cover bodies with clothing, even caps for hair and breathing masks, especially if mowing. It's best to have someone not allergic do the mowing.

- Keep windows closed during, and a few hours after, mowing.

- Begin allergy medication prior to your normal allergy season, follow directions through the season, and if severe consult a doctor or allergist.

- Choose low-allergen producing plants to begin with or to replace others in your landscape. Remember in general to avoid wind-pollinated plants, choosing insect-pollinated plants instead. Choose those with showy flowers, whether woody or herbaceous.

- Possibly avoid strongly scented flowers, as these may aggravate allergies.

- Beware of molds from compost and bark mulches, possibly substituting the latter with gravel.

- Avoid hedges, which can trap dust, pollen, and mold. Keep existing ones thinned.

For more information, you may wish to consult the book *Allergy-free Gardening* by Thomas Ogren. Websites with useful information are those of the American Lung Association, the American Academy of Allergy, Asthma and Immunology, and the Intellicast weather site among others. These and more can be found through a search on an internet search engine such as Google. Also keep watch in your local daily broadcast and print media during the season for pollen counts and garden when the counts are lower.

Chapter 51

Preventing Allergic Reactions away from Home

Chapter Contents

Section 51.1

Day-Care Settings Are a
Significant Source of Indoor Allergens

From the National Institute of Environmental Health Sciences
(www.niehs.nih.gov), part of the National Institutes of Health,
June 1, 2005.

Researchers studying day care facilities in the South have found the facilities to be a significant source for indoor allergen levels. A new study of 89 day care settings in two central North Carolina counties found detectable levels of seven common allergens from fungus, cats, cockroaches, dogs, dust mites, and mice in each facility tested. The levels were similar to those found in Southern homes.

"Because children spend a significant portion of time in day care settings, it is important that parents understand the risks of allergen exposure and know where these allergens can be found," said David A. Schwartz, M.D., the new Director of the National Institute of Environmental Health Sciences (NIEHS), the part of the National Institutes of Health that supported the study. The study will be available online in the *Journal of Allergy and Clinical Immunology* on June 1, 2005.

According to the U.S. Census Bureau, 63 percent of children under five spend 37 hours per week in child care. Exposure to indoor allergens has been shown in previous studies to increase the likelihood of developing asthma or allergic diseases, especially in vulnerable children.

Both licensed family day care homes and child care centers are represented in the study. The researchers used a three-pronged data collection approach to evaluate allergens in each care facility, including administering a questionnaire to each manager, observing the room where the children spent most of their time, and collecting dust samples from that room.

Dust was collected from up to four, one square meter areas of floor on both carpet and hard surfaces. Twenty facilities had dust collected from both surfaces.

Detectable levels of each allergen were found in every facility where dust samples were collected. Concentrations were the highest for allergens from cats, dogs, and a fungus known as *Alternaria*.

"Interestingly, similar to other studies, dog and cat allergens were detected in nearly all the facilities tested, although no dog or cat was observed in most," said Samuel Arbes, Ph.D., a NIEHS researcher and lead author on the study. "It is likely the pet allergens are brought in on the children's clothing."

The study also found significant differences between carpeted and non-carpeted surfaces. Concentrations for five of the allergens were lower on the non-carpeted surfaces.

The researchers compared the day care allergen levels to concentrations found in Southern homes collected previously as part of the National Survey of Lead and Allergens in Housing (NSLAH). The NSLAH collected samples from 831 homes representing various regions and settings across the country. Five of the seven allergen levels were statistically similar with only one of two dust mite allergens and mouse allergen being slightly higher in the NSLAH.

"The similarities in allergen levels between the day care centers and Southern home living rooms means children and the day care workers may be getting prolonged exposure to allergens," said Dr. Arbes. "More research needs to be conducted to determine the effects of allergen exposures outside of the home."

NIEHS, a component of the National Institutes of Health, supports research to understand the effects of the environment on human health. For more information about indoor allergens and other environmental health topics, please visit the NIEHS website at http://www.niehs.nih.gov.

Section 51.2

Choosing Child Care for Children with Allergies

"Childcare Center: What Parents Need to Know," reprinted courtesy of Allergy & Asthma Network Mothers of Asthmatics (AANMA), 800-878-4403, www.breatherville.org. The date of this document is unknown. Reviewed by David A. Cooke, M.D., January 5, 2007.

Looking for a child-care provider who understands the special needs of little ones with allergies and asthma?

Whether you need child-care services for an hour or by the week, with patience and a strategic plan, you can find quality child-care services.

Allergies and asthma are serious, potentially life-threatening conditions. Chronic ear infections can impact your baby's language development and learning skills. Eczema, hives, rashes, coughing, excess mucus—these and related conditions and symptoms present special challenges in the child-care setting.

While every child-care provider should be certified to perform CPR (cardiopulmonary resuscitation) in the event your child's heart stops beating, there is no certification program for child-care providers to know **your** child's special health needs.

That's because asthma and allergies wear a thousand different changing faces. It's like living at the base of a smoldering volcano; you don't know when the next eruption will send you running for help.

So what can you do as parents and child-care providers?

Start by identifying the health needs of the child during the hours he or she is away from home. Create a strategy that allows your child room to explore his boundaries without risking his or her health.

Provide a smoke- and pet-free environment and reduce or eliminate exposures to known food allergens preventively.

Parents and child-care providers must coordinate the child's needs as a team. It takes extra effort, time, and attention for all parties to ensure the baby's health needs are met while parents are at work.

Moms and dads need to organize medications as well as diapers, bottles, and food. If the nebulizer travels to and from the child-care center and home, both parents have to remember to put it in the car.

Child-care providers may need to remind parents to refill medications or replace nebulizer supplies periodically. They'll need to remember to tell mom or dad any early warning signs they may have noticed during the day—almost in the same manner as remembering to tell the parents that their baby is learning to share or speak a second language.

Section 51.3

Travel Tips for People with Allergies

"Flying with a Food Allergy," © 2006. Used with permission from The Food Allergy & Anaphylaxis Network (FAAN).

Flying with a Peanut Allergy

Individuals with peanut allergy often worry about reactions occurring on board commercial flights. A published study showed that severe, or anaphylactic, reactions caused by peanuts occurred on such flights from ingestion of peanut-containing food. Other reactions from exposure via skin contact or inhalation were generally less severe.

Many peanut-allergic individuals have safely flown without incident. It is always important, however, to exercise caution while flying and to have emergency medication available. Airlines are required to have epinephrine as part of their emergency medical kits, but flight attendants may not be properly trained to administer the medicine to a passenger. Generally, the flight crew will ask if there is a doctor or other type of medical professional on board the flight who would be willing to respond to the passenger's needs.

The Food Allergy & Anaphylaxis Network (FAAN) recommends that you talk with your physician, and assess the risks involved in your specific case. Below are current policies, tips, and strategies to help you take reasonable precautions and enjoy your trip.

Current Airline Policies regarding Peanut Snacks

To avoid possible inhalation or skin contact reactions due to large numbers of people opening their peanut snacks, most peanut-allergic passengers are well-advised to fly on one of the following airlines that don't serve peanut snacks: American, United, Northwest, Jet Blue, Spirit, AirTran, US Airways, America West, and ATA.

Continental continues to serve peanuts and makes no accommodations for peanut-allergic passengers. Delta and its related carrier, Delta Shuttle, now serve a choice of five snacks, including a peanut snack on many of their flights. Delta Connection serves some of those choices, but passengers cannot find out in advance which ones will be served. Delta also provides a peanut-free buffer zone. Alaska Airlines/Horizon Air serves peanuts but, according to its website, will also provide peanut-free buffer zones.

Southwest, long noted for its peanut-related advertising, "will make every attempt not to serve packaged peanuts" upon request. The longer the lead time you give an airline, the more likely that it will be able to honor any special requests.

The international carriers that do not serve peanut snacks include Aer Lingus, Al Italia, and British Air.

Flying with a Tree Nut Allergy

FAAN receives many questions from those allergic to tree nuts. The most common question is which airlines don't serve tree nuts? AirTran is the only airline that doesn't serve tree nuts at any time. Some airlines only serve them in first class (United), others in snacks sold on board (Northwest), and still others only at certain times of the year (Jet Blue). To find out for sure, ask the customer service representative who books your ticket.

Chapter 52

Choosing Skin-Safe Cosmetics

What are cosmetics? How are they different from over-the-counter (OTC) drugs?

Cosmetics are put on the body to:

- cleanse it;
- make it beautiful;
- make it attractive; or
- change its appearance or the way it looks.

Cosmetic products include:

- skin creams;
- lotions;
- perfumes;
- lipsticks;
- fingernail polishes;
- eye and face makeup products;
- permanent waves;
- hair dyes;

Excerpted from "Cosmetics and Your Health," a publication of the National Women's Health Information Center (www.4women.gov), part of the National Institutes of Health, November 2004.

- toothpastes; and
- deodorants.

Unlike drugs, which are used to treat or prevent disease in the body, cosmetics do not change or affect the body's structure or functions.

What's in cosmetics?

Fragrances and preservatives are the main ingredients in cosmetics. Fragrances are the most common cause of skin problems. More than 5,000 different kinds are used in products. Products marked "fragrance-free" or "without perfume" means that no fragrances have been added to make the product smell good.

Preservatives in cosmetics are the second most common cause of skin problems. They prevent bacteria and fungus from growing in the product and protect products from damage caused by air or light. But preservatives can also cause the skin to become irritated and infected. Some examples of preservatives are:

- paraben;
- imidazolidinyl urea;
- Quaternium-15;
- DMDM [1,3-dimethylol-5,5-dimethyl] hydantoin;
- phenoxyethanol; and
- formaldehyde.

The ingredients below cannot be used, or their use is limited, in cosmetics. They may cause cancer or other serious health problems.

- bithionol
- mercury compounds
- vinyl chloride
- halogenated salicylanilides
- zirconium complexes in aerosol sprays
- chloroform
- methylene chloride
- chlorofluorocarbon propellants
- hexachlorophene

What are hypoallergenic cosmetics?

Hypoallergenic cosmetics are products that makers claim cause fewer allergic reactions than other products. Women with sensitive skin, and even those with "normal" skin, may think these products will be gentler. But there are no federal standards for using the term hypoallergenic. The term can mean whatever a company wants it to mean. Cosmetic makers do not have to prove their claims to the FDA.

Some products that have "natural" ingredients can cause allergic reactions. If you have an allergy to certain plants or animals, you could have an allergic reaction to cosmetics with those things in them. For example, lanolin from sheep wool is found in many lotions. But it's a common cause of allergies, too.

Are tattoos and permanent makeup safe?

FDA is looking into the safety of tattoos and permanent makeup since they are now more popular. The inks, or dyes, used for tattoos are color additives. Right now, no color additives have been approved for tattoos, including those used in permanent makeup.

You should be aware of these risks of tattoos and permanent makeup:

- Tattoo needles and supplies can transmit diseases, such as hepatitis C and HIV. Be sure all needles and supplies are sterile before they are used on you.

- Tattoos and permanent makeup are not easy to take off. Removal may cause a permanent change in color.

- Think carefully before getting a tattoo. You could have an allergic reaction.

- You cannot make blood donations for a year after getting a tattoo or permanent makeup.

Are cosmetic products with alpha hydroxy acids safe?

Alpha hydroxy acids (AHAs) come from fruit and milk sugars. They are found in many creams and lotions. Many people buy products with AHAs, because they claim to reduce wrinkles, spots, sun-damaged skin, and other signs of aging. Some studies suggest they may work.

But are these products safe? FDA has received reports of reactions in people using AHA products. Their complaints include:

- severe redness;
- swelling (especially in the area of the eyes);
- burning;
- blistering;
- bleeding;
- rash;
- itching; and
- skin discoloration.

AHAs may also increase your skin's risk of sunburn. To find out if a product contains an AHA, look on the list of ingredients. By law, all cosmetics have ingredients on their outer label. AHAs may be called other names, like glycolic acid and lactic acid.

What precautions should I follow when using AHA products?

If you want to use AHA products, follow these safety tips:

- Always protect your skin before going out during the day. Use a sunscreen with a SPF (sun protection factor) of at least 15. Wear a hat with a brim. Cover up with lightweight, loose-fitting, long-sleeved shirts, and pants.
- Buy products with good label information:
  - a list of ingredients to see which AHA or other chemical acids are in the product
  - the name and address of the maker
  - a statement about the product's AHA and pH levels

The first two have to be on the label. The third is one is by choice. You can call or write the maker to find about a product's AHA and pH levels.

- Buy only products with an AHA level of 10 percent or less and a pH of 3.5 or more.
- Test a small area of skin to see if it is sensitive to any AHA product before using a lot of it.

- Stop using the product right away if you have a reaction, such as stinging, redness, or bleeding.

- Talk with your doctor or dermatologist (a doctor that treats skin problems) if you have a problem.

Are hair dyes safe?

The decision to change your hair color may be a hard one. Some studies have linked hair dyes with a higher risk of certain cancers, while other studies have not found this link. Most hair dyes also don't have to go through safety testing that other cosmetic color additives do before hitting store shelves. Women are often on their own trying to figure out whether hair dyes are safe.

When hair dyes first came out, the main ingredient in coal-tar hair dye caused allergic reactions in some people. Most hair dyes are now made from petroleum sources. But FDA still considers them to be coal-tar dyes. This is because they have some of the same compounds found in these older dyes.

Cosmetic makers have stopped using things known to cause cancer in animals. For example, 4-methoxy-m-phenylenediamine (4MMPD) or 4-methoxy-m-phenylenediamine sulfate (4MMPD sulfate) is no longer used. But chemicals made almost the same way have replaced some of the cancer-causing compounds. Some experts feel that these newer ingredients aren't very different from the things they're replacing.

Experts suggest that you may reduce your risk of cancer by using less hair dye over time. You may also reduce your risk by not dyeing your hair until it starts to gray.

What precautions should I take when I dye my hair?

You should follow these safety tips when dyeing your hair:

- Don't leave the dye on your head any longer than needed.

- Rinse your scalp thoroughly with water after use.

- Wear gloves when applying hair dye.

- Carefully follow the directions in the hair dye package.

- Never mix different hair dye products.

- Be sure to do a patch test for allergic reactions before applying the dye to your hair. Almost all hair dye products include instructions for doing a patch test. It's important to do this each time you dye your hair. Your hairdresser should also do the patch test before dyeing your hair. To test, put a dab of hair dye behind your ear, and don't wash it off for two days. If you don't have any signs of allergic reaction, such as itching, burning, or redness at the test spot, you can be somewhat sure that you won't have a reaction to the dye applied to your hair. If you do react to the patch test, do the same test with different brands or colors until you find one to which you're not allergic.

- Never dye your eyebrows or eyelashes. An allergic reaction to dye could cause swelling or increase risk of infection in the eye area. This can harm the eye and even cause blindness. Spilling dye into the eye by accident could also cause permanent damage. FDA bans the use of hair dyes for eyelash and eyebrow tinting or dyeing even in beauty salons.

Are lead acetates safe in hair dyes?

Lead acetate is used as a color additive in "progressive" hair dye products. These products are put on over a period of time to produce a gradual coloring effect. You can safely use these products if you follow the directions carefully. This warning statement must appear on the product labels of lead acetate hair dyes: "Caution: Contains lead acetate. For external use only. Keep this product out of children's reach. Do not use on cut or abraded scalp. If skin irritation develops, discontinue use. Do not use to color mustaches, eyelashes, eyebrows, or hair on parts of the body other than the scalp. Do not get in eyes. Follow instructions carefully and wash hands thoroughly after use."

Part Seven

Additional Help and Information

Chapter 53

Glossary of Terms Related to Allergies

acute: Symptoms or signs that begin and worsen quickly; not chronic.

adrenal gland: A gland located on each kidney that secretes hormones regulating metabolism, sexual function, water balance, and stress.

adrenaline: A hormone and neurotransmitter. Also called epinephrine.

allergen: Any substance that causes an allergic reaction. Examples include pollen, molds, and certain foods.

allergenic: Describes a substance that produces an allergic reaction.

allergic response: A hypersensitive immune reaction to a substance that normally is harmless or would not cause an immune response in everyone. An allergic response may cause harmful symptoms such as itching or inflammation or tissue injury.

allergic salute: In a child, persistent upward rubbing of the nose that causes a crease mark on the nose.

allergic shiners: Dark circles under the eyes caused by increased blood flow near the sinuses.

This glossary contains terms excerpted from glossaries and documents produced by the following government agencies: Centers for Disease Control and Prevention (CDC); National Cancer Institute (NCI); National Institute of Allergy and Infectious Diseases (NIAID); National Institute of Environmental Health Sciences (NIEHS); and the U.S. Food and Drug Administration.

allergy: A harmful response of the immune system to normally harmless substances.

alternative medicine: Practices used instead of standard treatments. They generally are not recognized by the medical community as standard or conventional medical approaches. Alternative medicine includes dietary supplements, megadose vitamins, herbal preparations, special teas, acupuncture, massage therapy, magnet therapy, spiritual healing, and meditation.

amino acids: Any of the 26 building blocks of proteins.

anaphylaxis: A violent allergic reaction involving a number of parts of the body simultaneously. Like less serious allergic reactions, anaphylaxis usually occurs after a person is exposed to an allergen to which he or she was sensitized by previous exposure (that is, it does not usually occur the first time a person eats a particular food). Although any food can trigger anaphylaxis (also known as anaphylactic shock), peanuts, tree nuts, shellfish, milk, eggs, and fish are the most common culprits.

angioedema: Tissue swelling.

antibiotic: A drug used to treat infections caused by bacteria and other microorganisms.

antibodies: Molecules (also called immunoglobulins) produced by a B cell in response to an antigen. When an antibody attaches to an antigen, it helps the body destroy or inactivate the antigen.

antigen: A substance or molecule that is recognized by the immune system. The molecule can be from foreign material such as bacteria or viruses.

antihistamine: A type of drug that blocks the action of histamines, which can cause fever, itching, sneezing, a runny nose, and watery eyes. Antihistamines are used to prevent fevers in patients receiving blood transfusions and to treat allergies, coughs, and colds.

anti-inflammatory: Having to do with reducing inflammation.

antimicrobial: A substance that kills microorganisms such as bacteria or mold or stops them from growing and causing disease.

asthma: A chronic disease in which the bronchial airways in the lungs become narrowed and swollen, making it difficult to breathe. Symptoms include wheezing, coughing, tightness in the chest, shortness of breath, and rapid breathing. An attack may be brought on by pet hair, dust, smoke, pollen, mold, exercise, cold air, or stress.

autoantibodies: Antibodies that react against a person's own tissue.

autoimmune disease: Disease that results when the immune system mistakenly attacks the body's own tissues. Examples include multiple sclerosis, type 1 diabetes, rheumatoid arthritis, and systemic lupus erythematosus.

B cells: Small white blood cells crucial to the immune defenses. Also know as B lymphocytes, they come from bone marrow and develop into blood cells called plasma cells, which are the source of antibodies.

bacteria: Microscopic organisms composed of a single cell. Some cause disease.

basophils: White blood cells that contribute to inflammatory reactions. Along with mast cells, basophils are responsible for the symptoms of allergy.

biological response modifiers: Substances, either natural or synthesized, that boost, direct, or restore normal immune defenses. They include interferons, interleukins, thymus hormones, and monoclonal antibodies.

blood vessels: Arteries, veins, and capillaries that carry blood to and from the heart and body tissues.

bone marrow: Soft tissue located in the cavities of the bones. Bone marrow is the source of all blood cells.

bronchi: The large air passages that lead from the trachea (windpipe) to the lungs.

bronchial: Having to do with the bronchi, which are the larger air passages of the lungs, including those that lead from the trachea (windpipe) to the lungs and those within the lungs.

bronchiole: A tiny branch of air tubes in the lungs.

bronchitis: Inflammation (swelling and reddening) of the bronchi.

bronchodilator: A type of drug that causes small airways in the lungs to open up. Bronchodilators are inhaled and are used to treat breathing disorders, such as asthma or emphysema.

Celiac disease: A digestive disease that is caused by an immune response to a protein called gluten, which is found in wheat, rye, barley, and oats. Celiac disease damages the lining of the small intestine and interferes with the absorption of nutrients from food. A person with celiac disease may become malnourished no matter how much food is consumed.

chemokines: Certain proteins that stimulate both specific and general immune cells and help coordinate immune responses and inflammation.

chronic: A disease or condition that persists or progresses over a long period of time.

clinical: Having to do with the examination and treatment of patients.

complement: A complex series of blood proteins whose action "complements" the work of antibodies. Complement destroys bacteria, produces inflammation, and regulates immune reactions.

complement cascade: A precise sequence of events, usually triggered by antigen-antibody complexes, in which each component of the complement system is activated in turn.

complementary medicine: Practices often used to enhance or complement standard treatments. They generally are not recognized by the medical community as standard or conventional medical approaches. Complementary medicine may include dietary supplements, megadose vitamins, herbal preparations, special teas, acupuncture, massage therapy, magnet therapy, spiritual healing, and meditation.

complete blood count (CBC): A test to check the number of red blood cells, white blood cells, and platelets in a sample of blood. Also called blood cell count.

conjunctivitis: Inflammation of the lining of the eyelid, causing red-rimmed, swollen eyes, and crusting of the eyelids.

corticosteroid: Any steroid hormone made in the adrenal cortex (the outer part of the adrenal gland). They are also made in the laboratory. Corticosteroids have many different effects in the body, and are used to treat many different conditions. They may be used as hormone replacement, to suppress the immune system, and to treat some side effects of cancer and its treatment.

cortisone: A natural steroid hormone produced in the adrenal gland. It can also be made in the laboratory. Cortisone reduces swelling and can suppress immune responses.

cytokines: Powerful chemical substances secreted by cells that enable the body's cells to communicate with one another. Cytokines include lymphokines produced by lymphocytes and monokines produced by monocytes and macrophages.

deoxyribonucleic acid (DNA): The molecules inside cells that carry genetic information and pass it from one generation to the next.

dermatitis: Inflammation of the skin.

dermis: The lower or inner layer of the two main layers of tissue that make up the skin.

diagnosis: The process of identifying a disease by the signs and symptoms.

dust mite: Microscopic organisms that live in the dust found in all dwellings and workplaces. Dust mites are perhaps the most common cause of perennial allergic rhinitis. House dust mite allergy usually produces symptoms similar to pollen allergy and also can produce symptoms of asthma.

eczema: A group of conditions in which the skin becomes inflamed, forms blisters, and becomes crusty, thick, and scaly. Eczema causes burning and itching, and may occur over a long period of time. Atopic dermatitis is the most common type of eczema.

ELISA: Enzyme-linked immunosorbent assay. A blood test used to check for allergies.

enzyme: A protein produced by living cells that promotes the chemical processes of life without itself being altered.

eosinophils: White blood cells that contain granules filled with chemicals damaging to parasites, and enzymes that affect inflammatory reactions.

epinephrine: A hormone and neurotransmitter. Also called adrenaline.

epithelial cells: Cells making up the epithelium, the covering for internal and external body surfaces.

extract: Concentrated liquid preparation containing minute parts of specific foods.

family history: A record of a person's current and past illnesses, and those of his or her parents, brothers, sisters, children, and other family members. A family history shows the pattern of certain diseases in a family, and helps to determine risk factors for those and other diseases.

food challenge: Health care providers use food challenges to diagnose food allergy. This testing has come to be the "gold standard" of allergy testing. The health care provider will give a person individual opaque capsules containing various foods, some of which are suspected of starting an allergic reaction. The person swallows a capsule and is watched to see if a reaction occurs. The advantage of such a challenge is that if the person reacts only to suspected foods and not to other foods tested, it confirms the diagnosis.

food intolerance: Unlike food allergy, the problem is not with the body's immune system, but, rather, with its metabolism. The body cannot adequately digest a portion of the offending food, usually because of some chemical deficiency. For example, persons who have difficulty digesting milk (lactose intolerance) often are deficient in the intestinal enzyme lactase, which is needed to digest milk sugar (lactose). The deficiency can cause cramps and diarrhea if milk is consumed.

fungus: A plant-like organism that does not make chlorophyll. Mushrooms, yeasts, and molds are examples. The plural is fungi.

gastrointestinal (GI) tract: Area of the body that includes the stomach and intestines.

genes: Units of genetic material that carry the directions a cell uses to perform a specific function.

granules: Small particles; in cells the particles typically include enzymes and other chemicals.

granulocytes: Phagocytic white blood cells filled with granules organisms. Neutrophils, eosinophils, basophils, and mast cells are examples of granulocytes.

hay fever: Pollen allergy. Pollen is made by trees, grasses, and weeds. During the spring, summer, and fall some plants release pollen into the air. Symptoms may include sneezing, runny or clogged nose, coughing, itchy eyes, nose and throat, watery eyes, and red, swollen eyes.

helper T cells (Th cells): A subset of T cells that carry the CD4 surface marker and are essential for turning on antibody production, activating cytotoxic T cells, and initiating many other immune functions.

histamine: Substance present in certain foods that causes a reaction like an allergic reaction. For example, histamine can reach high levels in cheese, some wines, and certain kinds of fish such as tuna and mackerel.

hygiene: The science of health, and the practice of cleanliness that promotes good health and well-being.

hypersensitivity: An exaggerated response by the immune system to a drug or other substance.

idiopathic: Describes a disease of unknown cause.

immune response: The activity of the immune system against foreign substances (antigens).

immune system: A complex network of specialized cells, tissues, and organs that defends the body against attacks by disease-causing organisms.

immunoglobulins: A family of large protein molecules, also known as antibodies, produced by B cells.

immunology: The study of the body's immune system.

immunosuppressive: Capable of reducing immune responses.

immunotherapy: Treatment to stimulate or restore the ability of the immune system to fight cancer, infections, and other diseases (such as allergies). Also called biological therapy, biotherapy, biological response modifier therapy, and BRM therapy.

inflammation: Redness, swelling, pain, and/or a feeling of heat in an area of the body. This is a protective reaction to injury, disease, or irritation of the tissues.

inflammatory response: Redness, warmth, and swelling produced in response to infection, as the result of increased blood flow and an influx of immune cells and secretions.

injectable epinephrine: A synthetic version of a naturally occurring hormone also known as adrenaline. For treatment of an anaphylactic reaction, it is injected directly into a thigh muscle or vein. It works directly on the cardiovascular and respiratory systems, causing rapid constriction of blood vessels, reversing throat swelling, relaxing lung muscles to improve breathing, and stimulating the heartbeat.

interferons: Proteins produced by cells that stimulate antivirus immune responses or alter the physical properties of immune cells.

latex: The product manufactured from a milky fluid derived from the rubber tree, *Hevea brasiliensis*. Several types of synthetic rubber are also referred to as latex, but these do not release the proteins that cause allergic reactions.

latex allergy: An allergic reaction to certain proteins in latex rubber.

leukocytes: All white blood cells.

lymph nodes: Small bean-shaped organs of the immune system, distributed widely throughout the body and linked by lymphatic vessels. Lymph nodes are garrisons of B, T, and other immune cells.

lymph: A transparent, slightly yellow fluid that carries lymphocytes, bathes the body tissues, and drains into the lymphatic vessels.

lymphatic vessels: A body-wide network of channels, similar to the blood vessels, which transport lymph to the immune organs and into the bloodstream.

lymphocytes: Small white blood cells produced in the lymphoid organs and paramount in the immune defenses. B cells and T cells are lymphocytes.

lymphoid organs: The organs of the immune system, where lymphocytes develop and congregate. They include the bone marrow, thymus, lymph nodes, spleen, and various other clusters of lymphoid tissue. Blood vessels and lymphatic vessels are also lymphoid organs.

lymphokines: Powerful chemical substances secreted by lymphocytes. These molecules help direct and regulate the immune responses.

macrophage: A large and versatile immune cell that devours invading pathogens and other intruders. Macrophages stimulate other immune cells by presenting them with small pieces of the invaders.

mast cell: A granulocyte found in tissue. The contents of mast cells, along with those of basophils, are responsible for the symptoms of allergy.

memory cells: A subset of T cells and B cells that have been exposed to antigens and can then respond more readily when the immune system encounters those same antigens again.

microbes: Microscopic living organisms, including bacteria, viruses, fungi, and protozoa, which sometimes cause disease.

microorganisms: Microscopic organisms, including bacteria, virus, fungi, plants, and parasites.

mold: Part of the fungus family. Molds are made of many cells that grow as branching threads called hyphae. The seeds or reproductive pieces of fungi are called spores. Spores differ in size, shape, and color among types of mold. Each spore that germinates can give rise to new mold growth, which in turn can produce millions of spores.

molecule: The smallest amount of a specific chemical substance. Large molecules such as proteins, fats, carbohydrates, and nucleic acids are the building blocks of a cell, and a gene determines how each molecule is produced.

monoclonal antibodies: Antibodies produced by a single cell or its identical progeny, specific for a given antigen. As tools for binding to specific protein molecules, they are invaluable in research, medicine, and industry.

monocytes: Large phagocytic white blood cells which, when entering tissue, develop into macrophages.

monokines: Powerful chemical substances secreted by monocytes and macrophages. These molecules help direct and regulate the immune responses.

multiple chemical sensitivities syndrome (MCSS): Also known as idiopathic environmental intolerance (IEI), which can be defined as a chronic, recurring disease caused by a person's inability to tolerate an environmental chemical or class of foreign chemicals.

natural killer (NK) cells: Large granule-containing lymphocytes that recognize and kill cells lacking self antigens. Their target recognition molecules are different from T cells.

neutrophil: White blood cell that is an abundant and important phagocyte.

nutritionist: A health professional with special training in nutrition who can help with dietary choices. Also called a dietitian.

ophthalmic: Having to do with the eye.

organism: An individual living thing.

parasites: Plants or animals that live, grow, and feed on or within another living organism.

pathogen: A disease-causing organism.

phagocytes: Large white blood cells that contribute to the immune defenses by ingesting microbes or other cells and foreign particles.

phagocytosis: Process by which one cell engulfs another cell or large particle.

plasma cells: Large antibody-producing cells that develop from B cells.

pollen: Tiny round or oval grains produced when plants reproduce. In some species, the plant uses the pollen from its own flowers to fertilize itself. The types of pollen that most commonly cause allergic reactions are produced by the plain-looking plants (trees, grasses, and weeds) that do not have showy flowers.

polyp: A growth that protrudes from a mucous membrane.

RAST: Radioallergosorbent test. A blood test used to test for allergies.

rhinitis: Inflammation of the nasal passages, which can cause a runny nose.

sinuses: Sinuses are hollow air spaces, or cavities, in the human body. These cavities, located within the skull or bones of the head surrounding the nose, include frontal sinuses over the eyes in the brow area; maxillary sinuses inside each cheekbone; ethmoid sinuses just behind the bridge of the nose and between the eyes; and sphenoid sinuses behind the ethmoids in the upper region of the nose and behind the eyes.

sinusitis: Sinusitis means the sinuses are infected or inflamed. Health expert classify sinusitis as acute, which last for 4 weeks or less; subacute, which lasts 4 to 8 weeks; chronic, which usually last up to 8 weeks but can continue for months or even years; or recurrent, which are several acute attacks within a year, and may be caused by different organisms.

spleen: A lymphoid organ in the abdominal cavity that is an important center for immune system activities.

sputum: Matter ejected from the lungs and windpipe through the mouth.

stem cells: Immature cells from which all cells derive. The bone marrow is rich in stem cells, which become specialized blood cells.

sulfites: Sulfites, a food additive, are used primarily as antioxidants to prevent or reduce discoloration of light-colored fruits and vegetables, such as dried apples and potatoes, and to inhibit the growth of microorganisms in fermented foods such as wine.

T cells: Small white blood cells (also known as T lymphocytes) that recognize antigen fragments bound to cell surfaces by specialized antibody-like receptors. "T" stands for thymus, where T cells acquire their receptors.

thymus: A primary lymphoid organ, high in the chest, where T lymphocytes proliferate and mature.

tissues: Groups of similar cells joined to perform the same function.

tolerance: A state of immune nonresponsiveness to a particular antigen or group of antigens.

tonsils and adenoids: Prominent oval masses of lymphoid tissues on either side of the throat.

toxins: Poisonous agents produced by plants and bacteria, normally very damaging to human cells.

trigger: In medicine, a specific event that starts a process or that causes a particular outcome. For example, in allergies, exposure to mold, pollen, or dust may trigger sneezing, watery eyes, and coughing.

upper respiratory tract: Area of the body which includes the nasal passages, mouth, and throat.

urticaria: Hives.

vaccine therapy: A type of treatment that uses a substance or group of substances to stimulate the immune system to destroy a tumor or infectious microorganisms such as bacteria or viruses.

vaccines: Preparations that stimulate an immune response that can prevent an infection or create resistance to an infection. They do not cause disease.

viruses: Microorganisms composed of a piece of genetic material—RNA or DNA—surrounded by a protein coat. Viruses can reproduce only in living cells.

Chapter 54

Directory of Government and Private Resources That Provide Information about Allergies and Immunology

Government Agencies That Provide Information about Allergies

Centers for Disease Control and Prevention
National Institute for Occupational Safety and Health
1600 Clifton Road
Atlanta, GA 30333
Toll-Free: 800-311-3435
Phone: 404-639-3311
Website: www.cdc.gov/niosh
E-mail: cdcinfo@cdc.gov

Healthfinder®
U.S. Department of Health and Human Services
P.O. Box 1133
Washington, DC 20013-1133
Website: www.healthfinder.gov
E-mail: healthfinder@nhic.org

Indoor Air Quality Information Clearinghouse
Environmental Protection Agency
P.O. Box 37133
Washington DC 20013-7133
Toll-Free: 800-438-4318
Fax: 703-356-5386
Website: www.epa.gov/iaq/iaqxline.html
E-mail: iaqinfo@aol.com

Resources in this chapter were compiled from several sources deemed reliable; all contact information was verified and updated in December 2006.

543

National Cancer Institute
Cancer Information Service
6116 Executive Boulevard
Room 3036A
Bethesda, MD 20892-8322
Toll-Free: 800-4-CANCER
(422-6237)
TTY Toll-Free: 800-332-8615
Website: www.cancer.gov
E-mail:
cancergovstaff@mail.nih.gov

***National Center for
Complementary and
Alternative Medicine***
NCCAM Clearinghouse
P.O. Box 7923
Gaithersburg, MD 20898-7923
Toll-Free: 888-644-6226
Phone: 301-519-3153
TTY: 866-464-3615
Website: nccam.nih.gov
E-mail: info@nccam.nih.gov

***National Center for Health
Statistics***
3311 Toledo Road
Hyattsville, MD 20782
Toll-Free: 866-441-NCHS
(441-6247)
Phone: 301-458-4000
Phone: 301-458-4636
Website: www.cdc.gov/nchs
E-mail: nchsquery@cdc.gov

***National Digestive Diseases
Information Clearinghouse***
2 Information Way
Bethesda, MD 20892-3570
Toll-Free: 800-891-5389
Fax: 703-738-4929
Website: digestive.niddk.nih.gov
E-mail: nddic@info.niddk.nih.gov

***National Heart, Lung, and
Blood Institute Health
Information Center***
P.O. Box 30105
Bethesda, MD 20824-0105
Phone: 301-592-8573
TTY: 240-629-3255
Fax: 240-629-3246
Website: www.nhlbi.nih.gov
E-mail: nhlbiinfo@nhlbi.nih.gov

***National Institute of
Allerg   d Infectious
Diseas   (NIAID)***
6610 Rockledge Drive, MSC 6612
Bethesda, MD 20892-6612
Phone: 301-496-5717
TDD: 800-877-8339
Fax: 301-402-3573
Website: www3.niaid.nih.gov

***National Institute of
Arthritis and Musculo-
skeletal and Skin Diseases***
1 AMS Circle
Bethesda, Maryland 20892-3675
Toll-Free: 877-22-NIAMS
(226-4267)
Phone: 301-495-4484
TTY: 301-565-2966
Fax: 301-718-6366
Website: www.niams.nih.gov
E-mail: niamsinfo@mail.nih.gov

National Institute of Environmental Health Sciences
P.O. Box 12233
Research Triangle Park
NC 27709
Phone: 919-541-3345
TTY: 919-541-0731
Website: www.niehs.nih.gov
E-mail:
webcenter@niehs.nih.gov

National Institute on Aging
Building 31C, Room 5C27
31 Center Drive, MSC 2292
Bethesda, MD 20892
Publications Toll-Free:
800-222-2225
Phone: 301-496-1752
TTY: 800-222-4225
Fax: 301-496-1072
Website: www.nia.nih.gov
Publications Website: www
.niapublications.org
E-mail: niainfo@nia.nih.gov

National Institutes of Health
9000 Rockville Pike
Bethesda, MD 20892
Phone: 301-496-4000
TTY: 301-402-9612
Website: www.nih.gov
E-mail: NIHinfo@od.nih.gov

National Institutes of Health Clinical Trials
National Library of Medicine
8600 Rockville Pike
Bethesda, MD 20894
Toll-Free: 888-346-3656
Phone: 301-594-5983
Fax: 301-496-2809
Website: www.clinicaltrials.gov

National Women's Health Information Center
8270 Willow Oaks Corporate Dr.
Fairfax, VA 22031
Toll-Free: 800-994-WOMAN
(994-9662)
TTY: 888-220-5446
Website: www.4woman.gov

U.S. Department of Agriculture
1400 Independence Ave., S.W.
Washington, DC 20250
Website: www.usda.gov

U.S. Department of Health and Human Services
200 Independence Avenue, S.W.
Washington, DC 20201
Toll-Free: 877-696-6775
Phone: 202-619-0257
Website: www.hhs.gov

U.S. Food and Drug Administration
5600 Fishers Lane
HFE-50
Rockville, MD 20857-0001
Toll-Free: 888-463-6332
Phone: 301-827-4420
Fax: 301-443-9767
Website: www.fda.gov

U.S. National Library of Medicine
8600 Rockville Pike
Bethesda, MD 20894
Toll-Free: 888-346-3656
Phone: 301-594-5983
Website: www.nlm.nih.gov
E-mail: custserv@nlm.nih.gov

Private Organizations That Provide Information about Allergies

AllergicChild.com
425 W Rockrimmon Blvd.
Suite 202
Colorado Springs, CO 80919
Website: www.allergicchild.com

Allergic Living
2100 Bloor Street West
Suite 6-168
Toronto, Ontario M6S 5A5
Canada
Phone: 416-604-0110
Toll-Free: 888-771-7747
Website: www.allergicliving.com
E-mail: info@allergicliving.com

Allergy and Asthma Network Mothers of Asthmatics
2751 Prosperity Avenue
Suite 150
Fairfax, VA 22031
Toll-Free: 800-878-4403
Fax: 703-573-7794
Website: www.aanma.org

Allergy Asthma Information Association
Vaughan Professional Centre
1-111 Zenway Boulevard
Vaughan, ON L4H 3H9
Canada
Toll-Free: 800-611-7011
Phone: 905-265-3322
Fax: 905-850-2070
Website: www.aaia.ca

Allergy Society of South Africa
P.O. Box 88
Observatory 7935
Cape Town
South Africa
Phone: +27 21 447 9019
Fax: +27 21 448 0846
Website: www.allergysa.org
E-mail: harris@zingsolutions.com

Allergy UK
3 White Oak Square
London Road
Swanley, Kent BR8 7AG
United Kingdom
Helpline: +13 22 619898
Fax: +13 22 663480
Website: www.allergyuk.org
E-mail: info@allergyuk.org

American Academy of Allergy, Asthma, and Immunology
555 East Wells Street, Suite 1100
Milwaukee, WI 53202-3823
Toll-Free: 800-822-2762
Phone: 414-272-6071
Fax: 414-272-6070
General Website: www.aaaai.org
National Allergy Bureau:
www.aaaai.org/nab/index.cfm
E-mail: info@aaaai.org

American Academy of Dermatology
P.O. Box 4014
Schaumburg, IL 60618-4014
Toll-Free: 866-503-SKIN
(503-7546)
Phone: 847-240-1280
Website: www.aad.org
E-mail: MRC@aad.org

American Academy of Family Physicians
11400 Tomahawk Creek Pkwy.
Leawood, KS 66211-2672
Toll-Free: 800-274-2237
Phone: 913-906-6000
Website: www.aafp.org
E-mail: fp@aafp.org

American Academy of Ophthalmology
P.O. Box 7424
San Francisco, CA 94120-7424
Phone: 415-561-8500
Fax: 415-561-8533
Website: www.aao.org

American Academy of Otolaryngic Allergy
1990 M Street, NW, Suite 680
Washington, DC 20036
Phone: 202-955-5010
Fax: 202-955-5016
Website: www.aaoaf.org

American Academy of Otolaryngology-Head and Neck Surgery
One Prince Street
Alexandria, VA 22314-3357
Phone: 703-836-4444
Website: www.entnet.org

American Academy of Pediatrics
141 Northwest Point Boulevard
Elk Grove Village, IL, 60007
Phone: 847-434-4000
Fax: 847-434-8000
Website: www.aap.org
E-mail: kidsdocs@aap.org

American Association for Clinical Chemistry
1850 K Street, NW Suite 625
Washington, DC 20006
Toll-Free: 800-892-1400
Phone: 202-857-0717
Fax: 202-887-5093
Websites: www.aacc.org;
www.labtestsonline.org

American Association for Respiratory Care
9425 N. MacArthur Blvd.
Suite 100
Irving, TX 75063-4706
Phone: 972-243-2272
Fax: 972-484-2720
Website: www.aarc.org
E-mail: info@aarc.org

American Association of Immunologists
9650 Rockville Pike
Bethesda, MD 20814
Phone: 301-634-7178
Fax: 301-634-7887
Website: www.aai.org
E-mail: infoaai@aai.org

American Board of Allergy and Immunology
111 S. Independence Mall East
Suite 701
Philadelphia, PA 19106
Toll-Free: 866-264-5568
Phone: 215-592-9466
Fax: 215-592-9411
Website: www.abai.org
E-mail: abai@abai.org

American College of Allergy, Asthma and Immunology
85 West Algonquin Road
Suite 550
Arlington Heights, IL 60005
Phone: 847-427-1200
Fax: 847-427-1294
Website: www.acaai.org
E-mail: mail@acaai.org

American College of Chest Physicians
3300 Dundee Road
Northbrook, IL 60062-2348
Toll-Free: 800-343-2227
Phone: 847-498-1400
Fax: 847-498-5460
Website: www.chestnet.org

American College of Emergency Physicians
1125 Executive Circle
Irving, TX 75038-2522
Toll-Free: 800-798-1822
Phone: 972-550-0911
Fax: 972-580-2816
Website: www.acep.org

American Dietetic Association
120 South Riverside Plaza
Suite 2000
Chicago, IL 60606-6995
Toll-Free: 800-877-1600
Website: www.eatright.org
E-mail: knowledge@eatright.org

American Latex Allergy Association
P.O. Box 198
Slinger, WI 53086
Toll-Free: 888-972-5378
Website: www
.latexallergyresources.org
E-mail:
alert@latexallergyresources.org

American Lung Association
61 Broadway, 6th Floor
New York, NY 10006
Toll-Free: 800-LUNGUSA
(586-4872)
Helpline: 800-548-8252
Phone: 212-315-8700
Website: www.lungusa.org

American Medical Association/Medem
649 Mission Street, 2nd Floor
San Francisco, CA 94105
Toll-Free: 877-926-3336
Phone: 415-644-3800
Fax: 415-644-3950
Website: www.medem.com
E-mail: info@medem.com

American Osteopathic College of Allergy and Immunology
7025 E. McDowell Road
Suite 1B
Scottsdale, AZ 85257
Phone: 480-585-1580

American Partnership for Eosinophilic Disorders (APFED)
3419 Whispering Way Drive
Richmond, TX 77469
Phone: 713-498-8216
Website: www.apfed.org
E-mail: mail@apfed.org

American Rhinologic Society
9 Sunset Terrace
Warwick, NY 10990
Phone: 845-988-1631
Fax: 845-986-1527
Website: www.
american-rhinologic.org
E-mail:
arsinfo@american-rhinologic.org

American Thoracic Society
61 Broadway
New York, NY 10006-2755
Phone: 212-315-8600
Fax: 212-315-6498
Website: www.thoracic.org

Anaphylaxis Campaign
P.O. Box 275
Farnborough GU14 6SX
United Kingdom
Phone: +12 52 546100
Helpline: +12 52 542029
Fax: +12 52 377140
Website:
www.anaphylaxis.org.uk
E-mail: info@anaphylaxis.org.uk

Asthma and Allergy Foundation of America
1233 20th Street, NW
Suite 402
Washington, DC 20036
Toll-Free: 800-727-8462
Website: www.aafa.org
E-mail: info@aafa.org

Canadian Food Inspection Agency
59 Camelot Drive
Ottawa, Ontario K1A 0Y9
Canada
Phone: 613-225-2342
Toll-Free: 1-800-442-2342
Website: www.inspection.gc.ca
E-mail:
cfiamaster@inspection.gc.ca

Cleveland Clinic
9500 Euclid Avenue
Cleveland, OH 44195
Toll-Free: 800-223-2273
Phone: 216-444-2200
TTY: 216-444-0261
Website:
www.clevelandclinic.org

European Federation of Asthma and Allergy Associations
Avenue Louise 327
1050 Brussels
Belgium
Phone: +32 2 646 9945
Fax: +32 2 646 4116
Website: www.efanet.org
E-mail: info@efanet.org

Food Allergy and Anaphylaxis Network
11781 Lee Jackson Highway
Suite 160
Fairfax, VA 22033-3309
Toll-Free: 800-929-4040
Fax: 703-691-2713
Website: www.foodallergy.org
E-mail: faan@foodallergy.org

Food Allergy Initiative
1414 Avenue of the Americas,
Suite 1804
New York, NY 10019
Phone: 212-207-1974
Fax: 212-572-8429
Website:
www.foodallergyinitiative.org
E-mail:
info@foodallergyinitiative.org

Immune Deficiency Foundation
40 W. Chesapeake Avenue
Suite 308
Towson, MD 21204
Toll-Free: 800-296-4433
Phone: 410-321-6647
Fax: 410-321-9165
Website:
www.primaryimmune.org
E-mail: idf@primaryimmune.org

International Food Information Council
1100 Connecticut Avenue, NW,
Suite 430
Washington, DC 20036
Phone: 202-296-6540
Fax: 202-296-6547
Website: www.ific.org
E-mail: foodinfo@ific.org

Joint Council of Allergy, Asthma and Immunology
50 North Brockway, Suite 3-3
Palatine, IL 60067
Phone: 847-934-1918
Website: www.jcaai.org
E-mail: info@jcaai.org

Kidswithfoodallergies.org
73 Old Dublin Pike
Suite 10, #163
Doylestown, PA 18901
Phone: 215-230-5394
Fax: 215-340-7674
Website:
www.kidswithfoodallergies.org

Mayo Foundation for Medical Education and Research
200 First Street SW
Rochester, MN 55905
Website: www.mayoclinic.com
E-mail:
comments@mayoclinic.com

National Air Filtration Association
P.O. Box 68639
Virginia Beach, VA 23471
Phone: 757-313-7400
Fax: 757-497-1895
Website: www.nafahq.org
E-mail: nafa@nafahq.org

National Eczema Association for Science and Education
4460 Redwood Hwy., Suite 16-D
San Rafael, CA 94903-1953
Toll-Free: 800-818-7546
Phone: 415-499-3474
Fax: 415-472-5345
Website:
www.nationaleczema.org
E-mail: info@nationaleczema.org

National Eczema Society
Hill House
Highgate Hill
London N19 5NA
United Kingdom
Phone: +20 7281 3553
Helpline: +0870 241 3604
Fax: +20 7281 6395
Website: www.eczema.org
E-mail: helpline@eczema.org

National Jewish Medical and Research Center
1400 Jackson Street
Denver, CO 80206
Toll-Free: 800-222-LUNG (222-5864)
Phone: 303-388-4461
Website: www.njc.org

Nemours Foundation Center for Children's Health Media
1600 Rockland Road
Wilmington, DE 19803
Phone: 302-651-4000
Fax: 302-651-4055
Website: www.kidshealth.org
E-mail: info@kidshealth.org

Practical Allergy Research Foundation
P.O. Box 60
Buffalo, NY 14223
Toll-Free: 800-787-8780
Phone: 805-356-2109
Fax: 805-650-0524
Website: www.drrapp.com

Safe4Kids
Website: www.safe4kids.ca

SchoolAsthmaAllergy.com
Schering-Plough
3070 Route 22 West
Branchburg, NJ 08876
Website:
www.schoolasthmaallergy.com
E-mail:
editor@schoolasthmaallergy.com

University of Pittsburgh Medical Center Eye & Ear Institute
200 Lothrop Street
Pittsburgh, PA 15213
Phone: 412-647-2345
Website: eyeandear.upmc.com

World Allergy Organization
555 East Wells Street
Suite 1100
Milwaukee, WI 53202-3823
Phone: 414-276-1791
Fax: 414-276-3349
Website: www.worldallergy.org
E-mail: info@worldallergy.org

Chapter 55

Additional Reading for People with Allergies and Their Families

Books about Allergies

Allergy Self-Help Cookbook: Over 325 Natural Foods Recipes, Free of All Common Food Allergens, Revised Edition. By Marjorie Hurt Jones, January 2001. ISBN: 157954276X.

Asthma and Allergy Action Plan for Kids: A Complete Program to Help Your Child Live a Full and Active Life. By Allen J. Dozor and Kate Kelly, April 2004. ISBN: 064173316X.

Caring for Your Child with Severe Food Allergies: Emotional Support and Practical Advice from a Parent Who's Been There. By Lisa Cipriano Collins, January 2000. ISBN: 047134785X.

Complete Peanut Allergy Handbook. By Scott H. Sicherer and Terry Malloy, August 2005. ISBN: 0425204413.

Dairy-Free Cookbook: Over 250 Recipes For People With Lactose Intolerance Or Milk Allergy, Revised Edition. By Jane Zukin, May 1998. ISBN: 0761514678.

Resources listed in this chapter were compiled from several sources. Inclusion does not constitute endorsement. This list is not considered complete; it is merely intended to serve as a starting point for readers interested in pursuing additional information. Websites were verified and accessed in January 2007.

Food Allergies and Food Intolerance: The Complete Guide to Their Identification and Treatment. By Jonathan Brostoff and Linda Gamlin, May 2000. ISBN: 0892818751.

Gluten-Free Kitchen: Over 135 Delicious Recipes for People with Gluten Intolerance or Wheat Allergy. By Roben Ryberg, April 2000. ISBN: 0761522727.

Kid Friendly Food Allergy Cookbook. By Leslie Hammond and Lynne Marie Rominger, February 2004. ISBN: 1592330541.

Let's Eat out!: Your Passport to Living Gluten and Allergy Free. By Kim M. Koeller and Robert La France, September 2005. ISBN: 0976484501.

Mold Survival Guide: For Your Home and for Your Health. By Jeffrey C. May and Connie L. May, April 2004. ISBN: 0801879388.

My House Is Killing Me!: The Home Guide for Families with Allergies and Asthma. By Jeffrey C. May and Jonathan M. Samet, October 2001. ISBN: 0801867304.

Parent's Guide to Food Allergies: Clear and Complete Advice from the Experts on Raising Your Food Allergic Child. By Marianne S. Barber, Maryanne Bartoszek Scott, and Elinor Greenberg, January 2001. ISBN: 0805066004.

Peanut Allergy Answer Book. By Michael C. Young, August 2006. ISBN: 1592332331.

Understanding and Managing Your Child's Food Allergies. By Scott H. Sicherer, November 2006. ISBN: 0801884926.

What Your Doctor May Not Tell You about Children's Allergies and Asthma: Simple Steps to Help Stop Attacks and Improve Your Child's Health. By Paul Ehrlich and Larry Chiaramonte, October 2003. ISBN: 0446679887.

Whole Foods Allergy Cookbook: 200 Gourmet & Homestyle Recipes for the Food Allergic Family. By Cybele Pascal, September 2005. ISBN: 1890612456.

Magazines, Journals, and Newsletters That Publish Information about Allergies

Allergology International
http://ai.jsaweb.jp

Allergy
http://www.blackwellpublishing.com/journal.asp?ref=0105-4538

Allergy & Asthma ADVOCATE: *A Patient Newsletter of the American Academy of Allergy, Asthma and Immunology*
http://www.aaaai.org/patients/advocate/

Allergy & Clinical Immunology International: *Journal of the World Allergy Organization*
http://verlag.hanshuber.com/ezm/index.php?ezm=ACI&la=e

Annals of Allergy, Asthma and Immunology: *The official publication of the American College of Allergy, Asthma, & Immunology*
http://caliban.annallergy.org/vl=9330690/cl=12/nw=1/rpsv/home.htm

Anti-Inflammatory & Anti-Allergy Agents in Medicinal Chemistry
http://bentham.org/cmcaiaa/index.htm

Asthma and Allergy Proceedings
http://www.ingentaconnect.com/content/ocean/aap

Chronicle of Skin & Allergy
http://skin.chronicle.ca

Clinical and Experimental Allergy
http://www.blackwellpublishing.com/journal.asp?ref=0954-7894&site=1

Clinical and Molecular Allergy
http://www.clinicalmolecularallergy.com/home/

Clinical Reviews in Allergy & Immunology
http://www.clinicalmolecularallergy.com/home/

Current Allergy and Asthma Reports
http://www.current-reports.com/home_journal.cfm?JournalID=AL

Current Opinion in Allergy and Clinical Immunology
http://www.co-allergy.com

FreshAAIR: A Newsletter by the Asthma and Allergy Foundation of America
http://www.aafa.org/subscribe.cfm?item=freshaair

Immunology and Allergy Clinics of North America
http://www.us.elsevierhealth.com/product.jsp?isbn=08898561

International Archives of Allergy and Immunology
http://content.karger.com/ProdukteDB/
produkte.asp?Aktion=JournalHome&ProduktNr=224161&ContentOnly
=false

Internet Journal of Asthma, Allergy and Immunology
http://www.ispub.com/ostia/index.php?xmlFilePath=journals/ijaai/
front.xml

Journal of Allergy and Clinical Immunology
http://journals.elsevierhealth.com/periodicals/ymai

Journal of Asthma
http://journalsonline.tandf.co.uk/(su2xt355flgp1r55ku5gnaze)/app/
home/journal.asp?referrer=parent&backto=linkingpublication
results,1:107839,1&linkin=

Pediatric Allergy and Immunology
http://journals.elsevierhealth.com/periodicals/ymai

Pediatric Asthma, Allergy & Immunology
http://www.liebertpub.com/publication.aspx?pub_id=48

Skin & Allergy News
http://www.sdefderm.com/SkinAllergyLink.aspx

Year Book of Allergy, Asthma and Clinical Immunology
http://www.us.elsevierhealth.com/product.jsp?isbn=10829776

Organizations That Provide Referrals to Allergists

American Academy of Allergy, Asthma & Immunology
Toll-Free: 800-822-2762
Phone: 414-272-6071
Website: www.aaaai.org
E-mail: info@aaaai.org

American College of Allergy, Asthma & Immunology
Phone: 847-427-1200
Website: www.acaai.org
E-mail: mail@acaai.org

Pollen Counts and Maps

National Allergy Bureau
Phone: 414-272-6071
Website: www.aaaai.org/nab/index.cfm

Index

Index

Page numbers followed by 'n' indicate a footnote. Page numbers in *italics* indicate a table or illustration.

cold remedies, described 447
cold therapy
  eczema 187
  urticaria 124
colophony, facial contact
  dermatitis 136
combination medications
  described 446–47
  side effects *447*
complement
  defined 534
  described 9–10
complementary medicine, defined 534
  see also alternative medicine
complement cascade
  defined 534
  described 10
complement proteins, described 10
complete blood count (CBC)
  allergies 427
  defined 534
"Complications of Nasal and Sinus
  Surgery" (American Rhinologic
  Society) 111n
computed axial tomography scan
  (CAT scan; CT scan), fungal
  sinusitis 99
congestion, described 446
conjunctivitis, defined 534
Contac 446
contact dermatitis
  defined 128
  described 413
  overview 128–34
  statistics 17
  see also facial contact dermatitis
"Contact Dermatitis" (World Allergy
  Organization) 128n
"Contact Dermatitis: Sometimes It's
  In Your Face" (American Academy
  of Dermatology) 135n
contact eczema, described 149
Cooke, David A. 24n, 31n, 65n, 81n,
  94n, 141n, 217n, 276n, 278n, 285n,
  372n, 398n, 405n, 467n, 520n
COPD *see* chronic obstructive
  pulmonary disease
Co-Pyronil 446
corn allergy 222

corticosteroids
  adverse effects *75*
  allergic conjunctivitis 119
  atopic dermatitis 156–57
  contact dermatitis 134
  defined 534
  described 73
  eczema 169, 184–85
  facial contact dermatitis 137
  overview 449–53
  pregnancy 472
  recommended dosages *453*
  urushiol 143–44
"Corticosteroids" (Asthma
  and Allergy Foundation of
  America) 449n
cortisone
  defined 535
  described 449
cosmetics
  facial contact dermatitis 136
  overview 523–28
"Cosmetics and Your Health"
  (National Women's Health
  Information Center) 523n
cow milk allergy
  children 40
  food labels 303–4
  infants 231–34
Creticos, Peter 356
Crixivan (indinavir) 191
Crohn disease, hygiene
  hypothesis 62–63
cromolyn
  allergic rhinitis 74, *75*, 436, 439
  non-sedating property 68
  pregnancy concerns 472, 473
  sinus problems 96
cromolyn sodium 347
cross contamination
  egg allergy 226
  food labels 310–12
  school lunches 327
  seafood allergy 250–51
  wheat allergy 258
cross reactions
  children 41–42
  food allergy 205, 222
crustaceans *see* seafood allergy

intoxication syndrome, described 381
intracellular parasites, described 11
intracutaneous skin tests, described
   422
intranasal influenza vaccine 230
"Introducing Cereal to Infants:
   Delaying Past 6 Months May
   Increase the Risk of Allergy"
   (Nemours Foundation) 316n
ipratropium 471–72
irritant contact dermatitis
   described 128
   symptoms 129
irritational syndromes,
   described 381
"Is It a Cold or an Allergy?"
   (NIAID) 331n
Isoclor 447
isoetharine 471
isoniazid 191
Isoptin (verapamil) 191
"The Itch That Won't Quit"
   (American Academy of
   Dermatology) 138n
itraconazole 191

J

Johnson, Christine C. 48
Johnson, Steven B. 392n
Joint Council of Allergy, Asthma
   and Immunology, contact
   information 551
*Journal of Allergy and Clinical
   Immunology*, website address 556
Journal of Asthma, website address
   556

K

keratosis pilaris, atopic
   dermatitis 150
ketoconazole 191
Kidswithfoodallergies.org,
   contact information 551
killer T cells, described 8
   see also natural killer cells

kinins, allergic rhinitis 73
Ko, Hon-Sum 142
Kugathasan, Subra 61–64

L

lactose intolerance
   blood test 427
   described 207, 536
Langerhans cells, atopic
   dermatitis 162–63
Lanier, Bobby 22–23
laser therapy, described 163
latex allergy
   defined 538
   described 16
   overview 405–7
latex, defined 538
lead acetate, safety concerns 528
Lebwohl, Mark 178–80
Leeder, Steve 384n
legislation
   Americans with Disabilities
      Act 484–87
   EpiPens 481
   food labels 300, 313–14
   sulfites 280–81
leukocytes, defined 538
leukotriene antagonists, asthma
   treatment 438
leukotrienes
   allergic reaction 334
   allergic rhinitis 73
Levaquin 440
lichenification, atopic dermatitis
   150
"Looking for Relief? New Treatments
   Successfully Target Biology Behind
   Common Skin Conditions"
   (American Academy of
   Dermatology) 178n
loratadine 67, 74, 75, 76, 473
   see also Claritin
Luvox (fluvoxamine) 191
lymphatic vessels
   defined 538
   described 4–5
lymph, defined 538

577

terbutaline 471
tests
    allergies 20–21, 341–42, 417–20
    allergists 414
    chemical sensitivity 383–84
    childhood food allergy 323
    contact dermatitis 132–33
    eczema 165, 174
    ELISA (enzyme-linked
        immunosorbent assay)
        defined 535
    eosinophilic esophagitis 291–93
    food allergies 209–11, 215, 219–20
    food challenge
        defined 536
        described 430–33
    immunotherapy 456
    milk allergy 232–33
    nut allergies 238
    ragweed allergy 353–54
    RAST (radioallergosorbent test) 540
    sulfites 280
Th cells *see* helper T cells
theophylline 471, 474
thiurams, allergic contact
    dermatitis 130–31
thrush (oral candidiasis)
    inhaled corticosteroids 450
    nasal steroids 436
thymus
    defined 541
    described 4
thyroid disease, urticaria 127
Tiazac (diltiazem) 191
Tilade (nedocromil) 472
Tilex 497–98
TIM *see* topical immunomodulators
tissues, defined 541
tissue transplantation, antigens 4
T lymphocytes *see* T cells
tobacco smoke, described 494
    see also environmental
        tobacco smoke
tolerance, defined 541
tonsils
    defined 541
    described 6
topical immunomodulators
    (TIM) 178–79

Tornalate (bitolterol) 471
toxins, defined 541
travel concerns
    childhood food allergy 326
    peanut allergy 521–22
    sinusitis 93
tree nut allergies
    children 40–41, 325
    food labels 307–8
    oral allergy syndrome 285–88
    overview 236–46
    statistics 17
triamcinolone 472, 473
triamcinolone acetonide *83*, *453*
Triaminic 447
triggers
    allergic conjunctivitis 116
    atopic dermatitis 155–56
    avoidance 25
    childhood allergies 38
    defined 541
    eczema 165
    home allergies 492–96
    migraine headache 97
    outdoor 508–15
trimethoprim-sulfamethoxazole 109
Trinalin 447
Tri-Nasal (triamcinolone)
    81, *83*, 473
tripelennamine 473
troleandomycin 191
Trottier, Marie 485–86
Turbuhaler, recommended
    dosages *453*
Turvey, Stuart E. 464
Twinject 480
tyramine, migraine headache 97

U

"Understanding the Immune System:
    How It Works" (NIAID) 3n
Uniphyl 440
University of Pittsburgh Medical
    Center Eye and Ear Institute,
    contact information 552
University of Texas, insect sting
    allergies publication 394n

Health Reference Series
COMPLETE CATALOG

List price $87 per volume. **School and library price $78 per volume.**

Adolescent Health Sourcebook, 2nd Edition

Basic Consumer Health Information about the Physical, Mental, and Emotional Growth and Development of Adolescents, Including Medical Care, Nutritional and Physical Activity Requirements, Puberty, Sexual Activity, Acne, Tanning, Body Piercing, Common Physical Illnesses and Disorders, Eating Disorders, Attention Deficit Hyperactivity Disorder, Depression, Bullying, Hazing, and Adolescent Injuries Related to Sports, Driving, and Work

Along with Substance Abuse Information about Nicotine, Alcohol, and Drug Use, a Glossary, and Directory of Additional Resources

Edited by Joyce Brennfleck Shannon. 683 pages. 2006. 978-0-7808-0943-7.

"It is written in clear, nontechnical language aimed at general readers. . . . Recommended for public libraries, community colleges, and other agencies serving health care consumers."
— *American Reference Books Annual, 2003*

"Recommended for school and public libraries. Parents and professionals dealing with teens will appreciate the easy-to-follow format and the clearly written text. This could become a 'must have' for every high school teacher." — *E-Streams, Jan '03*

"A good starting point for information related to common medical, mental, and emotional concerns of adolescents." — *School Library Journal, Nov '02*

"This book provides accurate information in an easy to access format. It addresses topics that parents and caregivers might not be aware of and provides practical, useable information."
— *Doody's Health Sciences Book Review Journal, Sep-Oct '02*

"Recommended reference source."
— *Booklist, American Library Association, Sep '02*

AIDS Sourcebook, 3rd Edition

Basic Consumer Health Information about Acquired Immune Deficiency Syndrome (AIDS) and Human Immunodeficiency Virus (HIV) Infection, Including Facts about Transmission, Prevention, Diagnosis, Treatment, Opportunistic Infections, and Other Complications, with a Section for Women and Children, Including Details about Associated Gynecological Concerns, Pregnancy, and Pediatric Care

Along with Updated Statistical Information, Reports on Current Research Initiatives, a Glossary, and Directories of Internet, Hotline, and Other Resources

Edited by Dawn D. Matthews. 664 pages. 2003. 978-0-7808-0631-3.

"The 3rd edition of the *AIDS Sourcebook*, part of Omnigraphics' *Health Reference Series*, is a welcome update. . . . This resource is highly recommended for academic and public libraries."
— *American Reference Books Annual, 2004*

"Excellent sourcebook. This continues to be a highly recommended book. There is no other book that provides as much information as this book provides."
— *AIDS Book Review Journal, Dec-Jan '00*

"Recommended reference source."
— *Booklist, American Library Association, Dec '99*

Alcoholism Sourcebook, 2nd Edition

Basic Consumer Health Information about Alcohol Use, Abuse, and Dependence, Featuring Facts about the Physical, Mental, and Social Health Effects of Alcohol Addiction, Including Alcoholic Liver Disease, Pancreatic Disease, Cardiovascular Disease, Neurological Disorders, and the Effects of Drinking during Pregnancy

Along with Information about Alcohol Treatment, Medications, and Recovery Programs, in Addition to Tips for Reducing the Prevalence of Underage Drinking, Statistics about Alcohol Use, a Glossary of Related Terms, and Directories of Resources for More Help and Information

Edited by Amy L. Sutton. 653 pages. 2006. 978-0-7808-0942-0.

"This title is one of the few reference works on alcoholism for general readers. For some readers this will be a welcome complement to the many self-help books on the market. Recommended for collections serving general readers and consumer health collections."
— *E-Streams, Mar '01*

"This book is an excellent choice for public and academic libraries."
— *American Reference Books Annual, 2001*

"Recommended reference source."
— *Booklist, American Library Association, Dec '00*

"Presents a wealth of information on alcohol use and abuse and its effects on the body and mind, treatment, and prevention." — *SciTech Book News, Dec '00*

"Important new health guide which packs in the latest consumer information about the problems of alcoholism." — *Reviewer's Bookwatch, Nov '00*

SEE ALSO Drug Abuse Sourcebook

Allergies Sourcebook, 3rd Edition

Basic Consumer Health Information about Allergic Disorders, Such as Anaphylaxis, Hives, Eczema, Rhinitis, Sinusitis, and Conjunctivitis, and Their Triggers, Including Pollen, Mold, Dust Mites, Animal Dander, Insects, Chemicals, Food, Food Additives, and Medications;

Along with Advice about the Diagnosis and Treatment of Allergy Symptoms, a Glossary of Related Terms, a Directory of Resources for Help and Information, and Suggestions for Additional Reading

Edited by Amy L. Sutton. 616 pages. 2007. 978-0-7808-0950-5.

"This book brings a great deal of useful material together. . . . This is an excellent addition to public and consumer health library collections." — *American Reference Books Annual, 2003*

"This second edition would be useful to laypersons with little or advanced knowledge of the subject matter. This book would also serve as a resource for nursing and other health care professions students. It would be useful in public, academic, and hospital libraries with consumer health collections." — *E-Streams, Jul '02*

■

Alternative Medicine Sourcebook

SEE Complementary & Alternative Medicine Sourcebook

■

Alzheimer's Disease Sourcebook, 3rd Edition

Basic Consumer Health Information about Alzheimer's Disease, Other Dementias, and Related Disorders, Including Multi-Infarct Dementia, AIDS Dementia Complex, Dementia with Lewy Bodies, Huntington's Disease, Wernicke-Korsakoff Syndrome (Alcohol-Related Dementia), Delirium, and Confusional States

Along with Information for People Newly Diagnosed with Alzheimer's Disease and Caregivers, Reports Detailing Current Research Efforts in Prevention, Diagnosis, and Treatment, Facts about Long-Term Care Issues, and Listings of Sources for Additional Information

Edited by Karen Bellenir. 645 pages. 2003. 978-0-7808-0666-5.

"This very informative and valuable tool will be a great addition to any library serving consumers, students and health care workers." — *American Reference Books Annual, 2004*

"This is a valuable resource for people affected by dementias such as Alzheimer's. It is easy to navigate and includes important information and resources." — *Doody's Review Service, Feb '04*

"Recommended reference source." — *Booklist, American Library Association, Oct '99*

***SEE ALSO** Brain Disorders Sourcebook*

Arthritis Sourcebook, 2nd Edition

Basic Consumer Health Information about Osteoarthritis, Rheumatoid Arthritis, Other Rheumatic Disorders, Infectious Forms of Arthritis, and Diseases with Symptoms Linked to Arthritis, Featuring Facts about Diagnosis, Pain Management, and Surgical Therapies

Along with Coping Strategies, Research Updates, a Glossary, and Resources for Additional Help and Information

Edited by Amy L. Sutton. 593 pages. 2004. 978-0-7808-0667-2.

"This easy-to-read volume is recommended for consumer health collections within public or academic libraries." — *E-Streams, May '05*

"As expected, this updated edition continues the excellent reputation of this series in providing sound, usable health information. . . . Highly recommended." — *American Reference Books Annual, 2005*

"Excellent reference." — *The Bookwatch, Jan '05*

■

Asthma Sourcebook, 2nd Edition

Basic Consumer Health Information about the Causes, Symptoms, Diagnosis, and Treatment of Asthma in Infants, Children, Teenagers, and Adults, Including Facts about Different Types of Asthma, Common Co-Occurring Conditions, Asthma Management Plans, Triggers, Medications, and Medication Delivery Devices

Along with Asthma Statistics, Research Updates, a Glossary, a Directory of Asthma-Related Resources, and More

Edited by Karen Bellenir. 609 pages. 2006. 978-0-7808-0866-9.

"A worthwhile reference acquisition for public libraries and academic medical libraries whose readers desire a quick introduction to the wide range of asthma information." — *Choice, Association of College & Research Libraries, Jun '01*

"Recommended reference source." — *Booklist, American Library Association, Feb '01*

"Highly recommended." — *The Bookwatch, Jan '01*

"There is much good information for patients and their families who deal with asthma daily." — *American Medical Writers Association Journal, Winter '01*

"This informative text is recommended for consumer health collections in public, secondary school, and community college libraries and the libraries of universities with a large undergraduate population." — *American Reference Books Annual, 2001*

■

Attention Deficit Disorder Sourcebook

Basic Consumer Health Information about Attention Deficit/Hyperactivity Disorder in Children and Adults,

Including Facts about Causes, Symptoms, Diagnostic Criteria, and Treatment Options Such as Medications, Behavior Therapy, Coaching, and Homeopathy

Along with Reports on Current Research Initiatives, Legal Issues, and Government Regulations, and Featuring a Glossary of Related Terms, Internet Resources, and a List of Additional Reading Material

Edited by Dawn D. Matthews. 470 pages. 2002. 978-0-7808-0624-5.

"Recommended reference source."
— *Booklist, American Library Association, Jan '03*

"This book is recommended for all school libraries and the reference or consumer health sections of public libraries." — *American Reference Books Annual, 2003*

■

Back & Neck Sourcebook, 2nd Edition

Basic Consumer Health Information about Spinal Pain, Spinal Cord Injuries, and Related Disorders, Such as Degenerative Disk Disease, Osteoarthritis, Scoliosis, Sciatica, Spina Bifida, and Spinal Stenosis, and Featuring Facts about Maintaining Spinal Health, Self-Care, Pain Management, Rehabilitative Care, Chiropractic Care, Spinal Surgeries, and Complementary Therapies

Along with Suggestions for Preventing Back and Neck Pain, a Glossary of Related Terms, and a Directory of Resources

Edited by Amy L. Sutton. 633 pages. 2004. 978-0-7808-0738-9.

"Recommended . . . an easy to use, comprehensive medical reference book." — *E-Streams, Sep '05*

"The strength of this work is its basic, easy-to-read format. Recommended." — *Reference and User Services Quarterly, American Library Association, Winter '97*

■

Blood & Circulatory Disorders Sourcebook, 2nd Edition

Basic Consumer Health Information about the Blood and Circulatory System and Related Disorders, Such as Anemia and Other Hemoglobin Diseases, Cancer of the Blood and Associated Bone Marrow Disorders, Clotting and Bleeding Problems, and Conditions That Affect the Veins, Blood Vessels, and Arteries, Including Facts about the Donation and Transplantation of Bone Marrow, Stem Cells, and Blood and Tips for Keeping the Blood and Circulatory System Healthy

Along with a Glossary of Related Terms and Resources for Additional Help and Information

Edited by Amy L. Sutton. 659 pages. 2005. 978-0-7808-0746-4.

"Highly recommended pick for basic consumer health reference holdings at all levels."
— *The Bookwatch, Aug '05*

"Recommended reference source."
— *Booklist, American Library Association, Feb '99*

"An important reference sourcebook written in simple language for everyday, non-technical users. "
— *Reviewer's Bookwatch, Jan '99*

■

Brain Disorders Sourcebook, 2nd Edition

Basic Consumer Health Information about Acquired and Traumatic Brain Injuries, Infections of the Brain, Epilepsy and Seizure Disorders, Cerebral Palsy, and Degenerative Neurological Disorders, Including Amyotrophic Lateral Sclerosis (ALS), Dementias, Multiple Sclerosis, and More

Along with Information on the Brain's Structure and Function, Treatment and Rehabilitation Options, Reports on Current Research Initiatives, a Glossary of Terms Related to Brain Disorders and Injuries, and a Directory of Sources for Further Help and Information

Edited by Sandra J. Judd. 625 pages. 2005. 978-0-7808-0744-0.

"Highly recommended pick for basic consumer health reference holdings at all levels."
— *The Bookwatch, Aug '05*

"Belongs on the shelves of any library with a consumer health collection." — *E-Streams, Mar '00*

"Recommended reference source."
— *Booklist, American Library Association, Oct '99*

SEE ALSO Alzheimer's Disease Sourcebook

■

Breast Cancer Sourcebook, 2nd Edition

Basic Consumer Health Information about Breast Cancer, Including Facts about Risk Factors, Prevention, Screening and Diagnostic Methods, Treatment Options, Complementary and Alternative Therapies, Post-Treatment Concerns, Clinical Trials, Special Risk Populations, and New Developments in Breast Cancer Research

Along with Breast Cancer Statistics, a Glossary of Related Terms, and a Directory of Resources for Additional Help and Information

Edited by Sandra J. Judd. 595 pages. 2004. 978-0-7808-0668-9.

"This book will be an excellent addition to public, community college, medical, and academic libraries."
— *American Reference Books Annual, 2006*

"It would be a useful reference book in a library or on loan to women in a support group."
— *Cancer Forum, Mar '03*

"Recommended reference source."
— *Booklist, American Library Association, Jan '02*

"This reference source is highly recommended. It is quite informative, comprehensive and detailed in nature, and yet it offers practical advice in easy-to-read language. It could be thought of as the 'bible' of breast cancer for the consumer." — *E-Streams, Jan '02*

"From the pros and cons of different screening methods and results to treatment options, *Breast Cancer Sourcebook* provides the latest information on the subject." — *Library Bookwatch, Dec '01*

"This thoroughgoing, very readable reference covers all aspects of breast health and cancer. . . . Readers will find much to consider here. Recommended for all public and patient health collections." — *Library Journal, Sep '01*

SEE ALSO Cancer Sourcebook for Women, Women's Health Concerns Sourcebook

■

Breastfeeding Sourcebook

Basic Consumer Health Information about the Benefits of Breastmilk, Preparing to Breastfeed, Breastfeeding as a Baby Grows, Nutrition, and More, Including Information on Special Situations and Concerns Such as Mastitis, Illness, Medications, Allergies, Multiple Births, Prematurity, Special Needs, and Adoption

Along with a Glossary and Resources for Additional Help and Information

Edited by Jenni Lynn Colson. 388 pages. 2002. 978-0-7808-0332-9.

"Particularly useful is the information about professional lactation services and chapters on breastfeeding when returning to work. . . . *Breastfeeding Sourcebook* will be useful for public libraries, consumer health libraries, and technical schools offering nurse assistant training, especially in areas where Internet access is problematic." — *American Reference Books Annual, 2003*

SEE ALSO Pregnancy & Birth Sourcebook

■

Burns Sourcebook

Basic Consumer Health Information about Various Types of Burns and Scalds, Including Flame, Heat, Cold, Electrical, Chemical, and Sun Burns

Along with Information on Short-Term and Long-Term Treatments, Tissue Reconstruction, Plastic Surgery, Prevention Suggestions, and First Aid

Edited by Allan R. Cook. 604 pages. 1999. 978-0-7808-0204-9.

"This is an exceptional addition to the series and is highly recommended for all consumer health collections, hospital libraries, and academic medical centers." — *E-Streams, Mar '00*

"This key reference guide is an invaluable addition to all health care and public libraries in confronting this ongoing health issue." —*American Reference Books Annual, 2000*

"Recommended reference source." —*Booklist, American Library Association, Dec '99*

SEE ALSO Dermatological Disorders Sourcebook

Cancer Sourcebook, 5th Edition

Basic Consumer Health Information about Major Forms and Stages of Cancer, Featuring Facts about Head and Neck Cancers, Lung Cancers, Gastrointestinal Cancers, Genitourinary Cancers, Lymphomas, Blood Cell Cancers, Endocrine Cancers, Skin Cancers, Bone Cancers, Metastatic Cancers, and More

Along with Facts about Cancer Treatments, Cancer Risks and Prevention, a Glossary of Related Terms, Statistical Data, and a Directory of Resources for Additional Information

Edited by Karen Bellenir. 1,133 pages. 2007. 978-0-7808-0947-5.

"With cancer being the second leading cause of death for Americans, a prodigious work such as this one, which locates centrally so much cancer-related information, is clearly an asset to this nation's citizens and others." — *Journal of the National Medical Association, 2004*

"This title is recommended for health sciences and public libraries with consumer health collections." — *E-Streams, Feb '01*

". . . can be effectively used by cancer patients and their families who are looking for answers in a language they can understand. Public and hospital libraries should have it on their shelves." — *American Reference Books Annual, 2001*

"Recommended reference source." — *Booklist, American Library Association, Dec '00*

SEE ALSO Breast Cancer Sourcebook, Cancer Sourcebook for Women, Pediatric Cancer Sourcebook, Prostate Cancer Sourcebook

■

Cancer Sourcebook for Women, 3rd Edition

Basic Consumer Health Information about Leading Causes of Cancer in Women, Featuring Facts about Gynecologic Cancers and Related Concerns, Such as Breast Cancer, Cervical Cancer, Endometrial Cancer, Uterine Sarcoma, Vaginal Cancer, Vulvar Cancer, and Common Non-Cancerous Gynecologic Conditions, in Addition to Facts about Lung Cancer, Colorectal Cancer, and Thyroid Cancer in Women

Along with Information about Cancer Risk Factors, Screening and Prevention, Treatment Options, and Tips on Coping with Life after Cancer Treatment, a Glossary of Cancer Terms, and a Directory of Resources for Additional Help and Information

Edited by Amy L. Sutton. 715 pages. 2006. 978-0-7808-0867-6.

"An excellent addition to collections in public, consumer health, and women's health libraries." —*American Reference Books Annual, 2003*

"Overall, the information is excellent, and complex topics are clearly explained. As a reference book for the consumer it is a valuable resource to assist them to make informed decisions about cancer and its treatments." — *Cancer Forum, Nov '02*

"Highly recommended for academic and medical reference collections." — *Library Bookwatch, Sep '02*

"This is a highly recommended book for any public or consumer library, being reader friendly and containing accurate and helpful information."
— *E-Streams, Aug '02*

"Recommended reference source."
— *Booklist, American Library Association, Jul '02*

SEE ALSO Breast Cancer Sourcebook, Women's Health Concerns Sourcebook

■

Cancer Survivorship Sourcebook

Basic Consumer Health Information about the Physical, Educational, Emotional, Social, and Financial Needs of Cancer Patients from Diagnosis, through Cancer Treatment, and Beyond, Including Facts about Researching Specific Types of Cancer and Learning about Clinical Trials and Treatment Options, and Featuring Tips for Coping with the Side Effects of Cancer Treatments and Adjusting to Life after Cancer Treatment Concludes

Along with Suggestions for Caregivers, Friends, and Family Members of Cancer Patients, a Glossary of Cancer Care Terms, and Directories of Related Resources

Edited by Karen Bellenir. 6561 pages. 2007. 978-0-7808-0985-7.

■

Cardiovascular Diseases & Disorders Sourcebook, 3rd Edition

Basic Consumer Health Information about Heart and Vascular Diseases and Disorders, Such as Angina, Heart Attacks, Arrhythmias, Cardiomyopathy, Valve Disease, Atherosclerosis, and Aneurysms, with Information about Managing Cardiovascular Risk Factors and Maintaining Heart Health, Medications and Procedures Used to Treat Cardiovascular Disorders, and Concerns of Special Significance to Women

Along with Reports on Current Research Initiatives, a Glossary of Related Medical Terms, and a Directory of Sources for Further Help and Information

Edited by Sandra J. Judd. 713 pages. 2005. 978-0-7808-0739-6.

"This updated sourcebook is still the best first stop for comprehensive introductory information on cardiovascular diseases."
— *American Reference Books Annual, 2006*

"Recommended for public libraries and libraries supporting health care professionals."
— *E-Streams, Sep '05*

"This should be a standard health library reference."
— *The Bookwatch, Jun '05*

"Recommended reference source."
— *Booklist, American Library Association, Dec '00*

". . . comprehensive format provides an extensive overview on this subject."
— *Choice, Association of College & Research Libraries*

■

Caregiving Sourcebook

Basic Consumer Health Information for Caregivers, Including a Profile of Caregivers, Caregiving Responsibilities and Concerns, Tips for Specific Conditions, Care Environments, and the Effects of Caregiving

Along with Facts about Legal Issues, Financial Information, and Future Planning, a Glossary, and a Listing of Additional Resources

Edited by Joyce Brennfleck Shannon. 600 pages. 2001. 978-0-7808-0331-2.

"Essential for most collections."
— *Library Journal, Apr 1, 2002*

"An ideal addition to the reference collection of any public library. Health sciences information professionals may also want to acquire the *Caregiving Sourcebook* for their hospital or academic library for use as a ready reference tool by health care workers interested in aging and caregiving." — *E-Streams, Jan '02*

"Recommended reference source."
— *Booklist, American Library Association, Oct '01*

■

Child Abuse Sourcebook

Basic Consumer Health Information about the Physical, Sexual, and Emotional Abuse of Children, with Additional Facts about Neglect, Munchausen Syndrome by Proxy (MSBP), Shaken Baby Syndrome, and Controversial Issues Related to Child Abuse, Such as Withholding Medical Care, Corporal Punishment, and Child Maltreatment in Youth Sports, and Featuring Facts about Child Protective Services, Foster Care, Adoption, Parenting Challenges, and Other Abuse Prevention Efforts

Along with a Glossary of Related Terms and Resources for Additional Help and Information

Edited by Dawn D. Matthews. 620 pages. 2004. 978-0-7808-0705-1.

"A valuable and highly recommended resource for school, academic and public libraries whether used on its own or as a starting point for more in-depth research." — *E-Streams, Apr '05*

"Every week the news brings cases of child abuse or neglect, so it is useful to have a source that supplies so much helpful information. . . . Recommended. Public and academic libraries, and child welfare offices."
— *Choice, Association of College & Research Libraries, Mar '05*

"Packed with insights on all kinds of issues, from foster care and adoption to parenting and abuse prevention."
— *The Bookwatch, Nov '04*

SEE ALSO: Domestic Violence Sourcebook

Childhood Diseases & Disorders Sourcebook

Basic Consumer Health Information about Medical Problems Often Encountered in Pre-Adolescent Children, Including Respiratory Tract Ailments, Ear Infections, Sore Throats, Disorders of the Skin and Scalp, Digestive and Genitourinary Diseases, Infectious Diseases, Inflammatory Disorders, Chronic Physical and Developmental Disorders, Allergies, and More

Along with Information about Diagnostic Tests, Common Childhood Surgeries, and Frequently Used Medications, with a Glossary of Important Terms and Resource Directory

Edited by Chad T. Kimball. 662 pages. 2003. 978-0-7808-0458-6.

"This is an excellent book for new parents and should be included in all health care and public libraries."
—*American Reference Books Annual, 2004*

SEE ALSO: *Healthy Children Sourcebook*

Colds, Flu & Other Common Ailments Sourcebook

Basic Consumer Health Information about Common Ailments and Injuries, Including Colds, Coughs, the Flu, Sinus Problems, Headaches, Fever, Nausea and Vomiting, Menstrual Cramps, Diarrhea, Constipation, Hemorrhoids, Back Pain, Dandruff, Dry and Itchy Skin, Cuts, Scrapes, Sprains, Bruises, and More

Along with Information about Prevention, Self-Care, Choosing a Doctor, Over-the-Counter Medications, Folk Remedies, and Alternative Therapies, and Including a Glossary of Important Terms and a Directory of Resources for Further Help and Information

Edited by Chad T. Kimball. 638 pages. 2001. 978-0-7808-0435-7.

"A good starting point for research on common illnesses. It will be a useful addition to public and consumer health library collections."
—*American Reference Books Annual, 2002*

"Will prove valuable to any library seeking to maintain a current, comprehensive reference collection of health resources. . . . Excellent reference."
— *The Bookwatch, Aug '01*

"Recommended reference source."
— *Booklist, American Library Association, Jul '01*

Communication Disorders Sourcebook

Basic Information about Deafness and Hearing Loss, Speech and Language Disorders, Voice Disorders, Balance and Vestibular Disorders, and Disorders of Smell, Taste, and Touch

Edited by Linda M. Ross. 533 pages. 1996. 978-0-7808-0077-9.

"This is skillfully edited and is a welcome resource for the layperson. It should be found in every public and medical library." — *Booklist Health Sciences Supplement, American Library Association, Oct '97*

Complementary & Alternative Medicine Sourcebook, 3rd Edition

Basic Consumer Health Information about Complementary and Alternative Medical Therapies, Including Acupuncture, Ayurveda, Traditional Chinese Medicine, Herbal Medicine, Homeopathy, Naturopathy, Biofeedback, Hypnotherapy, Yoga, Art Therapy, Aromatherapy, Clinical Nutrition, Vitamin and Mineral Supplements, Chiropractic, Massage, Reflexology, Crystal Therapy, Therapeutic Touch, and More

Along with Facts about Alternative and Complementary Treatments for Specific Conditions Such as Cancer, Diabetes, Osteoarthritis, Chronic Pain, Menopause, Gastrointestinal Disorders, Headaches, and Mental Illness, a Glossary, and a Resource List for Additional Help and Information

Edited by Sandra J. Judd. 657 pages. 2006. 978-0-7808-0864-5.

"Recommended for public, high school, and academic libraries that have consumer health collections. Hospital libraries that also serve the public will find this to be a useful resource." — *E-Streams, Feb '03*

"Recommended reference source."
—*Booklist, American Library Association, Jan '03*

"An important alternate health reference."
— *MBR Bookwatch, Oct '02*

"A great addition to the reference collection of every type of library." — *American Reference Books Annual, 2000*

Congenital Disorders Sourcebook, 2nd Edition

Basic Consumer Health Information about Nonhereditary Birth Defects and Disorders Related to Prematurity, Gestational Injuries, Congenital Infections, and Birth Complications, Including Heart Defects, Hydrocephalus, Spina Bifida, Cleft Lip and Palate, Cerebral Palsy, and More

Along with Facts about the Prevention of Birth Defects, Fetal Surgery and Other Treatment Options, Research Initiatives, a Glossary of Related Terms, and Resources for Additional Information and Support

Edited by Sandra J. Judd. 647 pages. 2006. 978-0-7808-0945-1.

"Recommended reference source."
— *Booklist, American Library Association, Oct '97*

SEE ALSO *Pregnancy & Birth Sourcebook*

Contagious Diseases Sourcebook

Basic Consumer Health Information about Infectious Diseases Spread by Person-to-Person Contact through

Direct Touch, Airborne Transmission, Sexual Contact, or Contact with Blood or Other Body Fluids, Including Hepatitis, Herpes, Influenza, Lice, Measles, Mumps, Pinworm, Ringworm, Severe Acute Respiratory Syndrome (SARS), Streptococcal Infections, Tuberculosis, and Others

Along with Facts about Disease Transmission, Antimicrobial Resistance, and Vaccines, with a Glossary and Directories of Resources for More Information

Edited by Karen Bellenir. 643 pages. 2004. 978-0-7808-0736-5.

"This easy-to-read volume is recommended for consumer health collections within public or academic libraries." — E-Streams, May '05

"This informative book is highly recommended for public libraries, consumer health collections, and secondary schools and undergraduate libraries."
— American Reference Books Annual, 2005

"Excellent reference." — The Bookwatch, Jan '05

Death & Dying Sourcebook, 2nd Edition

Basic Consumer Health Information about End-of-Life Care and Related Perspectives and Ethical Issues, Including End-of-Life Symptoms and Treatments, Pain Management, Quality-of-Life Concerns, the Use of Life Support, Patients' Rights and Privacy Issues, Advance Directives, Physician-Assisted Suicide, Caregiving, Organ and Tissue Donation, Autopsies, Funeral Arrangements, and Grief

Along with Statistical Data, Information about the Leading Causes of Death, a Glossary, and Directories of Support Groups and Other Resources

Edited by Joyce Brennfleck Shannon. 653 pages. 2006. 978-0-7808-0871-3.

"Public libraries, medical libraries, and academic libraries will all find this sourcebook a useful addition to their collections."
— American Reference Books Annual, 2001

"An extremely useful resource for those concerned with death and dying in the United States."
— Respiratory Care, Nov '00

"Recommended reference source."
— Booklist, American Library Association, Aug '00

"This book is a definite must for all those involved in end-of-life care." — Doody's Review Service, 2000

Dental Care & Oral Health Sourcebook, 2nd Edition

Basic Consumer Health Information about Dental Care, Including Oral Hygiene, Dental Visits, Pain Management, Cavities, Crowns, Bridges, Dental Implants, and Fillings, and Other Oral Health Concerns, Such as Gum Disease, Bad Breath, Dry Mouth, Genetic and Developmental Abnormalities, Oral Cancers, Orthodontics, and Temporomandibular Disorders

Along with Updates on Current Research in Oral Health, a Glossary, a Directory of Dental and Oral Health Organizations, and Resources for People with Dental and Oral Health Disorders

Edited by Amy L. Sutton. 609 pages. 2003. 978-0-7808-0634-4.

"This book could serve as a turning point in the battle to educate consumers in issues concerning oral health."
— American Reference Books Annual, 2004

"Unique source which will fill a gap in dental sources for patients and the lay public. A valuable reference tool even in a library with thousands of books on dentistry. Comprehensive, clear, inexpensive, and easy to read and use. It fills an enormous gap in the health care literature." — Reference & User Services Quarterly, American Library Association, Summer '98

"Recommended reference source."
— Booklist, American Library Association, Dec '97

Depression Sourcebook

Basic Consumer Health Information about Unipolar Depression, Bipolar Disorder, Postpartum Depression, Seasonal Affective Disorder, and Other Types of Depression in Children, Adolescents, Women, Men, the Elderly, and Other Selected Populations

Along with Facts about Causes, Risk Factors, Diagnostic Criteria, Treatment Options, Coping Strategies, Suicide Prevention, a Glossary, and a Directory of Sources for Additional Help and Information

Edited by Karen Bellenir. 602 pages. 2002. 978-0-7808-0611-5.

"Depression Sourcebook is of a very high standard. Its purpose, which is to serve as a reference source to the lay reader, is very well served."
— Journal of the National Medical Association, 2004

"Invaluable reference for public and school library collections alike." — Library Bookwatch, Apr '03

"Recommended for purchase."
— American Reference Books Annual, 2003

Dermatological Disorders Sourcebook, 2nd Edition

Basic Consumer Health Information about Conditions and Disorders Affecting the Skin, Hair, and Nails, Such as Acne, Rosacea, Rashes, Dermatitis, Pigmentation Disorders, Birthmarks, Skin Cancer, Skin Injuries, Psoriasis, Scleroderma, and Hair Loss, Including Facts about Medications and Treatments for Dermatological Disorders and Tips for Maintaining Healthy Skin, Hair, and Nails

Along with Information about How Aging Affects the Skin, a Glossary of Related Terms, and a Directory of Resources for Additional Help and Information

Edited by Amy L. Sutton. 645 pages. 2005. 978-0-7808-0795-2.

"... comprehensive, easily read reference book."
—*Doody's Health Sciences Book Reviews, Oct '97*

SEE ALSO *Burns Sourcebook*

∎

Diabetes Sourcebook, 3rd Edition

Basic Consumer Health Information about Type 1 Diabetes (Insulin-Dependent or Juvenile-Onset Diabetes), Type 2 Diabetes (Noninsulin-Dependent or Adult-Onset Diabetes), Gestational Diabetes, Impaired Glucose Tolerance (IGT), and Related Complications, Such as Amputation, Eye Disease, Gum Disease, Nerve Damage, and End-Stage Renal Disease, Including Facts about Insulin, Oral Diabetes Medications, Blood Sugar Testing, and the Role of Exercise and Nutrition in the Control of Diabetes

Along with a Glossary and Resources for Further Help and Information

Edited by Dawn D. Matthews. 622 pages. 2003. 978-0-7808-0629-0.

"This edition is even more helpful than earlier versions. . . . It is a truly valuable tool for anyone seeking readable and authoritative information on diabetes."
— *American Reference Books Annual, 2004*

"An invaluable reference." — *Library Journal, May '00*

Selected as one of the 250 "Best Health Sciences Books of 1999." — *Doody's Rating Service, Mar-Apr '00*

"Provides useful information for the general public."
— *Healthlines, University of Michigan Health Management Research Center, Sep/Oct '99*

". . . provides reliable mainstream medical information . . . belongs on the shelves of any library with a consumer health collection." — *E-Streams, Sep '99*

"Recommended reference source."
— *Booklist, American Library Association, Feb '99*

∎

Diet & Nutrition Sourcebook, 3rd Edition

Basic Consumer Health Information about Dietary Guidelines and the Food Guidance System, Recommended Daily Nutrient Intakes, Serving Proportions, Weight Control, Vitamins and Supplements, Nutrition Issues for Different Life Stages and Lifestyles, and the Needs of People with Specific Medical Concerns, Including Cancer, Celiac Disease, Diabetes, Eating Disorders, Food Allergies, and Cardiovascular Disease

Along with Facts about Federal Nutrition Support Programs, a Glossary of Nutrition and Dietary Terms, and Directories of Additional Resources for More Information about Nutrition

Edited by Joyce Brennfleck Shannon. 633 pages. 2006. 978-0-7808-0800-3.

"This book is an excellent source of basic diet and nutrition information." — *Booklist Health Sciences Supplement, American Library Association, Dec '00*

"This reference document should be in any public library, but it would be a very good guide for beginning students in the health sciences. If the other books in this publisher's series are as good as this, they should all be in the health sciences collections."
— *American Reference Books Annual, 2000*

"This book is an excellent general nutrition reference for consumers who desire to take an active role in their health care for prevention. Consumers of all ages who select this book can feel confident they are receiving current and accurate information." — *Journal of Nutrition for the Elderly, Vol. 19, No. 4, 2000*

SEE ALSO *Digestive Diseases & Disorders Sourcebook, Eating Disorders Sourcebook, Gastrointestinal Diseases & Disorders Sourcebook, Vegetarian Sourcebook*

∎

Digestive Diseases & Disorders Sourcebook

Basic Consumer Health Information about Diseases and Disorders that Impact the Upper and Lower Digestive System, Including Celiac Disease, Constipation, Crohn's Disease, Cyclic Vomiting Syndrome, Diarrhea, Diverticulosis and Diverticulitis, Gallstones, Heartburn, Hemorrhoids, Hernias, Indigestion (Dyspepsia), Irritable Bowel Syndrome, Lactose Intolerance, Ulcers, and More

Along with Information about Medications and Other Treatments, Tips for Maintaining a Healthy Digestive Tract, a Glossary, and Directory of Digestive Diseases Organizations

Edited by Karen Bellenir. 335 pages. 2000. 978-0-7808-0327-5.

"This title would be an excellent addition to all public or patient-research libraries."
— *American Reference Books Annual, 2001*

"This title is recommended for public, hospital, and health sciences libraries with consumer health collections." — *E-Streams, Jul-Aug '00*

"Recommended reference source."
— *Booklist, American Library Association, May '00*

SEE ALSO *Eating Disorders Sourcebook, Gastrointestinal Diseases & Disorders Sourcebook*

∎

Disabilities Sourcebook

Basic Consumer Health Information about Physical and Psychiatric Disabilities, Including Descriptions of Major Causes of Disability, Assistive and Adaptive Aids, Workplace Issues, and Accessibility Concerns

Along with Information about the Americans with Disabilities Act, a Glossary, and Resources for Additional Help and Information

Edited by Dawn D. Matthews. 616 pages. 2000. 978-0-7808-0389-3.

"It is a must for libraries with a consumer health section." — *American Reference Books Annual, 2002*

"A much needed addition to the Omnigraphics *Health Reference Series*. A current reference work to provide people with disabilities, their families, caregivers or those who work with them, a broad range of information in one volume, has not been available until now. . . . It is recommended for all public and academic library reference collections." — *E-Streams, May '01*

"An excellent source book in easy-to-read format covering many current topics; highly recommended for all libraries." — *Choice, Association of College & Research Libraries, Jan '01*

"Recommended reference source." — *Booklist, American Library Association, Jul '00*

■

Domestic Violence Sourcebook, 2nd Edition

Basic Consumer Health Information about the Causes and Consequences of Abusive Relationships, Including Physical Violence, Sexual Assault, Battery, Stalking, and Emotional Abuse, and Facts about the Effects of Violence on Women, Men, Young Adults, and the Elderly, with Reports about Domestic Violence in Selected Populations, and Featuring Facts about Medical Care, Victim Assistance and Protection, Prevention Strategies, Mental Health Services, and Legal Issues

Along with a Glossary of Related Terms and Resources for Additional Help and Information

Edited by Dawn D. Matthews. 628 pages. 2004. 978-0-7808-0669-6.

"Educators, clergy, medical professionals, police, and victims and their families will benefit from this realistic and easy-to-understand resource." — *American Reference Books Annual, 2005*

"Recommended for all collections supporting consumer health information. It should also be considered for any collection needing general, readable information on domestic violence." — *E-Streams, Jan '05*

"This sourcebook complements other books in its field, providing a one-stop resource . . . Recommended." — *Choice, Association of College & Research Libraries, Jan '05*

"Interested lay persons should find the book extremely beneficial. . . . A copy of *Domestic Violence and Child Abuse Sourcebook* should be in every public library in the United States." — *Social Science & Medicine, No. 56, 2003*

"This is important information. The Web has many resources but this sourcebook fills an important societal need. I am not aware of any other resources of this type." — *Doody's Review Service, Sep '01*

"Recommended reference source." — *Booklist, American Library Association, Apr '01*

"Important pick for college-level health reference libraries." — *The Bookwatch, Mar '01*

"Because this problem is so widespread and because this book includes a lot of issues within one volume, this work is recommended for all public libraries." — *American Reference Books Annual, 2001*

SEE ALSO *Child Abuse Sourcebook*

■

Drug Abuse Sourcebook, 2nd Edition

Basic Consumer Health Information about Illicit Substances of Abuse and the Misuse of Prescription and Over-the-Counter Medications, Including Depressants, Hallucinogens, Inhalants, Marijuana, Stimulants, and Anabolic Steroids

Along with Facts about Related Health Risks, Treatment Programs, Prevention Programs, a Glossary of Abuse and Addiction Terms, a Glossary of Drug-Related Street Terms, and a Directory of Resources for More Information

Edited by Catherine Ginther. 607 pages. 2004. 978-0-7808-0740-2.

"Commendable for organizing useful, normally scattered government and association-produced data into a logical sequence." — *American Reference Books Annual, 2006*

"This easy-to-read volume is recommended for consumer health collections within public or academic libraries." — *E-Streams, Sep '05*

"An excellent library reference." — *The Bookwatch, May '05*

"Containing a wealth of information, this book will be useful to the college student just beginning to explore the topic of substance abuse. This resource belongs in libraries that serve a lower-division undergraduate or community college clientele as well as the general public." — *Choice, Association of College & Research Libraries, Jun '01*

"Recommended reference source." — *Booklist, American Library Association, Feb '01*

SEE ALSO *Alcoholism Sourcebook*

■

Ear, Nose & Throat Disorders Sourcebook, 2nd Edition

Basic Consumer Health Information about Disorders of the Ears, Hearing Loss, Vestibular Disorders, Nasal and Sinus Problems, Throat and Vocal Cord Disorders, and Otolaryngologic Cancers, Including Facts about Ear Infections and Injuries, Genetic and Congenital Deafness, Sensorineural Hearing Disorders, Tinnitus, Vertigo, Ménière Disease, Rhinitis, Sinusitis, Snoring, Sore Throats, Hoarseness, and More

Along with Reports on Current Research Initiatives, a Glossary of Related Medical Terms, and a Directory of Sources for Further Help and Information

Edited by Sandra J. Judd. 659 pages. 2006. 978-0-7808-0872-0.

"Overall, this sourcebook is helpful for the consumer seeking information on ENT issues. It is recommended for public libraries."
—*American Reference Books Annual, 1999*

"Recommended reference source."
—*Booklist, American Library Association, Dec '98*

Eating Disorders Sourcebook, 2nd Edition

Basic Consumer Health Information about Anorexia Nervosa, Bulimia Nervosa, Binge Eating, Compulsive Exercise, Female Athlete Triad, and Other Eating Disorders, Including Facts about Body Image and Other Cultural and Age-Related Risk Factors, Prevention Efforts, Adverse Health Effects, Treatment Options, and the Recovery Process

Along with Guidelines for Healthy Weight Control, a Glossary, and Directories of Additional Resources

Edited by Joyce Brennfleck Shannon. 585 pages. 2007. 978-0-7808-0948-2.

"Recommended for health science libraries that are open to the public, as well as hospital libraries. This book is a good resource for the consumer who is concerned about eating disorders." —*E-Streams, Mar '02*

"This volume is another convenient collection of excerpted articles. Recommended for school and public library patrons; lower-division undergraduates; and two-year technical program students."
—*Choice, Association of College & Research Libraries, Jan '02*

"Recommended reference source."
—*Booklist, American Library Association, Oct '01*

SEE ALSO *Diet & Nutrition Sourcebook, Digestive Diseases & Disorders Sourcebook, Gastrointestinal Diseases & Disorders Sourcebook*

Emergency Medical Services Sourcebook

Basic Consumer Health Information about Preventing, Preparing for, and Managing Emergency Situations, When and Who to Call for Help, What to Expect in the Emergency Room, the Emergency Medical Team, Patient Issues, and Current Topics in Emergency Medicine

Along with Statistical Data, a Glossary, and Sources of Additional Help and Information

Edited by Jenni Lynn Colson. 494 pages. 2002. 978-0-7808-0420-3.

"Handy and convenient for home, public, school, and college libraries. Recommended."
—*Choice, Association of College & Research Libraries, Apr '03*

"This reference can provide the consumer with answers to most questions about emergency care in the United States, or it will direct them to a resource where the answer can be found."
—*American Reference Books Annual, 2003*

"Recommended reference source."
—*Booklist, American Library Association, Feb '03*

Endocrine & Metabolic Disorders Sourcebook

Basic Information for the Layperson about Pancreatic and Insulin-Related Disorders Such as Pancreatitis, Diabetes, and Hypoglycemia; Adrenal Gland Disorders Such as Cushing's Syndrome, Addison's Disease, and Congenital Adrenal Hyperplasia; Pituitary Gland Disorders Such as Growth Hormone Deficiency, Acromegaly, and Pituitary Tumors; Thyroid Disorders Such as Hypothyroidism, Graves' Disease, Hashimoto's Disease, and Goiter; Hyperparathyroidism; and Other Diseases and Syndromes of Hormone Imbalance or Metabolic Dysfunction

Along with Reports on Current Research Initiatives

Edited by Linda M. Shin. 574 pages. 1998. 978-0-7808-0207-0.

"Omnigraphics has produced another needed resource for health information consumers."
—*American Reference Books Annual, 2000*

"Recommended reference source."
—*Booklist, American Library Association, Dec '98*

Environmental Health Sourcebook, 2nd Edition

Basic Consumer Health Information about the Environment and Its Effect on Human Health, Including the Effects of Air Pollution, Water Pollution, Hazardous Chemicals, Food Hazards, Radiation Hazards, Biological Agents, Household Hazards, Such as Radon, Asbestos, Carbon Monoxide, and Mold, and Information about Associated Diseases and Disorders, Including Cancer, Allergies, Respiratory Problems, and Skin Disorders

Along with Information about Environmental Concerns for Specific Populations, a Glossary of Related Terms, and Resources for Further Help and Information

Edited by Dawn D. Matthews. 673 pages. 2003. 978-0-7808-0632-0.

"This recently updated edition continues the level of quality and the reputation of the numerous other volumes in Omnigraphics' *Health Reference Series*."
—*American Reference Books Annual, 2004*

"An excellent updated edition."
—*The Bookwatch, Oct '03*

"Recommended reference source."
—*Booklist, American Library Association, Sep '98*

"This book will be a useful addition to anyone's library." —*Choice Health Sciences Supplement, Association of College & Research Libraries, May '98*

". . . a good survey of numerous environmentally induced physical disorders . . . a useful addition to anyone's library."
—*Doody's Health Sciences Book Reviews, Jan '98*

Ethnic Diseases Sourcebook

Basic Consumer Health Information for Ethnic and Racial Minority Groups in the United States, Including General Health Indicators and Behaviors, Ethnic Diseases, Genetic Testing, the Impact of Chronic Diseases, Women's Health, Mental Health Issues, and Preventive Health Care Services

Along with a Glossary and a Listing of Additional Resources

Edited by Joyce Brennfleck Shannon. 664 pages. 2001. 978-0-7808-0336-7.

"Recommended for health sciences libraries where public health programs are a priority."
— *E-Streams, Jan '02*

"Not many books have been written on this topic to date, and the *Ethnic Diseases Sourcebook* is a strong addition to the list. It will be an important introductory resource for health consumers, students, health care personnel, and social scientists. It is recommended for public, academic, and large hospital libraries."
— *American Reference Books Annual, 2002*

"Recommended reference source."
— *Booklist, American Library Association, Oct '01*

"Will prove valuable to any library seeking to maintain a current, comprehensive reference collection of health resources.... An excellent source of health information about genetic disorders which affect particular ethnic and racial minorities in the U.S."
— *The Bookwatch, Aug '01*

■

Eye Care Sourcebook, 2nd Edition

Basic Consumer Health Information about Eye Care and Eye Disorders, Including Facts about the Diagnosis, Prevention, and Treatment of Common Refractive Problems Such as Myopia, Hyperopia, Astigmatism, and Presbyopia, and Eye Diseases, Including Glaucoma, Cataract, Age-Related Macular Degeneration, and Diabetic Retinopathy

Along with a Section on Vision Correction and Refractive Surgeries, Including LASIK and LASEK, a Glossary, and Directories of Resources for Additional Help and Information

Edited by Amy L. Sutton. 543 pages. 2003. 978-0-7808-0635-1.

"... a solid reference tool for eye care and a valuable addition to a collection."
— *American Reference Books Annual, 2004*

■

Family Planning Sourcebook

Basic Consumer Health Information about Planning for Pregnancy and Contraception, Including Traditional Methods, Barrier Methods, Hormonal Methods, Permanent Methods, Future Methods, Emergency Contraception, and Birth Control Choices for Women at Each Stage of Life

Along with Statistics, a Glossary, and Sources of Additional Information

Edited by Amy Marcaccio Keyzer. 520 pages. 2001. 978-0-7808-0379-4.

"Recommended for public, health, and undergraduate libraries as part of the circulating collection."
— *E-Streams, Mar '02*

"Information is presented in an unbiased, readable manner, and the sourcebook will certainly be a necessary addition to those public and high school libraries where Internet access is restricted or otherwise problematic." — *American Reference Books Annual, 2002*

"Recommended reference source."
— *Booklist, American Library Association, Oct '01*

"Will prove valuable to any library seeking to maintain a current, comprehensive reference collection of health resources.... Excellent reference."
— *The Bookwatch, Aug '01*

SEE ALSO Pregnancy & Birth Sourcebook

■

Fitness & Exercise Sourcebook, 3rd Edition

Basic Consumer Health Information about the Physical and Mental Benefits of Fitness, Including Cardiorespiratory Endurance, Muscular Strength, Muscular Endurance, and Flexibility, with Facts about Sports Nutrition and Exercise-Related Injuries and Tips about Physical Activity and Exercises for People of All Ages and for People with Health Concerns

Along with Advice on Selecting and Using Exercise Equipment, Maintaining Exercise Motivation, a Glossary of Related Terms, and a Directory of Resources for More Help and Information

Edited by Amy L. Sutton. 663 pages. 2007. 978-0-7808-0946-8.

"This work is recommended for all general reference collections."
— *American Reference Books Annual, 2002*

"Highly recommended for public, consumer, and school grades fourth through college." — *E-Streams, Nov '01*

"Recommended reference source."
— *Booklist, American Library Association, Oct '01*

"The information appears quite comprehensive and is considered reliable.... This second edition is a welcomed addition to the series."
— *Doody's Review Service, Sep '01*

■

Food Safety Sourcebook

Basic Consumer Health Information about the Safe Handling of Meat, Poultry, Seafood, Eggs, Fruit Juices, and Other Food Items, and Facts about Pesticides, Drinking Water, Food Safety Overseas, and the Onset, Duration, and Symptoms of Foodborne Illnesses, Including Types of Pathogenic Bacteria, Parasitic Protozoa, Worms, Viruses, and Natural Toxins

Along with the Role of the Consumer, the Food Handler, and the Government in Food Safety; a Glossary, and Resources for Additional Help and Information

Edited by Dawn D. Matthews. 339 pages. 1999. 978-0-7808-0326-8.

"This book is recommended for public libraries and universities with home economic and food science programs." — *E-Streams, Nov '00*

"Recommended reference source."
— *Booklist, American Library Association, May '00*

"This book takes the complex issues of food safety and foodborne pathogens and presents them in an easily understood manner. [It does] an excellent job of covering a large and often confusing topic."
— *American Reference Books Annual, 2000*

Forensic Medicine Sourcebook

Basic Consumer Information for the Layperson about Forensic Medicine, Including Crime Scene Investigation, Evidence Collection and Analysis, Expert Testimony, Computer-Aided Criminal Identification, Digital Imaging in the Courtroom, DNA Profiling, Accident Reconstruction, Autopsies, Ballistics, Drugs and Explosives Detection, Latent Fingerprints, Product Tampering, and Questioned Document Examination

Along with Statistical Data, a Glossary of Forensics Terminology, and Listings of Sources for Further Help and Information

Edited by Annemarie S. Muth. 574 pages. 1999. 978-0-7808-0232-2.

"Given the expected widespread interest in its content and its easy to read style, this book is recommended for most public and all college and university libraries."
— *E-Streams, Feb '01*

"Recommended for public libraries."
— *Reference & User Services Quarterly, American Library Association, Spring 2000*

"Recommended reference source."
— *Booklist, American Library Association, Feb '00*

"A wealth of information, useful statistics, references are up-to-date and extremely complete. This wonderful collection of data will help students who are interested in a career in any type of forensic field. It is a great resource for attorneys who need information about types of expert witnesses needed in a particular case. It also offers useful information for fiction and nonfiction writers whose work involves a crime. A fascinating compilation. All levels."
— *Choice, Association of College & Research Libraries, Jan '00*

"There are several items that make this book attractive to consumers who are seeking certain forensic data. . . . This is a useful current source for those seeking general forensic medical answers."
— *American Reference Books Annual, 2000*

Gastrointestinal Diseases & Disorders Sourcebook, 2nd Edition

Basic Consumer Health Information about the Upper and Lower Gastrointestinal (GI) Tract, Including the Esophagus, Stomach, Intestines, Rectum, Liver, and Pancreas, with Facts about Gastroesophageal Reflux Disease, Gastritis, Hernias, Ulcers, Celiac Disease, Diverticulitis, Irritable Bowel Syndrome, Hemorrhoids, Gastrointestinal Cancers, and Other Diseases and Disorders Related to the Digestive Process

Along with Information about Commonly Used Diagnostic and Surgical Procedures, Statistics, Reports on Current Research Initiatives and Clinical Trials, a Glossary, and Resources for Additional Help and Information

Edited by Sandra J. Judd. 681 pages. 2006. 978-0-7808-0798-3.

". . . very readable form. The successful editorial work that brought this material together into a useful and understandable reference makes accessible to all readers information that can help them more effectively understand and obtain help for digestive tract problems."
— *Choice, Association of College & Research Libraries, Feb '97*

SEE ALSO *Diet & Nutrition Sourcebook, Digestive Diseases & Disorders Sourcebook, Eating Disorders Sourcebook*

Genetic Disorders Sourcebook, 3rd Edition

Basic Consumer Health Information about Hereditary Diseases and Disorders, Including Facts about the Human Genome, Genetic Inheritance Patterns, Disorders Associated with Specific Genes, Such as Sickle Cell Disease, Hemophilia, and Cystic Fibrosis, Chromosome Disorders, Such as Down Syndrome, Fragile X Syndrome, and Turner Syndrome, and Complex Diseases and Disorders Resulting from the Interaction of Environmental and Genetic Factors, Such as Allergies, Cancer, and Obesity

Along with Facts about Genetic Testing, Suggestions for Parents of Children with Special Needs, Reports on Current Research Initiatives, a Glossary of Genetic Terminology, and Resources for Additional Help and Information

Edited by Karen Bellenir. 777 pages. 2004. 978-0-7808-0742-6.

"This text is recommended for any library with an interest in providing consumer health resources."
— *E-Streams, Aug '05*

"This is a valuable resource for anyone wishing to have an understandable description of any of the topics or disorders included. The editor succeeds in making complex genetic issues understandable."
— *Doody's Book Review Service, May '05*

"A good acquisition for public libraries."
— *American Reference Books Annual, 2005*

■

Head Trauma Sourcebook

Basic Information for the Layperson about Open-Head and Closed-Head Injuries, Treatment Advances, Recovery, and Rehabilitation

Along with Reports on Current Research Initiatives

Edited by Karen Bellenir. 414 pages. 1997. 978-0-7808-0208-7.

Headache Sourcebook

Basic Consumer Health Information about Migraine, Tension, Cluster, Rebound and Other Types of Headaches, with Facts about the Cause and Prevention of Headaches, the Effects of Stress and the Environment, Headaches during Pregnancy and Menopause, and Childhood Headaches

Along with a Glossary and Other Resources for Additional Help and Information

Edited by Dawn D. Matthews. 362 pages. 2002. 978-0-7808-0337-4.

■

Healthy Aging Sourcebook

Basic Consumer Health Information about Maintaining Health through the Aging Process, Including Advice on Nutrition, Exercise, and Sleep, Help in Making Decisions about Midlife Issues and Retirement, and Guidance Concerning Practical and Informed Choices in Health Consumerism

Along with Data Concerning the Theories of Aging, Different Experiences in Aging by Minority Groups, and Facts about Aging Now and Aging in the Future; and Featuring a Glossary, a Guide to Consumer Help, Additional Suggested Reading, and Practical Resource Directory

Edited by Jenifer Swanson. 536 pages. 1999. 978-0-7808-0390-9.

SEE ALSO *Physical & Mental Issues in Aging Sourcebook*

■

Healthy Children Sourcebook

Basic Consumer Health Information about the Physical and Mental Development of Children between the Ages of 3 and 12, Including Routine Health Care, Preventative Health Services, Safety and First Aid,

Healthy Sleep, Dental Care, Nutrition, and Fitness, and Featuring Parenting Tips on Such Topics as Bedwetting, Choosing Day Care, Monitoring TV and Other Media, and Establishing a Foundation for Substance Abuse Prevention

Along with a Glossary of Commonly Used Pediatric Terms and Resources for Additional Help and Information.

Edited by Chad T. Kimball. 647 pages. 2003. 978-0-7808-0247-6.

SEE ALSO *Childhood Diseases & Disorders Sourcebook*

■

Healthy Heart Sourcebook for Women

Basic Consumer Health Information about Cardiac Issues Specific to Women, Including Facts about Major Risk Factors and Prevention, Treatment and Control Strategies, and Important Dietary Issues

Along with a Special Section Regarding the Pros and Cons of Hormone Replacement Therapy and Its Impact on Heart Health, and Additional Help, Including Recipes, a Glossary, and a Directory of Resources

Edited by Dawn D. Matthews. 336 pages. 2000. 978-0-7808-0329-9.

SEE ALSO *Cardiovascular Diseases & Disorders Sourcebook, Women's Health Concerns Sourcebook*

■

Hepatitis Sourcebook

Basic Consumer Health Information about Hepatitis A, Hepatitis B, Hepatitis C, and Other Forms of Hepatitis, Including Autoimmune Hepatitis, Alcoholic Hepatitis, Nonalcoholic Steatohepatitis, and Toxic Hepatitis, with

Facts about Risk Factors, Screening Methods, Diagnostic Tests, and Treatment Options

Along with Information on Liver Health, Tips for People Living with Chronic Hepatitis, Reports on Current Research Initiatives, a Glossary of Terms Related to Hepatitis, and a Directory of Sources for Further Help and Information

Edited by Sandra J. Judd. 597 pages. 2005. 978-0-7808-0749-5.

"Highly recommended."
— *American Reference Books Annual, 2006*

■

Household Safety Sourcebook

Basic Consumer Health Information about Household Safety, Including Information about Poisons, Chemicals, Fire, and Water Hazards in the Home

Along with Advice about the Safe Use of Home Maintenance Equipment, Choosing Toys and Nursery Furniture, Holiday and Recreation Safety, a Glossary, and Resources for Further Help and Information

Edited by Dawn D. Matthews. 606 pages. 2002. 978-0-7808-0338-1.

"This work will be useful in public libraries with large consumer health and wellness departments."
— *American Reference Books Annual, 2003*

"As a sourcebook on household safety this book meets its mark. It is encyclopedic in scope and covers a wide range of safety issues that are commonly seen in the home." — *E-Streams, Jul '02*

■

Hypertension Sourcebook

Basic Consumer Health Information about the Causes, Diagnosis, and Treatment of High Blood Pressure, with Facts about Consequences, Complications, and Co-Occurring Disorders, Such as Coronary Heart Disease, Diabetes, Stroke, Kidney Disease, and Hypertensive Retinopathy, and Issues in Blood Pressure Control, Including Dietary Choices, Stress Management, and Medications

Along with Reports on Current Research Initiatives and Clinical Trials, a Glossary, and Resources for Additional Help and Information

Edited by Dawn D. Matthews and Karen Bellenir. 613 pages. 2004. 978-0-7808-0674-0.

"Academic, public, and medical libraries will want to add the *Hypertension Sourcebook* to their collections."
— *E-Streams, Aug '05*

"The strength of this source is the wide range of information given about hypertension."
— *American Reference Books Annual, 2005*

■

Immune System Disorders Sourcebook, 2nd Edition

Basic Consumer Health Information about Disorders of the Immune System, Including Immune System Function and Response, Diagnosis of Immune Disorders, Information about Inherited Immune Disease, Acquired Immune Disease, and Autoimmune Diseases, Including Primary Immune Deficiency, Acquired Immunodeficiency Syndrome (AIDS), Lupus, Multiple Sclerosis, Type 1 Diabetes, Rheumatoid Arthritis, and Graves' Disease

Along with Treatments, Tips for Coping with Immune Disorders, a Glossary, and a Directory of Additional Resources.

Edited by Joyce Brennfleck Shannon. 671 pages. 2005. 978-0-7808-0748-8.

"Highly recommended for academic and public libraries." — *American Reference Books Annual, 2006*

"The updated second edition is a 'must' for any consumer health library seeking a solid resource covering the treatments, symptoms, and options for immune disorder sufferers. . . . An excellent guide."
— *MBR Bookwatch, Jan '06*

■

Infant & Toddler Health Sourcebook

Basic Consumer Health Information about the Physical and Mental Development of Newborns, Infants, and Toddlers, Including Neonatal Concerns, Nutrition Recommendations, Immunization Schedules, Common Pediatric Disorders, Assessments and Milestones, Safety Tips, and Advice for Parents and Other Caregivers

Along with a Glossary of Terms and Resource Listings for Additional Help

Edited by Jenifer Swanson. 585 pages. 2000. 978-0-7808-0246-9.

"As a reference for the general public, this would be useful in any library." — *E-Streams, May '01*

"Recommended reference source."
— *Booklist, American Library Association, Feb '01*

"This is a good source for general use."
— *American Reference Books Annual, 2001*

■

Infectious Diseases Sourcebook

Basic Consumer Health Information about Non-Contagious Bacterial, Viral, Prion, Fungal, and Parasitic Diseases Spread by Food and Water, Insects and Animals, or Environmental Contact, Including Botulism, E. Coli, Encephalitis, Legionnaires' Disease, Lyme Disease, Malaria, Plague, Rabies, Salmonella, Tetanus, and Others, and Facts about Newly Emerging Diseases, Such as Hantavirus, Mad Cow Disease, Monkeypox, and West Nile Virus

Along with Information about Preventing Disease Transmission, the Threat of Bioterrorism, and Current Research Initiatives, with a Glossary and Directory of Resources for More Information

Edited by Karen Bellenir. 634 pages. 2004. 978-0-7808-0675-7.

"This reference continues the excellent tradition of the *Health Reference Series* in consolidating a wealth of information on a selected topic into a format that is easy to use and accessible to the general public."
— *American Reference Books Annual, 2005*

"Recommended for public and academic libraries."
— *E-Streams, Jan '05*

■

Injury & Trauma Sourcebook

Basic Consumer Health Information about the Impact of Injury, the Diagnosis and Treatment of Common and Traumatic Injuries, Emergency Care, and Specific Injuries Related to Home, Community, Workplace, Transportation, and Recreation

Along with Guidelines for Injury Prevention, a Glossary, and a Directory of Additional Resources

Edited by Joyce Brennfleck Shannon. 696 pages. 2002. 978-0-7808-0421-0.

"This publication is the most comprehensive work of its kind about injury and trauma."
— *American Reference Books Annual, 2003*

"This sourcebook provides concise, easily readable, basic health information about injuries. . . . This book is well organized and an easy to use reference resource suitable for hospital, health sciences and public libraries with consumer health collections."
— *E-Streams, Nov '02*

"Practitioners should be aware of guides such as this in order to facilitate their use by patients and their families."
— *Doody's Health Sciences Book Review Journal, Sep-Oct '02*

"Recommended reference source."
— *Booklist, American Library Association, Sep '02*

"Highly recommended for academic and medical reference collections."
— *Library Bookwatch, Sep '02*

■

Kidney & Urinary Tract Diseases & Disorders Sourcebook

SEE *Urinary Tract & Kidney Diseases & Disorders Sourcebook*

■

Learning Disabilities Sourcebook, 2nd Edition

Basic Consumer Health Information about Learning Disabilities, Including Dyslexia, Developmental Speech and Language Disabilities, Non-Verbal Learning Disorders, Developmental Arithmetic Disorder, Developmental Writing Disorder, and Other Conditions That Impede Learning Such as Attention Deficit/Hyperactivity Disorder, Brain Injury, Hearing Impairment, Klinefelter Syndrome, Dyspraxia, and Tourette's Syndrome

Along with Facts about Educational Issues and Assistive Technology, Coping Strategies, a Glossary of Re-lated Terms, and Resources for Further Help and Information

Edited by Dawn D. Matthews. 621 pages. 2003. 978-0-7808-0626-9.

"The second edition of Learning Disabilities Sourcebook far surpasses the earlier edition in that it is more focused on information that will be useful as a consumer health resource."
— *American Reference Books Annual, 2004*

"Teachers as well as consumers will find this an essential guide to understanding various syndromes and their latest treatments. [An] invaluable reference for public and school library collections alike."
— *Library Bookwatch, Apr '03*

Named "Outstanding Reference Book of 1999."
— *New York Public Library, Feb '00*

"An excellent candidate for inclusion in a public library reference section. It's a great source of information. Teachers will also find the book useful. Definitely worth reading."
— *Journal of Adolescent & Adult Literacy, Feb 2000*

"Readable . . . provides a solid base of information regarding successful techniques used with individuals who have learning disabilities, as well as practical suggestions for educators and family members. Clear language, concise descriptions, and pertinent information for contacting multiple resources add to the strength of this book as a useful tool."
— *Choice, Association of College & Research Libraries, Feb '99*

"Recommended reference source."
— *Booklist, American Library Association, Sep '98*

"A useful resource for libraries and for those who don't have the time to identify and locate the individual publications."
— *Disability Resources Monthly, Sep '98*

■

Leukemia Sourcebook

Basic Consumer Health Information about Adult and Childhood Leukemias, Including Acute Lymphocytic Leukemia (ALL), Chronic Lymphocytic Leukemia (CLL), Acute Myelogenous Leukemia (AML), Chronic Myelogenous Leukemia (CML), and Hairy Cell Leukemia, and Treatments Such as Chemotherapy, Radiation Therapy, Peripheral Blood Stem Cell and Marrow Transplantation, and Immunotherapy

Along with Tips for Life During and After Treatment, a Glossary, and Directories of Additional Resources

Edited by Joyce Brennfleck Shannon. 587 pages. 2003. 978-0-7808-0627-6.

"Unlike other medical books for the layperson, . . . the language does not talk down to the reader. . . . This volume is highly recommended for all libraries."
— *American Reference Books Annual, 2004*

". . . a fine title which ranges from diagnosis to alternative treatments, staging, and tips for life during and after diagnosis."
— *The Bookwatch, Dec '03*

Liver Disorders Sourcebook

Basic Consumer Health Information about the Liver and How It Works; Liver Diseases, Including Cancer, Cirrhosis, Hepatitis, and Toxic and Drug Related Diseases; Tips for Maintaining a Healthy Liver; Laboratory Tests, Radiology Tests, and Facts about Liver Transplantation

Along with a Section on Support Groups, a Glossary, and Resource Listings

Edited by Joyce Brennfleck Shannon. 591 pages. 2000. 978-0-7808-0383-1.

"A valuable resource."
—American Reference Books Annual, 2001

"This title is recommended for health sciences and public libraries with consumer health collections."
—E-Streams, Oct '00

"Recommended reference source."
—Booklist, American Library Association, Jun '00

■

Lung Disorders Sourcebook

Basic Consumer Health Information about Emphysema, Pneumonia, Tuberculosis, Asthma, Cystic Fibrosis, and Other Lung Disorders, Including Facts about Diagnostic Procedures, Treatment Strategies, Disease Prevention Efforts, and Such Risk Factors as Smoking, Air Pollution, and Exposure to Asbestos, Radon, and Other Agents

Along with a Glossary and Resources for Additional Help and Information

Edited by Dawn D. Matthews. 678 pages. 2002. 978-0-7808-0339-8.

"This title is a great addition for public and school libraries because it provides concise health information on the lungs."
—American Reference Books Annual, 2003

"Highly recommended for academic and medical reference collections." *—Library Bookwatch, Sep '02*

SEE ALSO *Respiratory Diseases & Disorders Sourcebook*

■

Medical Tests Sourcebook, 2nd Edition

Basic Consumer Health Information about Medical Tests, Including Age-Specific Health Tests, Important Health Screenings and Exams, Home-Use Tests, Blood and Specimen Tests, Electrical Tests, Scope Tests, Genetic Testing, and Imaging Tests, Such as X-Rays, Ultrasound, Computed Tomography, Magnetic Resonance Imaging, Angiography, and Nuclear Medicine

Along with a Glossary and Directory of Additional Resources

Edited by Joyce Brennfleck Shannon. 654 pages. 2004. 978-0-7808-0670-2.

**"Recommended for hospital and health sciences

libraries with consumer health collections."**
—E-Streams, Mar '00

"This is an overall excellent reference with a wealth of general knowledge that may aid those who are reluctant to get vital tests performed."
—Today's Librarian, Jan '00

"A valuable reference guide."
—American Reference Books Annual, 2000

■

Men's Health Concerns Sourcebook, 2nd Edition

Basic Consumer Health Information about the Medical and Mental Concerns of Men, Including Theories about the Shorter Male Lifespan, the Leading Causes of Death and Disability, Physical Concerns of Special Significance to Men, Reproductive and Sexual Concerns, Sexually Transmitted Diseases, Men's Mental and Emotional Health, and Lifestyle Choices That Affect Wellness, Such as Nutrition, Fitness, and Substance Use

Along with a Glossary of Related Terms and a Directory of Organizational Resources in Men's Health

Edited by Robert Aquinas McNally. 644 pages. 2004. 978-0-7808-0671-9.

"A very accessible reference for non-specialist general readers and consumers." *—The Bookwatch, Jun '04*

"This comprehensive resource and the series are highly recommended."
—American Reference Books Annual, 2000

"Recommended reference source."
—Booklist, American Library Association, Dec '98

■

Mental Health Disorders Sourcebook, 3rd Edition

Basic Consumer Health Information about Mental and Emotional Health and Mental Illness, Including Facts about Depression, Bipolar Disorder, and Other Mood Disorders, Phobias, Post-Traumatic Stress Disorder (PTSD), Obsessive-Compulsive Disorder, and Other Anxiety Disorders, Impulse Control Disorders, Eating Disorders, Personality Disorders, and Psychotic Disorders, Including Schizophrenia and Dissociative Disorders

Along with Statistical Information, a Special Section Concerning Mental Health Issues in Children and Adolescents, a Glossary, and Directories of Resources for Additional Help and Information

Edited by Karen Bellenir. 661 pages. 2005. 978-0-7808-0747-1.

"Recommended for public libraries and academic libraries with an undergraduate program in psychology."
—American Reference Books Annual, 2006

"Recommended reference source."
—Booklist, American Library Association, Jun '00

Mental Retardation Sourcebook

Basic Consumer Health Information about Mental Retardation and Its Causes, Including Down Syndrome, Fetal Alcohol Syndrome, Fragile X Syndrome, Genetic Conditions, Injury, and Environmental Sources

Along with Preventive Strategies, Parenting Issues, Educational Implications, Health Care Needs, Employment and Economic Matters, Legal Issues, a Glossary, and a Resource Listing for Additional Help and Information

Edited by Joyce Brennfleck Shannon. 642 pages. 2000. 978-0-7808-0377-0.

"Public libraries will find the book useful for reference and as a beginning research point for students, parents, and caregivers."
— *American Reference Books Annual, 2001*

"The strength of this work is that it compiles many basic fact sheets and addresses for further information in one volume. It is intended and suitable for the general public. This sourcebook is relevant to any collection providing health information to the general public."
— *E-Streams, Nov '00*

"From preventing retardation to parenting and family challenges, this covers health, social and legal issues and will prove an invaluable overview."
— *Reviewer's Bookwatch, Jul '00*

■

Movement Disorders Sourcebook

Basic Consumer Health Information about Neurological Movement Disorders, Including Essential Tremor, Parkinson's Disease, Dystonia, Cerebral Palsy, Huntington's Disease, Myasthenia Gravis, Multiple Sclerosis, and Other Early-Onset and Adult-Onset Movement Disorders, Their Symptoms and Causes, Diagnostic Tests, and Treatments

Along with Mobility and Assistive Technology Information, a Glossary, and a Directory of Additional Resources

Edited by Joyce Brennfleck Shannon. 655 pages. 2003. 978-0-7808-0628-3.

". . . a good resource for consumers and recommended for public, community college and undergraduate libraries." — *American Reference Books Annual, 2004*

■

Muscular Dystrophy Sourcebook

Basic Consumer Health Information about Congenital, Childhood-Onset, and Adult-Onset Forms of Muscular Dystrophy, Such as Duchenne, Becker, Emery-Dreifuss, Distal, Limb-Girdle, Facioscapulohumeral (FSHD), Myotonic, and Ophthalmoplegic Muscular Dystrophies, Including Facts about Diagnostic Tests, Medical and Physical Therapies, Management of Co-Occurring Conditions, and Parenting Guidelines

Along with Practical Tips for Home Care, a Glossary, and Directories of Additional Resources

Edited by Joyce Brennfleck Shannon. 577 pages. 2004. 978-0-7808-0676-4.

"This book is highly recommended for public and academic libraries as well as health care offices that support the information needs of patients and their families."
— *E-Streams, Apr '05*

"Excellent reference." — *The Bookwatch, Jan '05*

■

Obesity Sourcebook

Basic Consumer Health Information about Diseases and Other Problems Associated with Obesity, and Including Facts about Risk Factors, Prevention Issues, and Management Approaches

Along with Statistical and Demographic Data, Information about Special Populations, Research Updates, a Glossary, and Source Listings for Further Help and Information

Edited by Wilma Caldwell and Chad T. Kimball. 376 pages. 2001. 978-0-7808-0333-6.

"The book synthesizes the reliable medical literature on obesity into one easy-to-read and useful resource for the general public."
— *American Reference Books Annual, 2002*

"This is a very useful resource book for the lay public."
— *Doody's Review Service, Nov '01*

"Well suited for the health reference collection of a public library or an academic health science library that serves the general population." — *E-Streams, Sep '01*

"Recommended reference source."
— *Booklist, American Library Association, Apr '01*

"Recommended pick both for specialty health library collections and any general consumer health reference collection." — *The Bookwatch, Apr '01*

■

Oral Health Sourcebook

SEE Dental Care & Oral Health Sourcebook

■

Osteoporosis Sourcebook

Basic Consumer Health Information about Primary and Secondary Osteoporosis and Juvenile Osteoporosis and Related Conditions, Including Fibrous Dysplasia, Gaucher Disease, Hyperthyroidism, Hypophosphatasia, Myeloma, Osteopetrosis, Osteogenesis Imperfecta, and Paget's Disease

Along with Information about Risk Factors, Treatments, Traditional and Non-Traditional Pain Management, a Glossary of Related Terms, and a Directory of Resources

Edited by Allan R. Cook. 584 pages. 2001. 978-0-7808-0239-1.

"This would be a book to be kept in a staff or patient library. The targeted audience is the layperson, but the therapist who needs a quick bit of information on a particular topic will also find the book useful."
— *Physical Therapy, Jan '02*

"This resource is recommended as a great reference source for public, health, and academic libraries, and is another triumph for the editors of Omnigraphics."
— *American Reference Books Annual, 2002*

"Recommended for all public libraries and general health collections, especially those supporting patient education or consumer health programs."
— *E-Streams, Nov '01*

"Will prove valuable to any library seeking to maintain a current, comprehensive reference collection of health resources. . . . From prevention to treatment and associated conditions, this provides an excellent survey."
— *The Bookwatch, Aug '01*

"Recommended reference source."
— *Booklist, American Library Association, Jul '01*

SEE ALSO *Healthy Aging Sourcebook, Physical & Mental Issues in Aging Sourcebook, Women's Health Concerns Sourcebook*

■

Pain Sourcebook, 2nd Edition

Basic Consumer Health Information about Specific Forms of Acute and Chronic Pain, Including Muscle and Skeletal Pain, Nerve Pain, Cancer Pain, and Disorders Characterized by Pain, Such as Fibromyalgia, Shingles, Angina, Arthritis, and Headaches

Along with Information about Pain Medications and Management Techniques, Complementary and Alternative Pain Relief Options, Tips for People Living with Chronic Pain, a Glossary, and a Directory of Sources for Further Information

Edited by Karen Bellenir. 670 pages. 2002. 978-0-7808-0612-2.

"A source of valuable information. . . . This book offers help to nonmedical people who need information about pain and pain management. It is also an excellent reference for those who participate in patient education."
— *Doody's Review Service, Sep '02*

"Highly recommended for academic and medical reference collections." — *Library Bookwatch, Sep '02*

"The text is readable, easily understood, and well indexed. This excellent volume belongs in all patient education libraries, consumer health sections of public libraries, and many personal collections."
— *American Reference Books Annual, 1999*

"The information is basic in terms of scholarship and is appropriate for general readers. Written in journalistic style . . . intended for non-professionals. Quite thorough in its coverage of different pain conditions and summarizes the latest clinical information regarding pain treatment." — *Choice, Association of College and Research Libraries, Jun '98*

"Recommended reference source."
— *Booklist, American Library Association, Mar '98*

■

Pediatric Cancer Sourcebook

Basic Consumer Health Information about Leukemias, Brain Tumors, Sarcomas, Lymphomas, and Other Cancers in Infants, Children, and Adolescents, Including Descriptions of Cancers, Treatments, and Coping Strategies

Along with Suggestions for Parents, Caregivers, and Concerned Relatives, a Glossary of Cancer Terms, and Resource Listings

Edited by Edward J. Prucha. 587 pages. 1999. 978-0-7808-0245-2.

"An excellent source of information. Recommended for public, hospital, and health science libraries with consumer health collections." — *E-Streams, Jun '00*

"Recommended reference source."
— *Booklist, American Library Association, Feb '00*

"A valuable addition to all libraries specializing in health services and many public libraries."
— *American Reference Books Annual, 2000*

SEE ALSO *Childhood Diseases & Disorders Sourcebook, Healthy Children Sourcebook*

■

Physical & Mental Issues in Aging Sourcebook

Basic Consumer Health Information on Physical and Mental Disorders Associated with the Aging Process, Including Concerns about Cardiovascular Disease, Pulmonary Disease, Oral Health, Digestive Disorders, Musculoskeletal and Skin Disorders, Metabolic Changes, Sexual and Reproductive Issues, and Changes in Vision, Hearing, and Other Senses

Along with Data about Longevity and Causes of Death, Information on Acute and Chronic Pain, Descriptions of Mental Concerns, a Glossary of Terms, and Resource Listings for Additional Help

Edited by Jenifer Swanson. 660 pages. 1999. 978-0-7808-0233-9.

"This is a treasure of health information for the layperson." — *Choice Health Sciences Supplement, Association of College & Research Libraries, May '00*

"Recommended for public libraries."
— *American Reference Books Annual, 2000*

"Recommended reference source."
— *Booklist, American Library Association, Oct '99*

SEE ALSO *Healthy Aging Sourcebook*

■

Podiatry Sourcebook, 2nd Edition

Basic Consumer Health Information about Disorders, Diseases, Deformities, and Injuries that Affect the Foot and Ankle, Including Sprains, Corns, Calluses, Bunions, Plantar Warts, Plantar Fasciitis, Neuromas, Clubfoot, Flat Feet, Achilles Tendonitis, and Much More

Along with Information about Selecting a Foot Care Specialist, Foot Fitness, Shoes and Socks, Diagnostic Tests and Corrective Procedures, Financial Assistance for Corrective Devices, a Glossary of Related Terms, and a Directory of Resources for Additional Help and Information

Edited by Ivy L. Alexander. 543 pages. 2007. 978-0-7808-0944-4.

"Recommended reference source."
— *Booklist, American Library Association, Feb '02*

"There is a lot of information presented here on a topic that is usually only covered sparingly in most larger comprehensive medical encyclopedias."
— *American Reference Books Annual, 2002*

■

Pregnancy & Birth Sourcebook, 2nd Edition

Basic Consumer Health Information about Conception and Pregnancy, Including Facts about Fertility, Infertility, Pregnancy Symptoms and Complications, Fetal Growth and Development, Labor, Delivery, and the Postpartum Period, as Well as Information about Maintaining Health and Wellness during Pregnancy and Caring for a Newborn

Along with Information about Public Health Assistance for Low-Income Pregnant Women, a Glossary, and Directories of Agencies and Organizations Providing Help and Support

Edited by Amy L. Sutton. 626 pages. 2004. 978-0-7808-0672-6.

"Will appeal to public and school reference collections strong in medicine and women's health. . . . Deserves a spot on any medical reference shelf."
— *The Bookwatch, Jul '04*

"A well-organized handbook. Recommended."
— *Choice, Association of College & Research Libraries, Apr '98*

"Recommended reference source."
— *Booklist, American Library Association, Mar '98*

"Recommended for public libraries."
— *American Reference Books Annual, 1998*

SEE ALSO *Breastfeeding Sourcebook, Congenital Disorders Sourcebook, Family Planning Sourcebook*

■

Prostate & Urological Disorders Sourcebook

Basic Consumer Health Information about Urogenital and Sexual Disorders in Men, Including Prostate and Other Andrological Cancers, Prostatitis, Benign Prostatic Hyperplasia, Testicular and Penile Trauma, Cryptorchidism, Peyronie Disease, Erectile Dysfunction, and Male Factor Infertility, and Facts about Commonly Used Tests and Procedures, Such as Prostatectomy, Vasectomy, Vasectomy Reversal, Penile Implants, and Semen Analysis

Along with a Glossary of Andrological Terms and a Directory of Resources for Additional Information

Edited by Karen Bellenir. 631 pages. 2005. 978-0-7808-0797-6.

Prostate Cancer Sourcebook

Basic Consumer Health Information about Prostate Cancer, Including Information about the Associated Risk Factors, Detection, Diagnosis, and Treatment of Prostate Cancer

Along with Information on Non-Malignant Prostate Conditions, and Featuring a Section Listing Support and Treatment Centers and a Glossary of Related Terms

Edited by Dawn D. Matthews. 358 pages. 2001. 978-0-7808-0324-4.

"Recommended reference source."
— *Booklist, American Library Association, Jan '02*

"A valuable resource for health care consumers seeking information on the subject. . . . All text is written in a clear, easy-to-understand language that avoids technical jargon. Any library that collects consumer health resources would strengthen their collection with the addition of the *Prostate Cancer Sourcebook.*"
— *American Reference Books Annual, 2002*

SEE ALSO *Men's Health Concerns Sourcebook*

■

Reconstructive & Cosmetic Surgery Sourcebook

Basic Consumer Health Information on Cosmetic and Reconstructive Plastic Surgery, Including Statistical Information about Different Surgical Procedures, Things to Consider Prior to Surgery, Plastic Surgery Techniques and Tools, Emotional and Psychological Considerations, and Procedure-Specific Information

Along with a Glossary of Terms and a Listing of Resources for Additional Help and Information

Edited by M. Lisa Weatherford. 374 pages. 2001. 978-0-7808-0214-8.

"An excellent reference that addresses cosmetic and medically necessary reconstructive surgeries. . . . The style of the prose is calm and reassuring, discussing the many positive outcomes now available due to advances in surgical techniques."
— *American Reference Books Annual, 2002*

"Recommended for health science libraries that are open to the public, as well as hospital libraries that are open to the patients. This book is a good resource for the consumer interested in plastic surgery."
— *E-Streams, Dec '01*

"Recommended reference source."
— *Booklist, American Library Association, Jul '01*

■

Rehabilitation Sourcebook

Basic Consumer Health Information about Rehabilitation for People Recovering from Heart Surgery, Spinal Cord Injury, Stroke, Orthopedic Impairments, Amputation, Pulmonary Impairments, Traumatic Injury, and More, Including Physical Therapy, Occupational Therapy, Speech/Language Therapy, Massage Therapy, Dance Therapy, Art Therapy, and Recreational Therapy

Along with Information on Assistive and Adaptive Devices, a Glossary, and Resources for Additional Help and Information

Edited by Dawn D. Matthews. 531 pages. 1999. 978-0-7808-0236-0.

"This is an excellent resource for public library reference and health collections."
— American Reference Books Annual, 2001

"Recommended reference source."
— Booklist, American Library Association, May '00

■

Respiratory Diseases & Disorders Sourcebook

Basic Information about Respiratory Diseases and Disorders, Including Asthma, Cystic Fibrosis, Pneumonia, the Common Cold, Influenza, and Others, Featuring Facts about the Respiratory System, Statistical and Demographic Data, Treatments, Self-Help Management Suggestions, and Current Research Initiatives

Edited by Allan R. Cook and Peter D. Dresser. 771 pages. 1995. 978-0-7808-0037-3.

"Designed for the layperson and for patients and their families coping with respiratory illness. . . . an extensive array of information on diagnosis, treatment, management, and prevention of respiratory illnesses for the general reader."
— Choice, Association of College & Research Libraries, Jun '96

"A highly recommended text for all collections. It is a comforting reminder of the power of knowledge that good books carry between their covers."
— Academic Library Book Review, Spring '96

"A comprehensive collection of authoritative information presented in a nontechnical, humanitarian style for patients, families, and caregivers."
— Association of Operating Room Nurses, Sep/Oct '95

SEE ALSO Lung Disorders Sourcebook

■

Sexually Transmitted Diseases Sourcebook, 3rd Edition

Basic Consumer Health Information about Chlamydial Infections, Gonorrhea, Hepatitis, Herpes, HIV/AIDS, Human Papillomavirus, Pubic Lice, Scabies, Syphilis, Trichomoniasis, Vaginal Infections, and Other Sexually Transmitted Diseases, Including Facts about Risk Factors, Symptoms, Diagnosis, Treatment, and the Prevention of Sexually Transmitted Infections

Along with Updates on Current Research Initiatives, a Glossary of Related Terms, and Resources for Additional Help and Information

Edited by Amy L. Sutton. 629 pages. 2006. 978-0-7808-0824-9.

"Recommended for consumer health collections in public libraries, and secondary school and community college libraries."
— American Reference Books Annual, 2002

"Every school and public library should have a copy of this comprehensive and user-friendly reference book."
— Choice, Association of College & Research Libraries, Sep '01

"This is a highly recommended book. This is an especially important book for all school and public libraries."
— AIDS Book Review Journal, Jul-Aug '01

"Recommended reference source."
— Booklist, American Library Association, Apr '01

■

Sleep Disorders Sourcebook, 2nd Edition

Basic Consumer Health Information about Sleep and Sleep Disorders, Including Insomnia, Sleep Apnea, Restless Legs Syndrome, Narcolepsy, Parasomnias, and Other Health Problems That Affect Sleep, Plus Facts about Diagnostic Procedures, Treatment Strategies, Sleep Medications, and Tips for Improving Sleep Quality

Along with a Glossary of Related Terms and Resources for Additional Help and Information

Edited by Amy L. Sutton. 567 pages. 2005. 978-0-7808-0743-3.

"This book will be useful for just about everybody, especially the 40 million Americans with sleep disorders."
— American Reference Books Annual, 2006

"Recommended for public libraries and libraries supporting health care professionals." — E-Streams, Sep '05

". . . key medical library acquisition."
— The Bookwatch, Jun '05

■

Smoking Concerns Sourcebook

Basic Consumer Health Information about Nicotine Addiction and Smoking Cessation, Featuring Facts about the Health Effects of Tobacco Use, Including Lung and Other Cancers, Heart Disease, Stroke, and Respiratory Disorders, Such as Emphysema and Chronic Bronchitis

Along with Information about Smoking Prevention Programs, Suggestions for Achieving and Maintaining a Smoke-Free Lifestyle, Statistics about Tobacco Use, Reports on Current Research Initiatives, a Glossary of Related Terms, and Directories of Resources for Additional Help and Information

Edited by Karen Bellenir. 621 pages. 2004. 978-0-7808-0323-7.

"Provides everything needed for the student or general reader seeking practical details on the effects of tobacco use."
— The Bookwatch, Mar '05

"Public libraries and consumer health care libraries will find this work useful."
— American Reference Books Annual, 2005

Sports Injuries Sourcebook, 3rd Edition

Basic Consumer Health Information about Sprains and Strains, Fractures, Growth Plate Injuries, Overtraining Injuries, and Injuries to the Head, Face, Shoulders, Elbows, Hands, Spinal Column, Knees, Ankles, and Feet, and with Facts about Heat-Related Illness, Steroids and Sport Supplements, Protective Equipment, Diagnostic Procedures, Treatment Options, and Rehabilitation

Along with a Glossary of Related Terms and a Directory of Resources for Additional Help and Information

Edited by Sandra J. Judd. 651 pages. 2007. 978-0-7808-0949-9.

"This is an excellent reference for consumers and it is recommended for public, community college, and undergraduate libraries."
— *American Reference Books Annual, 2003*

"Recommended reference source."
— *Booklist, American Library Association, Feb '03*

■

Stress-Related Disorders Sourcebook

Basic Consumer Health Information about Stress and Stress-Related Disorders, Including Stress Origins and Signals, Environmental Stress at Work and Home, Mental and Emotional Stress Associated with Depression, Post-Traumatic Stress Disorder, Panic Disorder, Suicide, and the Physical Effects of Stress on the Cardiovascular, Immune, and Nervous Systems

Along with Stress Management Techniques, a Glossary, and a Listing of Additional Resources

Edited by Joyce Brennfleck Shannon. 610 pages. 2002. 978-0-7808-0560-6.

"Well written for a general readership, the *Stress-Related Disorders Sourcebook* is a useful addition to the health reference literature."
— *American Reference Books Annual, 2003*

"I am impressed by the amount of information. It offers a thorough overview of the causes and consequences of stress for the layperson. . . . A well-done and thorough reference guide for professionals and nonprofessionals alike." — *Doody's Review Service, Dec '02*

■

Stroke Sourcebook

Basic Consumer Health Information about Stroke, Including Ischemic, Hemorrhagic, Transient Ischemic Attack (TIA), and Pediatric Stroke, Stroke Triggers and Risks, Diagnostic Tests, Treatments, and Rehabilitation Information

Along with Stroke Prevention Guidelines, Legal and Financial Information, a Glossary, and a Directory of Additional Resources

Edited by Joyce Brennfleck Shannon. 606 pages. 2003. 978-0-7808-0630-6.

"This volume is highly recommended and should be in every medical, hospital, and public library."
— *American Reference Books Annual, 2004*

"Highly recommended for the amount and variety of topics and information covered." — *Choice, Nov '03*

■

Surgery Sourcebook

Basic Consumer Health Information about Inpatient and Outpatient Surgeries, Including Cardiac, Vascular, Orthopedic, Ocular, Reconstructive, Cosmetic, Gynecologic, and Ear, Nose, and Throat Procedures and More

Along with Information about Operating Room Policies and Instruments, Laser Surgery Techniques, Hospital Errors, Statistical Data, a Glossary, and Listings of Sources for Further Help and Information

Edited by Annemarie S. Muth and Karen Bellenir. 596 pages. 2002. 978-0-7808-0380-0.

"Large public libraries and medical libraries would benefit from this material in their reference collections."
— *American Reference Books Annual, 2004*

"Invaluable reference for public and school library collections alike." — *Library Bookwatch, Apr '03*

■

Thyroid Disorders Sourcebook

Basic Consumer Health Information about Disorders of the Thyroid and Parathyroid Glands, Including Hypothyroidism, Hyperthyroidism, Graves Disease, Hashimoto Thyroiditis, Thyroid Cancer, and Parathyroid Disorders, Featuring Facts about Symptoms, Risk Factors, Tests, and Treatments

Along with Information about the Effects of Thyroid Imbalance on Other Body Systems, Environmental Factors That Affect the Thyroid Gland, a Glossary, and a Directory of Additional Resources

Edited by Joyce Brennfleck Shannon. 599 pages. 2005. 978-0-7808-0745-7.

"Recommended for consumer health collections."
— *American Reference Books Annual, 2006*

"Highly recommended pick for basic consumer health reference holdings at all levels."
— *The Bookwatch, Aug '05*

■

Transplantation Sourcebook

Basic Consumer Health Information about Organ and Tissue Transplantation, Including Physical and Financial Preparations, Procedures and Issues Relating to Specific Solid Organ and Tissue Transplants, Rehabilitation, Pediatric Transplant Information, the Future of Transplantation, and Organ and Tissue Donation

Along with a Glossary and Listings of Additional Resources

Edited by Joyce Brennfleck Shannon. 628 pages. 2002. 978-0-7808-0322-0.

"Along with these advances [in transplantation technology] have come a number of daunting questions for potential transplant patients, their families, and their health care providers. This reference text is the best single tool to address many of these questions. . . . It will be a much-needed addition to the reference collections in health care, academic, and large public libraries."
— *American Reference Books Annual, 2003*

"Recommended for libraries with an interest in offering consumer health information." — *E-Streams, Jul '02*

"This is a unique and valuable resource for patients facing transplantation and their families."
— *Doody's Review Service, Jun '02*

Traveler's Health Sourcebook

Basic Consumer Health Information for Travelers, Including Physical and Medical Preparations, Transportation Health and Safety, Essential Information about Food and Water, Sun Exposure, Insect and Snake Bites, Camping and Wilderness Medicine, and Travel with Physical or Medical Disabilities

Along with International Travel Tips, Vaccination Recommendations, Geographical Health Issues, Disease Risks, a Glossary, and a Listing of Additional Resources

Edited by Joyce Brennfleck Shannon. 613 pages. 2000. 978-0-7808-0384-8.

"Recommended reference source."
— *Booklist, American Library Association, Feb '01*

"This book is recommended for any public library, any travel collection, and especially any collection for the physically disabled."
— *American Reference Books Annual, 2001*

SEE ALSO Worldwide Health Sourcebook

Urinary Tract & Kidney Diseases & Disorders Sourcebook, 2nd Edition

Basic Consumer Health Information about the Urinary System, Including the Bladder, Urethra, Ureters, and Kidneys, with Facts about Urinary Tract Infections, Incontinence, Congenital Disorders, Kidney Stones, Cancers of the Urinary Tract and Kidneys, Kidney Failure, Dialysis, and Kidney Transplantation

Along with Statistical and Demographic Information, Reports on Current Research in Kidney and Urologic Health, a Summary of Commonly Used Diagnostic Tests, a Glossary of Related Terms, and a Directory of Resources for Additional Help and Information

Edited by Ivy L. Alexander. 649 pages. 2005. 978-0-7808-0750-1.

"A good choice for a consumer health information library or for a medical library needing information to refer to their patients."
— *American Reference Books Annual, 2006*

Vegetarian Sourcebook

Basic Consumer Health Information about Vegetarian Diets, Lifestyle, and Philosophy, Including Definitions of Vegetarianism and Veganism, Tips about Adopting Vegetarianism, Creating a Vegetarian Pantry, and Meeting Nutritional Needs of Vegetarians, with Facts Regarding Vegetarianism's Effect on Pregnant and Lactating Women, Children, Athletes, and Senior Citizens

Along with a Glossary of Commonly Used Vegetarian Terms and Resources for Additional Help and Information

Edited by Chad T. Kimball. 360 pages. 2002. 978-0-7808-0439-5.

"Organizes into one concise volume the answers to the most common questions concerning vegetarian diets and lifestyles. This title is recommended for public and secondary school libraries." — *E-Streams, Apr '03*

"Invaluable reference for public and school library collections alike." — *Library Bookwatch, Apr '03*

"The articles in this volume are easy to read and come from authoritative sources. The book does not necessarily support the vegetarian diet but instead provides the pros and cons of this important decision. The Vegetarian Sourcebook is recommended for public libraries and consumer health libraries."
— *American Reference Books Annual, 2003*

SEE ALSO Diet & Nutrition Sourcebook

Women's Health Concerns Sourcebook, 2nd Edition

Basic Consumer Health Information about the Medical and Mental Concerns of Women, Including Maintaining Health and Wellness, Gynecological Concerns, Breast Health, Sexuality and Reproductive Issues, Menopause, Cancer in Women, Leading Causes of Death and Disability among Women, Physical Concerns of Special Significance to Women, and Women's Mental and Emotional Health

Along with a Glossary of Related Terms and Directories of Resources for Additional Help and Information

Edited by Amy L. Sutton. 746 pages. 2004. 978-0-7808-0673-3.

"This is a useful reference book, which makes the reader knowledgeable about several issues that concern women's health. It is recommended for public libraries and home library collections." — *E-Streams, May '05*

"A useful addition to public and consumer health library collections."
— *American Reference Books Annual, 2005*

"A highly recommended title."
— *The Bookwatch, May '04*

"Handy compilation. There is an impressive range of diseases, devices, disorders, procedures, and other physical and emotional issues covered . . . well organized, illustrated, and indexed." — *Choice, Association of College & Research Libraries, Jan '98*

SEE ALSO *Breast Cancer Sourcebook, Cancer Sourcebook for Women, Healthy Heart Sourcebook for Women, Osteoporosis Sourcebook*

Workplace Health & Safety Sourcebook

Basic Consumer Health Information about Workplace Health and Safety, Including the Effect of Workplace Hazards on the Lungs, Skin, Heart, Ears, Eyes, Brain, Reproductive Organs, Musculoskeletal System, and Other Organs and Body Parts

Along with Information about Occupational Cancer, Personal Protective Equipment, Toxic and Hazardous Chemicals, Child Labor, Stress, and Workplace Violence

Edited by Chad T. Kimball. 626 pages. 2000. 978-0-7808-0231-5.

"As a reference for the general public, this would be useful in any library."   — *E-Streams, Jun '01*

"Provides helpful information for primary care physicians and other caregivers interested in occupational medicine. . . . General readers; professionals."
— *Choice, Association of College & Research Libraries, May '01*

"Recommended reference source."
— *Booklist, American Library Association, Feb '01*

"Highly recommended."   — *The Bookwatch, Jan '01*

Worldwide Health Sourcebook

Basic Information about Global Health Issues, Including Malnutrition, Reproductive Health, Disease Dispersion and Prevention, Emerging Diseases, Risky Health Behaviors, and the Leading Causes of Death

Along with Global Health Concerns for Children, Women, and the Elderly, Mental Health Issues, Research and Technology Advancements, and Economic, Environmental, and Political Health Implications, a Glossary, and a Resource Listing for Additional Help and Information

Edited by Joyce Brennfleck Shannon. 614 pages. 2001. 978-0-7808-0330-5.

"Named an Outstanding Academic Title."
— *Choice, Association of College & Research Libraries, Jan '02*

"Yet another handy but also unique compilation in the extensive *Health Reference Series*, this is a useful work because many of the international publications reprinted or excerpted are not readily available. Highly recommended."   — *Choice, Association of College & Research Libraries, Nov '01*

"Recommended reference source."
— *Booklist, American Library Association, Oct '01*

SEE ALSO *Traveler's Health Sourcebook*

Teen Health Series
Helping Young Adults Understand, Manage, and Avoid Serious Illness

List price $65 per volume. **School and library price $58 per volume.**

Alcohol Information for Teens
Health Tips about Alcohol and Alcoholism

Including Facts about Underage Drinking, Preventing Teen Alcohol Use, Alcohol's Effects on the Brain and the Body, Alcohol Abuse Treatment, Help for Children of Alcoholics, and More

Edited by Joyce Brennfleck Shannon. 370 pages. 2005. 978-0-7808-0741-9.

"Boxed facts and tips add visual interest to the well-researched and clearly written text."
— *Curriculum Connection, Apr '06*

Allergy Information for Teens
Health Tips about Allergic Reactions Such as Anaphylaxis, Respiratory Problems, and Rashes

Including Facts about Identifying and Managing Allergies to Food, Pollen, Mold, Animals, Chemicals, Drugs, and Other Substances

Edited by Karen Bellenir. 410 pages. 2006. 978-0-7808-0799-0.

Asthma Information for Teens
Health Tips about Managing Asthma and Related Concerns

Including Facts about Asthma Causes, Triggers, Symptoms, Diagnosis, and Treatment

Edited by Karen Bellenir. 386 pages. 2005. 978-0-7808-0770-9.

"Highly recommended for medical libraries, public school libraries, and public libraries."
— *American Reference Books Annual, 2006*

"It is so clearly written and well organized that even hesitant readers will be able to find the facts they need, whether for reports or personal information. . . . A succinct but complete resource."
— *School Library Journal, Sep '05*

Body Information for Teens
Health Tips about Maintaining Well-Being for a Lifetime

Including Facts about the Development and Functioning of the Body's Systems, Organs, and Structures and the Health Impact of Lifestyle Choices

Edited by Sandra Augustyn Lawton. 458 pages. 2007. 978-0-7808-0443-2.

Cancer Information for Teens
Health Tips about Cancer Awareness, Prevention, Diagnosis, and Treatment

Including Facts about Frequently Occurring Cancers, Cancer Risk Factors, and Coping Strategies for Teens Fighting Cancer or Dealing with Cancer in Friends or Family Members

Edited by Wilma R. Caldwell. 428 pages. 2004. 978-0-7808-0678-8.

"Recommended for school libraries, or consumer libraries that see a lot of use by teens."
— *E-Streams, May '05*

"A valuable educational tool."
— *American Reference Books Annual, 2005*

"Young adults and their parents alike will find this new addition to the *Teen Health Series* an important reference to cancer in teens."
— *Children's Bookwatch, Feb '05*

Complementary and Alternative Medicine Information for Teens
Health Tips about Non-Traditional and Non-Western Medical Practices

Including Information about Acupuncture, Chiropractic Medicine, Dietary and Herbal Supplements, Hypnosis, Massage Therapy, Prayer and Spirituality, Reflexology, Yoga, and More

Edited by Sandra Augustyn Lawton. 405 pages. 2006. 978-0-7808-0966-6.

Diabetes Information for Teens
Health Tips about Managing Diabetes and Preventing Related Complications

Including Information about Insulin, Glucose Control, Healthy Eating, Physical Activity, and Learning to Live with Diabetes

Edited by Sandra Augustyn Lawton. 410 pages. 2006. 978-0-7808-0811-9.

Diet Information for Teens, 2nd Edition

Health Tips about Diet and Nutrition

Including Facts about Dietary Guidelines, Food Groups, Nutrients, Healthy Meals, Snacks, Weight Control, Medical Concerns Related to Diet, and More

Edited by Karen Bellenir. 432 pages. 2006. 978-0-7808-0820-1.

"Full of helpful insights and facts throughout the book. . . . An excellent resource to be placed in public libraries or even in personal collections."
— *American Reference Books Annual, 2002*

"Recommended for middle and high school libraries and media centers as well as academic libraries that educate future teachers of teenagers. It is also a suitable addition to health science libraries that serve patrons who are interested in teen health promotion and education."
— *E-Streams, Oct '01*

"This comprehensive book would be beneficial to collections that need information about nutrition, dietary guidelines, meal planning, and weight control. . . . This reference is so easy to use that its purchase is recommended."
— *The Book Report, Sep-Oct '01*

"This book is written in an easy to understand format describing issues that many teens face every day, and then provides thoughtful explanations so that teens can make informed decisions. This is an interesting book that provides important facts and information for today's teens."
— *Doody's Health Sciences Book Review Journal, Jul-Aug '01*

"A comprehensive compendium of diet and nutrition. The information is presented in a straightforward, plain-spoken manner. This title will be useful to those working on reports on a variety of topics, as well as to general readers concerned about their dietary health."
— *School Library Journal, Jun '01*

Drug Information for Teens, 2nd Edition

Health Tips about the Physical and Mental Effects of Substance Abuse

Including Information about Marijuana, Inhalants, Club Drugs, Stimulants, Hallucinogens, Opiates, Prescription and Over-the-Counter Drugs, Herbal Products, Tobacco, Alcohol, and More

Edited by Sandra Augustyn Lawton. 468 pages. 2006. 978-0-7808-0862-1.

"A clearly written resource for general readers and researchers alike."
— *School Library Journal*

"This book is well-balanced. . . . a must for public and school libraries."
— *VOYA: Voice of Youth Advocates, Dec '03*

"The chapters are quick to make a connection to their teenage reading audience. The prose is straightforward and the book lends itself to spot reading. It should be useful both for practical information and for research, and it is suitable for public and school libraries."
— *American Reference Books Annual, 2003*

"Recommended reference source."
— *Booklist, American Library Association, Feb '03*

"This is an excellent resource for teens and their parents. Education about drugs and substances is key to discouraging teen drug abuse and this book provides this much needed information in a way that is interesting and factual." — *Doody's Review Service, Dec '02*

Eating Disorders Information for Teens

Health Tips about Anorexia, Bulimia, Binge Eating, and Other Eating Disorders

Including Information on the Causes, Prevention, and Treatment of Eating Disorders, and Such Other Issues as Maintaining Healthy Eating and Exercise Habits

Edited by Sandra Augustyn Lawton. 337 pages. 2005. 978-0-7808-0783-9.

"An excellent resource for teens and those who work with them."
— *VOYA: Voice of Youth Advocates, Apr '06*

"A welcome addition to high school and undergraduate libraries." — *American Reference Books Annual, 2006*

"This book covers the topic in a lucid manner but delves deeper into every aspect of an eating disorder. A solid addition for any nonfiction or reference collection." — *School Library Journal, Dec '05*

Fitness Information for Teens

Health Tips about Exercise, Physical Well-Being, and Health Maintenance

Including Facts about Aerobic and Anaerobic Conditioning, Stretching, Body Shape and Body Image, Sports Training, Nutrition, and Activities for Non-Athletes

Edited by Karen Bellenir. 425 pages. 2004. 978-0-7808-0679-5.

"Another excellent offering from Omnigraphics in their *Teen Health Series*. . . . This book will be a great addition to any public, junior high, senior high, or secondary school library."
— *American Reference Books Annual, 2005*

Learning Disabilities Information for Teens

Health Tips about Academic Skills Disorders and Other Disabilities That Affect Learning

Including Information about Common Signs of Learning Disabilities, School Issues, Learning to Live with a Learning Disability, and Other Related Issues

Edited by Sandra Augustyn Lawton. 337 pages. 2005. 978-0-7808-0796-9.

"This book provides a wealth of information for any reader interested in the signs, causes, and consequences of learning disabilities, as well as related legal rights and educational interventions. . . . Public and academic libraries should want this title for both students and general readers."

— *American Reference Books Annual, 2006*

■

Mental Health Information for Teens, 2nd Edition
Health Tips about Mental Wellness and Mental Illness

Including Facts about Mental and Emotional Health, Depression and Other Mood Disorders, Anxiety Disorders, Behavior Disorders, Self-Injury, Psychosis, Schizophrenia, and More

Edited by Karen Bellenir. 400 pages. 2006. 978-0-7808-0863-8.

"In both language and approach, this user-friendly entry in the *Teen Health Series* is on target for teens needing information on mental health concerns."

— *Booklist, American Library Association, Jan '02*

"Readers will find the material accessible and informative, with the shaded notes, facts, and embedded glossary insets adding appropriately to the already interesting and succinct presentation."

— *School Library Journal, Jan '02*

"This title is highly recommended for any library that serves adolescents and parents/caregivers of adolescents."

— *E-Streams, Jan '02*

"Recommended for high school libraries and young adult collections in public libraries. Both health professionals and teenagers will find this book useful."

— *American Reference Books Annual, 2002*

"This is a nice book written to enlighten the society, primarily teenagers, about common teen mental health issues. It is highly recommended to teachers and parents as well as adolescents."

— *Doody's Review Service, Dec '01*

■

Pregnancy Information for Teens
Health Tips about Teen Pregnancy and Teen Parenting

Including Facts about Prenatal Care, Pregnancy Complications, Labor and Delivery, Postpartum Care, Pregnancy-Related Lifestyle Concerns, and More

Edited by Robert Aquinas McNally. 425 pages. 2007. 978-0-7808-0984-0.

■

Sexual Health Information for Teens
Health Tips about Sexual Development, Human Reproduction, and Sexually Transmitted Diseases

Including Facts about Puberty, Reproductive Health, Chlamydia, Human Papillomavirus, Pelvic Inflam-matory Disease, Herpes, AIDS, Contraception, Pregnancy, and More

Edited by Deborah A. Stanley. 391 pages. 2003. 978-0-7808-0445-6.

"This work should be included in all high school libraries and many larger public libraries. . . . highly recommended."

— *American Reference Books Annual, 2004*

"*Sexual Health* approaches its subject with appropriate seriousness and offers easily accessible advice and information."

— *School Library Journal, Feb '04*

Skin Health Information for Teens
Health Tips about Dermatological Concerns and Skin Cancer Risks

Including Facts about Acne, Warts, Hives, and Other Conditions and Lifestyle Choices, Such as Tanning, Tattooing, and Piercing, That Affect the Skin, Nails, Scalp, and Hair

Edited by Robert Aquinas McNally. 429 pages. 2003. 978-0-7808-0446-3.

"This volume, as with others in the series, will be a useful addition to school and public library collections."

— *American Reference Books Annual, 2004*

"There is no doubt that this reference tool is valuable."

— *VOYA: Voice of Youth Advocates, Feb '04*

"This volume serves as a one-stop source and should be a necessity for any health collection."

— *Library Media Connection*

■

Sports Injuries Information for Teens
Health Tips about Sports Injuries and Injury Protection

Including Facts about Specific Injuries, Emergency Treatment, Rehabilitation, Sports Safety, Competition Stress, Fitness, Sports Nutrition, Steroid Risks, and More

Edited by Joyce Brennfleck Shannon. 405 pages. 2003. 978-0-7808-0447-0.

"This work will be useful in the young adult collections of public libraries as well as high school libraries."

— *American Reference Books Annual, 2004*

■

Suicide Information for Teens
Health Tips about Suicide Causes and Prevention

Including Facts about Depression, Risk Factors, Getting Help, Survivor Support, and More

Edited by Joyce Brennfleck Shannon. 368 pages. 2005. 978-0-7808-0737-2.

Tobacco Information for Teens

Health Tips about the Hazards of Using Cigarettes, Smokeless Tobacco, and Other Nicotine Products

Including Facts about Nicotine Addiction, Immediate and Long-Term Health Effects of Tobacco Use, Related Cancers, Smoking Cessation, Tobacco Use Prevention, and Tobacco Use Statistics

Edited by Karen Bellenir. 440 pages. 2007. 978-0-7808-0976-5.